Essentials of Disaster Anesthesia

Essentials of Disaster Anesthesia

Edited by

Joseph McIsaac
University of Connecticut

Kelly McQueen
University of Wisconsin

Corry Kucik
United States Navy

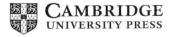
CAMBRIDGE
UNIVERSITY PRESS

CAMBRIDGE
UNIVERSITY PRESS

University Printing House, Cambridge CB2 8BS, United Kingdom

One Liberty Plaza, 20th Floor, New York, NY 10006, USA

477 Williamstown Road, Port Melbourne, VIC 3207, Australia

314–321, 3rd Floor, Plot 3, Splendor Forum, Jasola District Centre,
New Delhi – 110025, India

79 Anson Road, #06–04/06, Singapore 079906

Cambridge University Press is part of the University of Cambridge.

It furthers the University's mission by disseminating knowledge in the pursuit of
education, learning, and research at the highest international levels of excellence.

www.cambridge.org
Information on this title: www.cambridge.org/9781107498259
DOI: 10.1017/9781316181454

© Cambridge University Press 2020

First published 2020

Printed in the United Kingdom by TJ International Ltd, Padstow, Cornwall.

A catalogue record for this publication is available from the British Library.

Library of Congress Cataloging-in-Publication Data
Names: McIsaac, Joseph H., editor. | McQueen, Kelly, 1962– editor. | Kucik, Corry, editor.
Title: Essentials of disaster anesthesia / edited by Joseph McIsaac, Kelly McQueen, Corry Kucik.
Description: Cambridge, United Kingdom; New York, NY: Cambridge University Press, 2020. |
Includes bibliographical references and index.
Identifiers: LCCN 2019037718 (print) | LCCN 2019037719 (ebook) | ISBN 9781107498259 (paperback) |
ISBN 9781316181454 (ebook)
Subjects: MESH: Anesthesia | Disasters | Emergency Medicine
Classification: LCC RD81 (print) | LCC RD81 (ebook) | NLM WO 200 | DDC 617.9/6–dc23
LC record available at https://lccn.loc.gov/2019037718
LC ebook record available at https://lccn.loc.gov/2019037719

ISBN 978-1-107-49825-9 Paperback

....

Contents

Contributors

Mohammed Iqbal Ahmed, MD, FASA
Attending Anesthesiologist, Children's
Medical Center
University of Texas – Southwest
Dallas, TX

Jordan Anderson, MS
Clinical Engineer
Providence VA Medical Center
Providence, RI

David Besachio, DO
Commander, Medical Corps, US Navy
Staff Physician for Vascular, Interventional,
and Neuroradiology
Naval Medical Center Portsmouth, VA

Robert Bishop, MD
Attending Anesthesiologist
St Clares/Eastern Health
Torbay, Newfoundland and Labrador,
Canada

Phillip Blum, FANZCA
Deputy Director of Anaesthesia
Royal Darwin Hospital
Darwin, Australia

Steve J. Brasington, MD
Medical Executive Director and Pediatric
Psychiatrist
North Florida Evaluation and Treatment
Center
Florida Department of Children and
Families
Gainesville, FL

Carlton Brown, MD
Retired Attending Anesthesiologist
National Naval Medical Center
Walter Reed National Military Center
Bethesda, MD

Frederick W. Burgess, MD, PhD
Chief, Anesthesia Section
Providence VA Medical Center
Clinical Professor of Surgery
(Anesthesiology)
Warren Alpert Medical School of Brown
University

Christopher M. Burkle, MD, JD
Consultant, Department of Anesthesiology
and Perioperative Medicine
Professor of Anesthesiology
Mayo Clinic
Rochester, MN

Jeffrey M. Carness, MD
Lieutenant Commander, Medical Corps
US Navy
Attending Anesthesiologist
Naval Hospital Bremerton, WA

Johanna de Haan, MD
Program Director, Regional Anesthesia and
Acute Pain Fellowship
Assistant Anesthesiology Residency
Program Director
University of Texas Health
Science Center
Houston, TX

Proshad Efune, MD
Assistant Professor
Department of Anesthesiology and Pain
Management
University of Texas – Southwest
Dallas, TX

Kristin Falce, MD
Obstetric Anesthesiologist
Steward Health Care
St. Joseph's Medical Center
Houston, TX

Christos Giannou, MBBCh, Mch
International Health and Management of
Health Crises
National and Kapodistrian University
Athens, Greece

Martin Graves, BSc, MBBS, FANZCA
LTCOL, Royal Australian Army Medical
Corps
Anaesthetist, The Wollongong Hospital,
Australia
Senior Instructor in Defence Medicine,
University College Cork, Ireland

Simon Hendel, MBBS, MPH, FANZCA
Specialist Anaesthetist and Trauma
Consultant
Alfred Health
Melbourne, Australia

Nadia Hernandez, MD
Director, Acute Pain Medicine
Regional Anesthesia and Perioperative
Ultrasound
University of Texas Health Science Center
Houston, TX

Dan Holmes, MBChB, MHM, MRCP, FRCA, FANZCA
Clinical Director of Trauma
Deputy Director of Anaesthesia
Specialist Anaesthetist
Sunshine Coast University Hospital
Queensland, Australia

Tracey Jackson, MD
Physician and Consultant
Bright Heart Health
San Ramon, CA

Shaukat A. Khan, MD
Assistant Clinical Professor of Psychiatry
Yale University School of Medicine
Staff Psychiatrist, VA Connecticut Health
Care System
West Haven, CT

Ashlee Klevens Hayes, PharmD, MHA
Founder, Rx Ashlee
Huntington Beach, CA

Corry "Jeb" Kucik, MD, MA, DMCC, FASA, FCCP, FCCM,
FUHM, FACHE
Captain, Medical Corps, US Navy
Chief Medical Officer
Naval Medical Readiness and Training
Command Oak Harbor, WA
Associate Professor of Anesthesiology,
Rocky Vista University,
Parker, CO

Mark J. Lenart, MD, MPH, FASA
Captain, Medical Corps, US Navy
Branch Head, Surface Medicine
Bureau of Medicine and Surgery
Falls Church, VA
Associate Professor of Anesthesiology
Uniformed Services University of the
Health Sciences,
F. Edward Hebert School of Medicine
Bethesda, MD

Joseph McIsaac, MD, MS, MBA, CPE, FASA
Clinical Professor of Anesthesiology
University of Connecticut School of
Medicine
Farmington, CT
Chief of Trauma Anesthesia
Hartford Hospital
Hartford, CT
Director and Chair of Quality and
Practice
Integrated Anesthesiology
Associates, LLC
East Hartford, CT
Supervisory Medical Officer
National Disaster Medical System
US Department of Health and Human
Services
Washington, DC

Kelly McQueen, MD, MPH
Chair, Department of Anesthesiology
University of Wisconsin – Madison
Madison, WI

Michael J. Murray, MD, PhD
Colonel (Retired), Medical Corps,
US Army

Professor of Medicine and Anesthesiology
Geisinger Medical Center
Danville, PA

Bruce Paix, MBBS, FANZCA
Wing Commander, RAAF Reserve
Medical Retrieval Consultant
SAAS Medstar Emergency Medical
Retrieval
Adelaide, Australia

Matthew Pena, MD
Lieutenant Commander (Retired), Medical
Corps, US Navy
Associate Professor of Anesthesiology and
Pain Medicine
University of California – Davis
Sacramento, CA

Felicity Stone, MBBS
Consultant Anaesthetist
Royal Darwin Hospital
Darwin, Australia

Knut Ole Sundnes, MD
Colonel and Head of Anaesthesia
Norwegian Armed Forces Medical Services
Jar, Norway

Professor, Centre for Risk Management
and Societal Safety, University of Stavanger,
Norway

Daniel Sutton, MD
Commander, Medical Corps, US Navy
Attending Trauma and Critical Care
Surgeon
Naval Medical Center Portsmouth,
VA

Liza Weavind, MBBCh, MD
Professor of Anesthesiology and Critical
Care
Vanderbilt University
Nashville, TN

Kirsten M. Wilkins, MD
Attending Psychiatrist
Veterans Administration Healthcare
System
West Haven, CT

Marina Zuetell, MBA
Consultant, Radio Communications for
Healthcare
MHz Consulting Services
Seattle, WA

Preface

The primary thrust of our book is to quickly provide guidance and prepare those anesthesia and critical care providers who respond to a disaster – whether as a volunteer traveling to help at a disaster site or as a responder who has survived a disaster event at home.

The book intends to be a clinical guide to the essentials of anesthesia and critical care for disasters and austere environments. It can also serve as a guide for those doing mission work under austere conditions. It is not a comprehensive reference textbook but rather, a practical primer or refresher for the field.

No one practices medicine in a vacuum. All parts of the health care system as well as the greater incident response system must work together. Depending on the nature of your practice and location in the world, you may work as a generalist, a first responder, an emergency medicine physician, a nurse anesthetist, an operating room anesthesiologist, a pain management physician, an administrator, a surgical nurse, or a critical care physician. Maybe all of the above. Therefore, we have included material of a much wider scope than that of traditional clinical text. Only when the logistics and all of the components of the system work together can the anesthetist perform his or her function.

Chapters are short and to the point. The text is written by many authors with a host of different perspectives. We intend it to be readable in a short time to convey the major principles and techniques necessary to deliver anesthesia for surgical and critical care in a resource-poor environment. We hope you will agree.

Disclaimer

The views expressed in this work are those of the authors and do not necessarily reflect the official policy or position of any military department or government.

Disaster Anesthesia

Knut Ole Sundnes

A disaster is by definition a situation in which the resources available do not match the demands of the population impacted. This often forces serious modifications in standards of best practice, all coping activities, and expected outcomes. Generally in most disasters, if assistance from outside is unavailable, mortality rates and disabilities are much higher than during crises which are met with adequate resources. "Disaster medicine" is population based, which is vastly different to individual-based medicine. The goal of medical care applied during disasters is to provide the best for the many, to treat only those expected to survive with treatment, and to not waste scarce resources. This means reduced quality of health care, even with optimal use of all available resources. The term "health disaster" is also used as it indicates how a disaster deteriorates health indirectly through destruction of infrastructure and societal functions.

The term "disaster anesthesia" has not been systematically addressed in the anesthesia literature. In fact, a definition has not reached consensus within the community of anesthesiologists responding to disasters. Narrative presentations dominate, underlining the brutal meeting of high-tech users and a low-tech scenario. There are exceptions, but the bottom line is that this seems to have never been addressed in a conceptualized way. The first paper that surfaced is "The Anæsthetist in the Management of a Disaster" by Dobkin, Wyant, and Kilduff, dating back to 1957.[1] In a short editorial Hapuarachchi, in 2009, addressed "The Role of the Anaesthetist in Disaster Management," pointing out the multi-faceted nature of disasters and the wide scope of challenges anesthetists may face.[2]

Also, since the job descriptions for anesthetists vary extensively throughout the world, universally accepted descriptions of anesthetists' tasks and challenges will differ. Consequently, how anesthesia personnel from different "schools" handle and/or involve themselves in disasters will be different. What is applicable to certain European nations cannot automatically be applied to other countries, e.g. USA, India, and Japan. A book on disaster anesthesia must mirror the different scopes of the anesthesia specialty in different countries. In some countries anesthesia is confined to the operating theatre only, whereas in other countries the specialty of anesthesia includes pre-hospital care, intensive care, pain management, and emergency medicine, in addition to anesthesia in the operating room.

Disasters are a relative "thing." Three critically wounded patients in a small district hospital will often qualify for the term disaster. The shoot-out at a political youth camp in Norway, July 22, 2011, killing 69 and wounding 66, could, however, be dealt with within an acceptable time frame and with no reduction in expected outcome. As such it was a tragedy of unprecedented proportion but did not qualify for the term "disaster," after the killing had stopped. The situation will also vary according to where it takes place. An event in a rural district in a developing country may be very different from a situation taking place in an urban environment in an industrialized country. In this context, anesthesia has to find its place and be executed in a way that gives maximum outcome with the given resources, maintaining the best possible patient safety. More precisely, the anesthesiologist must optimize the use of his/her resources without reducing patient safety, compared to how they would have done it under normal circumstances, in spite of the increased numbers of patients needing to be treated.

In the little literature you find on this subject, disaster anesthesia is often seen as synonymous with anesthesia for mass trauma.[3] This is, as we see it, too narrow minded. Disaster anesthesia encompasses more than just trauma anesthesia. In the majority of situations trauma will probably dominate as a challenge, both in sheer numbers but also with regard to type of trauma. Trauma patients from disasters may present themselves with a wider range of pathophysiology that goes beyond the traditional emergency trauma patient. The time factor is not on the patient's side and the process of multiorgan failure may have started. For example, in cases of earthquakes (or otherwise collapsed buildings) delayed arrival at the hospital may give additional challenges as organ failure may already be present (e.g. renal failure due to crush syndrome and dehydration). In a mass shooting, hypotension due to blood loss is the dominating urgent problem, but the unpredictable internal ballistics will require extensive examination to identify all damaged organs and structures. In the absence of X-rays the slightest possibility of a pneumothorax will require a chest tube, prior to anesthesia, even without an X-ray and/or an ultrasound examination.

As such, disaster anesthesia comprises a mixture of many challenges, including mass casualties in civilian life (railroad accidents, fire accidents, naval tragedies), war surgery encompassing field anesthesia, including pre-hospital care (in many countries) and other non-surgical events. The Bhopal tragedy in India in 1984, with the release of methyl isocyanate, required ventilatory and medical support to an extent far beyond existing resources; a huge disaster without any need for surgery, but with permanent damage to health, even with optimal therapy.[4,5]

What contributes to these challenges may be listed, e.g. Box 1.1.

These challenges require additional elaboration and consideration. Anesthesia is no longer just a choice of anesthetics and how to handle patients. It starts with strategic thinking, hopefully done beforehand. How do you plan for the above? Thereafter, what tactical modifications are needed to make the hospital master plan function?[i] How to organize your hospital and yourself to get maximum numbers of patients treated? How to optimize safety with as little reduction as possible in patient comfort? This differs from country to country. In some countries one can increase the working hours for each employee. This works in countries with less than 50 work hours a week; however, it is less applicable to countries where hospital workers (e.g. physicians) already have rosters of 80 working hours a week. The basic objective is optimal patient flow, and this again demands that some "sacred cows" may be sacrificed. Two operating tables per anesthesia machine is normally unheard of, but will help tremendously in increasing patient flow. If a hospital has floor-fixed sockets, this is difficult. If the operating tables are on wheels, this is possible and reduces time between patients significantly. Set up your operating room in such a way that one anesthesia machine can serve two operating tables. A physician or nurse skilled in anesthesia can make the necessary preparations for the next patient while maintaining anesthesia on the patient currently undergoing surgery, even if alone and without a mechanical ventilator. This may save up to 15 minutes between patients, without

---

[i] "Plans are nothing. Planning is everything". Dwight D. Eisenhower

Box 1.1 Challenges Unique to Disaster Anesthesia

1. Surge activity: disasters produce more victims.
2. Lack of time.
3. Resources are reduced/unavailable:
   a. Destruction
      i. Equipment/consumables
      ii. Infrastructure/logistical system
   b. Logistical constraints (roads blocked, bridges down, air transport limited (rotary wing))
   c. Production facilities are down
   d. Other regions are given priority (e.g. production in a foreign country)
4. Vulnerable groups dominate:
   a. Children (Figure 1.1)
   b. Elderly
   c. Pregnant women
5. Characteristics of challenge; high numbers of:
   a. Trauma
      i. Blunt
         1. Crush syndrome
      ii. Penetrating
      iii. Burns
      iv. High pressure (explosions in closed rooms)
   b. Hypothermia
   c. Hyperthermia

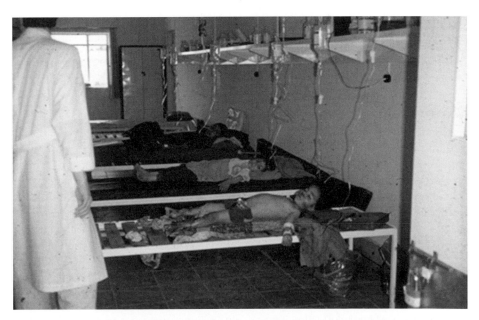

Figure 1.1 Children constitute a depressingly high proportion of patients. They are a vulnerable group and also present different challenges compared to adults.

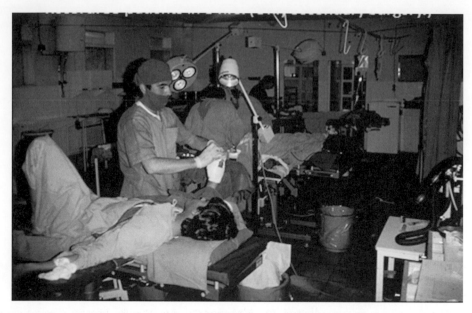

Figure 1.2 Operating room at the ICRC Hospital for War Wounded, Kabul, Afghanistan, 1992. Three operating tables served by one anesthesiologist (and one local staff technician before curfew). After curfew it was served by one expatriate anesthesiologist only. One anesthesia machine was placed between tables 1 and 2 and one oxygen bottle to which a self-expanding bag was attached was sited between tables 2 and 3. No ventilators were available. The maximum turnover (secondary surgery only) was 39 patients in 7–8 hours.

an increase in personnel. In a field hospital this is relatively easy to achieve. If your fixed installations are not originally designed for such flexibility, this may be more difficult. It is important to note that we have no indications that such an arrangement has jeopardized any patient's safety. At the ICRC Hospital for War Wounded in Kabul, Afghanistan, 1991–1992, this was the standard setup. No unfortunate incidents were registered, in spite of a patient flow of 4000–6000 per year divided between an average of three surgeons, three anesthesiologists, and three expatriate operating theatre nurses[ii] (Figure 1.2).

Anesthesia

For an anesthesiologist trained in modern medical centers, in high-income countries, responding to a disaster – at home or abroad – is not intuitive. Anesthesiologists must be trained to triage resources, to safely practice without best practice equipment and supplies, and to recognize futility for the sake of the many. *Key words for disaster anesthesia are "safe" and "simple"*. Disaster anesthesia is not a special form of anesthesia. It is the application of accumulated experience, using drugs and armamentarium in the most well-conceived, cost-effective, and time-efficient way, with the simple objective of helping as many as possible without reducing patient safety, but sometimes being forced to reduce patient comfort.

[ii] This is typical of situations forced through due to extreme situations. The production of good science in such circumstances is difficult, but not impossible. A standard registry used throughout would facilitate such research and evaluation. Maybe we will have that in the future. Today this is not the case and a lot of data and information is lost.

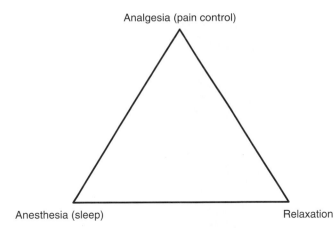

Analgesia (pain control)

Anesthesia (sleep)   Relaxation

Figure 1.3 The classic anesthesiological triangle. Some drugs have only one property (e.g. local anesthetics), some have two (e.g. ketamine), and some provide all three (volatile anesthetics).

A competent anesthesiologist capable of managing ruptured aortic aneurysms in elderly people with chronic obstructive lung disease and/or cardiac insufficiency should be more than capable of handling the different aspects of disaster anesthesia. The basic principles must always be adhered to. Also during disasters the three components, sleep, analgesia, and relaxation, will be the framework within which we operate (Figure 1.3). However, as the situation requires, one may be forced to sacrifice some procedures, either because they are resource consuming (equipment, consumables, or personnel) or time consuming. In a disaster setting, time is often your most precious "commodity." Those procedures that add little to safety may be the first to be sacrificed/omitted. A typical example at the ICRC Hospital for War Wounded in Kabul, Afghanistan from 1990–1992 was not to empty the stomach before surgery (which was standard procedure in most hospitals at that time). We just decided that patients requiring intubation should be induced with rapid sequence intubation (RSI). Spontaneously breathing patients under ketamine anesthesia, on the other hand, were only observed carefully. Regurgitation or vomiting was never observed. NB: Bowel obstruction will always require gastric emptying.

Concomitantly, the provider of the analgesia/anesthesia must take into account other side effects which may be more relevant than in a controlled normal hospital situation. Planning for post-operative care starts in the operating room. If you have two nurses to take care of 20–30 post-operative patients, including patients in critical or serious condition waiting for surgery, and subject to surveillance and retriage, post-operative pain control cannot be as perfect as you want it. You have to keep a good distance from respiratory depression. During surgery, but even more so post-operatively, too much pain treatment may cause respiratory depression, and, if not recognized, be fatal for the patient. Insufficient pain treatment, on the other side, causes significant stress and may also hamper the patient's situation and increase the risk of complications, both mentally and physically. The proper balance between patient safety and patient comfort is therefore an art in its own right (Figure 1.4).

Recurarization is another mechanism that may threaten a patient's life, if not considered peri-operatively and post-operatively. This requires a good collaboration between surgeon

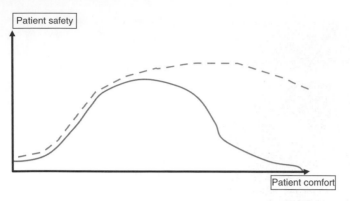

Figure 1.4 Patient comfort is crucial for patient safety and also treatment outcome. The comfort/safety window is, however, more narrow in a disaster. This generic curve pictures how patient comfort and safety are linked. Too little jeopardizes the patient's health and life, too much can also be fatal in the absence of proper monitoring and observation personnel. The dotted line symbolizes a normal situation compared to a similar patient under disaster conditions (solid line).

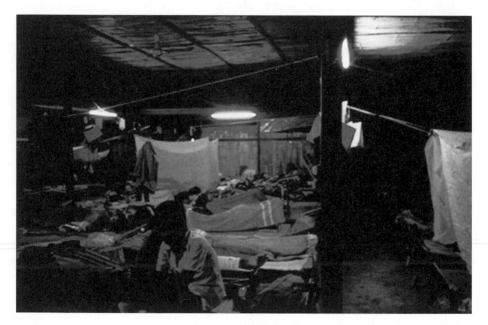

Figure 1.5 Surgical ward at the ICRC Hospital for War Wounded in Khao I Dang at the Thai-Cambodian border. Any patient with respiratory depression or any other post-operative complication will hardly be observed. The only option is to design the anesthetic procedure to eliminate/minimize this threat.

and anesthetist, fine-tuning the use of muscle-relaxing drugs (Figures 1.5 and 1.6). A muscle-relaxed patient blocking an operating table is incompatible with highly effective utilization of the operating theatre. She/he will also require special attention for up to one hour after arrival at the post-operative ward. The short-acting muscle-relaxing drugs developed over recent decades have reduced this problem somewhat, but not removed it completely. If the disaster takes place in a low-resource country (which it often does), you should be prepared that only cheaper, long-acting muscle-relaxing drugs are available, e.g. pancuronium bromide. Recurarization is a phenomenon that you cannot allow to happen!

Pulmonary shunting is another challenge and will be dealt with later.

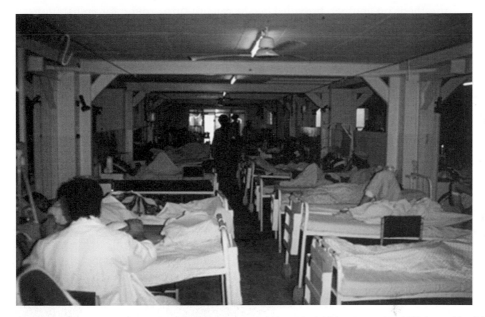

Figure 1.6 Surgical ward at the ICRC Hospital for War Wounded in Kabul, Afghanistan, 1992. With limited health care personnel here post-operative complications can be left unnoticed. Key to avoiding problems is the quality of work done in the operating room, by both surgeons and anesthetists.

Tactical Approach

The disaster anesthesia "teams" are often "one man deep" and therefore require competent and experienced anesthesiologists. On that background the key to managing a disaster scenario is more directed at identifying proper robust anesthetic equipment combined with simple and safe anesthetic procedures, not overly sophisticated, but with the prime focus on patient safety, with patient comfort being secondary. This means that organizing everything to optimum time-saving procedures is crucial. Equipment, consumables, and personnel are all below need. Consequently, as stated above, time has to be viewed as a precious "commodity" and has to be economized. Even saving one or two minutes for each procedure may accumulate to an hour or two at the end of the day, resulting in one or more extra patients treated or allowing for valuable extra sleep for health care workers. With this in mind the key essentials that will have to be addressed in planning for and executing patient management in a disaster scenario are:

- In-hospital flowcharts:
  - Easy access to triage area facilitating triage and retriage
  - Avoiding unnecessary movement of patients resulting in expedient patient treatment without loss of time
- Operating theatre/operating room:
  - Prepare patients outside the operating room with all that can be done beforehand
  - If possible, two operating tables for each anesthesia machine. Even a "one man deep" anesthesia team is able to prepare the next patient while he/she maintains

anesthesia on another, provided he/she can just turn around for preparation. (Also without mechanical ventilators.)
- Use large syringes that do not need to be discarded before the next patient
  - Focus on anesthesia drugs that do not foster bacterial growth. Drugs in fat emulsion are inappropriate for a disaster scenario.
- Choice of anesthetics adjusted to a situation where:
  - Post-operative care is limited
  - Monitoring equipment is limited
    - Respiratory depressions will often not be noticed
  - Patients are hemodynamically unstable.

Most anesthetic drugs are either bactericidal or bacteriostatic. To discard a syringe containing remaining drugs, because it has been used for another patient, is unnecessary and wrong in a disaster scenario, even if you have no back flow valves. The only exception is propofol. This drug is delivered in a fat emulsion which results in bacterial growth if contaminated and kept overnight. Consequently propofol is less compatible with a disaster scenario. Diazepam is in the same lipid solution, but since the whole contents of one ampoule normally is given to one patient (e.g. prior to ketamine) this constitutes less of a problem.

Anesthesia

With regard to anesthesia there are two competing challenges, each needing treatment which is counterproductive to the other.

Hypotensive resuscitation is the current paradigm for all patients suffering blood loss, with bleeding not yet under control. This paradigm will probably stay as the correct approach for non-controlled bleeding situations. Anesthetic components should therefore aim at keeping the blood pressure low until the bleeding is under control. However, if a patient is hypotensive, vasodilating drugs may result in an ultimate drop in blood-pressure leading to a cardiac arrest in very grave situations. Further, vasodilating drugs also increase pulmonary shunting. This must be taken into consideration if oxygenation is already threatened. *Ketamine increases blood pressure* and is considered safer than other drugs as it does not block the hypoxic pulmonary reflex which protects against pulmonary shunting. However, the down side is increased blood pressure, with more bleeding if a wound is not packed with compressive dressing or the bleeding is otherwise under control. Correctly used, ketamine also maintains respiration. Only during induction may ketamine cause respiratory depression, even respiratory arrest, if administered too quickly intravenously. As stated, pulmonary shunting is no problem. Congestive heart failure, however, is. Improper use of ketamine in these patients normally will ultimately result in worsening of the patient's cardiac condition. Induction with a combination of thiopental (<1 mg/kg) combined with ketamine 2 mg/kg usually puts the patient to sleep without any significant change in the blood pressure and could prove to be a "golden mixture."

General Anesthesia

As soon as bleeding is under control the use of vasodilating drugs should be reduced. This will reduce the need for extra oxygen. Ketamine and pentazocine (opioid agonist and antagonist) are probably the drugs that best meet with this requirement. However, even with standard use of volatile anesthetic gas (e.g. halothane (in developing countries), isoflurane, and sevoflorane) saturation in healthy patients can probably be maintained at 94–95%, if recruitment of alveoli is done regularly during anesthesia. This has been well demonstrated during live tissue training on anesthetized healthy pigs exposed to war wounds.[iii] Caution must be taken in elderly patients with increased pulmonary closing volume and other patients with a pre-morbid condition. In difficult situations, however, if surgery is urgently needed in critically wounded patients, and ventilation on room air only is possible, lifesaving surgery should not categorically be ruled out or postponed, just for the lack of supplemental oxygen. To reduce this problem, all anesthetic systems meant to function during disaster scenarios should have available draw-over anesthesia machines (low-pressure systems based on room air and an inlet for low-pressure oxygen provided by e.g. oxygen concentrators[iv]). This was not the case during the aftermath of the Haiti earthquake. Seemingly, much effort was invested in repairing and bringing the destroyed high-pressure anesthesia machines back into working condition.[6]

Dinitrous oxide (laughing gas) is obsolete in a disaster setting. It is a high-pressure gas and can only be used in combination with high-pressure oxygen. This will burden the logistical system unnecessarily. Equipment failure, which may appear more frequently under overwhelmingly difficult situations, like disasters, will add an additional threat to patient safety, if you use dinitrous oxide during anesthesia. Dinitrous oxide was completely removed from the anesthetic setup in the Norwegian Armed Forces from 1997. All anesthesia machines were rebuilt and now have only medical air and oxygen flow meters. In addition they are combined high-pressure–draw-over machines and the switch between the two systems takes less than 20 seconds.

Volatile anesthetics are excellent drugs as they can deliver pain control, sleep, and muscle relaxation without the use of other drugs e.g. muscle-relaxing drugs. The patients may even be on spontaneous ventilation and, as such, regulate themselves. Most colleagues would, however, be uncomfortable with that, as the muscle relaxation for e.g. large abdominal surgery would only be achieved with a patient so deep that respiration might be insufficient. If oxygen is to be rationed, this creates an uncomfortable situation. The only volatile drug that could work in such a situation, on room air, would be ether, as it does not block the pulmonary hypoxic response and stimulates both cardiac function and respiration, while still at the correct surgical depth. However, most colleagues in the industrialized world are today unfamiliar with the use of ether. Further, the very long induction time, potential vomiting, and long wake-up time makes it unsuitable for disaster anesthesia compared to other options available.

Combining volatile anesthetics with other iv analgesics and anesthetics e.g. pentazocine or ketamine are more optimal solutions.

Total intravenous anesthesia has reached a strong position amongst anesthesiologists, for good reasons, even more so in a disaster scenario. The drug of choice may differ somewhat, but drug number one in disaster settings is ketamine (Figure 1.7) It has its down sides, like every drug, but normally it is safe in the hands of less experienced personnel. Used poorly,

---

[iii] Evidence-based knowledge originating from double blind randomized trials on humans is not available on this topic (and will never be). These procedures are based on basic pathophysiology and pharmacology paired with experience acquired during long-term work under difficult field conditions, and must be considered as the current paradigm.

[iv] The oxygen concentrators require less than 350 watts of electricity per hour, which normally is available.

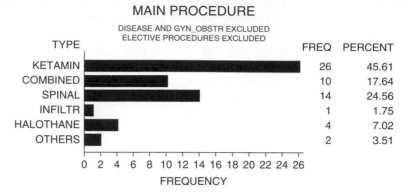

MAIN PROCEDURE

DISEASE AND GYN_OBSTR EXCLUDED
ELECTIVE PROCEDURES EXCLUDED

TYPE		FREQ	PERCENT
KETAMIN		26	45.61
COMBINED		10	17.64
SPINAL		14	24.56
INFILTR		1	1.75
HALOTHANE		4	7.02
OTHERS		2	3.51

0 2 4 6 8 10 12 14 16 18 20 22 24 26
FREQUENCY

Figure 1.7 Anesthetic procedures as executed at the ICRC hospital in Khao I Dang, Thailand, 1984. The predominant drug is ketamine. For combined anesthesia (abdominal surgery with muscle relaxation) ketamine and volatile anesthetics were used interchangeably. In Afghanistan, (Kabul, 1990–1992) with a significantly higher workload, ketamine dominated even more.

however, even ketamine has killing power. Respiratory depression following intravenous induction is typical, especially if injected too fast and in doses of 2 mg/kg and up. If observed, (as it should be) normal mask-bag ventilation (room air suffices) will bridge this period. After the first dose, however, this rarely happens, if at all. Muscle relaxation is, however, minimal and muscle-relaxing drugs during abdominal surgery can rarely be omitted.[v] Always remember anticholinergic drugs in children when ketamine is used.

Pre-hospital anesthesia may be required from time to time. In these situations ketamine is the only suitable drug. This is more frequent in single emergency trauma situations, but may also be necessary during disasters e.g. earthquakes.

Intravenous Lines

If intravenous access is difficult, especially in children, the full anesthetic dose for intra-muscular induction should be given without wasting time. As soon as the patient is asleep, establishing an iv is normally no problem. The only drawback is that priming of the "psychomimetic" receptors with benzodiazepine is suboptimal as it has to be given con-comitantly, eventually rectally as premedication if time and situation permit. Atropine must always be included in the first syringe. Ketamine-induced hyper-salivation may otherwise be significant and, in children, even life-threatening.[vi]

If access is difficult, extreme Trendelenburg position will practically always give access to the external jugular veins. Central venous lines also solve this problem, but may become an increasing obstacle as the coming generation of anesthesiologists are trained with use of ultrasound guidance and less used to anatomical landmarks. [Editor's note: Intraosseous access (before central access) should be considered if venepuncture is unsuccessful. This

---

[v] During service in Afghanistan it was observed that at district hospitals, caesarian section was done on patients on room air only, breathing spontaneously and anesthetized on ketamine as the sole drug. (Faryab province June 2006.) Records were not kept and overall mortality/morbidity could not be given.

[vi] Personal experience by the author during mission at the ICRC hospital in Khao I Dang in 1984.

route is equivalent to a small gauge central line in terms of rate of fluid delivery as well as time to enter the central circulation. If practiced, it can be performed faster than an intravenous line can be established.]

Local Anesthetic Techniques

If it is possible to use local anesthetics, they provide great benefits. Properly administered, this will save a significant amount of time. The patients breathe by themselves, normally room air only. Post-operative pain control with opioids will be less needed or at least postponed. The patients can be prepared in due time before surgery, without occupying an operating table.

1. Infiltration: always dilute the local anesthetic. Lidocaine functions down to 3 mg/ml and should never exceed 5 mg/ml. Epinephrine (adrenaline) can be added at 5 µg/ml to prolong the duration and reduce potential toxic side effects.
2. Regional blocks: require higher concentration and mostly bupivacaine 5 mg/ml or similar long-acting drugs.
3. Central blocks: require full control of any bleeding and a restored blood volume. Hemoglobin level is of lesser importance.
   a. Spinal: the method of choice. Gives best anesthesia and best surgical conditions and consumes less drug. Bupivacaine 5 mg/ml vials are identical to bupivacaine spinal and adhering to sterile techniques, one glass gives 5–7 spinal doses. However, this vial must be discarded after 24 hours as there are no preservatives. Bupivacaine heavy is only produced in ampoules. [Isobaric bupivacaine is safer in Trendelenburg.]
   b. Epidural has no advantage unless it can be used for post-operative pain control with an indwelling catheter. This requires, however, good hygienic conditions and experienced health care personnel, which is often not the case in a disaster scenario. A single shot epidural is inferior to spinal.

For central blocks prophylactic sympathicomimetica (e.g. ephedrine 50 mg im) is highly recommended as it will in nearly all cases prevent spinal hypotension and bradyarrhythmia.

Logistics

If a disaster unfolds in your vicinity and involves your own hospital directly, current disaster procedures and master plans should be activated and adhered to and, if needed, only be reinforced or modified. If infrastructure is destroyed, hampering logistics, all procedures and efforts minimizing the burdening of the logistical system must be implemented.

If this happens outside your own hospital district, (e.g. if deployed out in the field or even in a different country, like the Ebola epidemic in Western Africa), the situation changes. Procedures for procurement, transport, and warehousing/storage become much more of a challenge. As a basic rule, only essential drugs should be procured (see World Health Organization list) and in the highest concentration (e.g. ketamine 50 mg/ml and local anesthetic (lidocaine 20 mg/ml)). This will of course necessitate dilution for different requirements, but normally this takes very little time if it has been prepared for (Figure 1.8).

Also, focus on drugs that are not sensitive to heat variations. Alternatively, try to get drugs that are delivered as sterile, dry powder, e.g. thiopental, or cryoprecipitate to reduce your dependency on refrigerators and freezers.

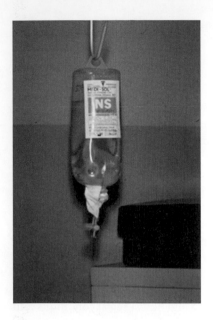

Figure 1.8 As all drugs were procured in only the highest concentration available the first thing to be done every morning was to prepare a "dilution bottle" comprising a 1000 ml bottle of normal saline, perforated with a large bore intravenous cannula and attached a three-way stop cock.

Oxygen constitutes its own "problem." If supplies are sufficient one may utilize it as normal. If a scarce commodity, economizing on oxygen is crucial. The questions are (1) to whom and (2) when should it be given? High-pressure oxygen can only be used once. If given to a patient who does not necessarily need it, just as safety precaution, it will not be available for patients who really need it. A healthy patient undergoing primary surgery, even if acute/urgent, will normally do absolutely fine on room air. Maintaining oxygen saturation of 94–96% suffices. For secondary surgery and for patients with pre-morbid conditions, the situation often changes. These patients will normally require or at least benefit from additional oxygen. The other crucial situation for which oxygen must be reserved is *rapid sequence intubation* with the use of succinylcholine. During the diesel embargo to Afghanistan by the Soviet Union in 1990–1991, there was not enough diesel to run electrical power plants, oxygen production facilities, heating, diesel-powered cars (ambulances), and so on. Oxygen became a scarce commodity and had to be reserved for the most critical oxygen consumption phase of anesthesia. A short pilot study (not published), demonstrated a fall in oxygen saturation from 95% down to 60% during the time needed for an uncomplicated rapid intubation. The RSI for this study had to be modified, i.e. the patients were mask ventilated on room air to maintain saturation above or equal to 95% as long as there were visible fasciculations. Sellick's maneuver was carried out rigorously and intubation was done when the patient was clinically relaxed. However, the oxygen-consuming microfasciculation (not visible) must have continued as there is no other explanation for this extraordinarily rapid fall in oxygen saturation. After identical results with eight patients, all of them intubated on room air only, it was decided to reserve oxygen for pre-oxygenation for RSI. Conversely, also when ventilated on room air only, oxygen saturation did not start to drop until after a minute when using a non-depolarizing agent (pancuronium-bromide) and it took up to 2 minutes before the saturation had dropped to 70%.[vii] During a three month mission giving more than 20 anesthetics daily, exclusively for the war wounded, only two patients needed extra oxygen to maintain saturation of 94% or above. This included thoracic-abdominal surgery.

A pulse-oximeter is key. It tells you about the patient's condition, including when added oxygen is wasted.

Conclusion

Disaster anesthesia constitutes no mystery requiring unique anesthetic procedures due to unknown pathophysiology. What is different is, per definition, the mismatch between resources (any kind) and the tasks ahead, and how and when the patients arrive at the hospital. Consequently, a disaster scenario will require an analysis of how to best serve the population exposed with the resources at hand. This includes pre-planned contingencies, an organizational setup, and flow charts, combined with an understanding of which standard procedures will have to be modified/sacrificed in order to cover the surge activity per se and the monitoring challenges that follow surgery/treatment. Remember, patient safety has priority over patient comfort.

Any capable anesthetist with some experience should be up to these challenges.

References

1. Dobkin AB, Wyant GM, Kilduff CJ. The anæsthetist in the management of a disaster. *Can Med Assoc J.* 1957;**76**(9):763–770.

2. Hapuarachchi S. The role of the anaesthetist in disaster management. *Sri Lankan J Anaesthesiol.* 2009;**17**(1):1–2.

3. Grande CM, Baskett PJ, Donchin Y, Wiener M, Bernhard WN. Trauma anesthesia for disasters. *Crit Care Clin.* 1991;7(2):339–361.

4. Dhara VR, Dhara R. The Union Carbide disaster in Bhopal: a review of health effects. *Arch Environ Health.* 2002;**57**(5):391–404.

5. Bowonder B. The Bhopal incident: implications for developing countries. *Environmentalist.* 1985;**5**(2):89–103.

6. Jama RS, Zakrison TL, Richards AT, Young Dh, Heir JS. Facilitating safer surgery and anesthesia in a disaster zone. *Am J Surg.* 2012;**204**:406–409.

[vii] After curfew the anesthesiologist was a one man deep anesthesia team. This latter test was done to identify the time available to leave the patient unventilated in the case that any item or supplementary drug had to be collected from e.g. storage adjacent to the operating theatre. The anesthetic machine was a draw-over machine without a ventilator. As such, all ventilations were done manually with a self-expanding bag.

Preparing to Deploy to a Remote Disaster

Joseph McIsaac

Type of Disaster Scenario

In order to prepare to respond to a disaster event, one must consider the type of disaster. Is it a one-time event, the result of weather, seismic activity, or a technological/transportation mishap? Is it an acute occurrence in a chronically affected area? What is the scale: large scale (widespread) vs limited in scope? The spectrum of medical and surgical disease that you will likely treat and approximate numbers of patients influences both preparation and logistics. Always count on a disproportionate number of children. The age spectrum is usually shifted to the left in developing countries, kids have a higher likelihood of being injured than adults, but they are often more resilient. When will you arrive? The first 48 hours will see mainly acute injuries. Only local resources that survive the event will be available. As time passes, acute injuries will decrease and more secondary effects will emerge, along with common acute and chronic surgical disease. After about 2 weeks, the usual spectrum of surgical disease will predominate, along with re-operation of injuries, wound revisions, new acute injuries (especially of relief workers), and possibly reconstructive surgeries.

Who will you be deploying with? One should never self-deploy. Always go with an established, experienced group. Will you be part of an organized, self-contained surgical team joining an existing hospital or part of a deploying surgical hospital? The core of a surgical hospital consists of a preop/ER, at least one OR, a PACU/ICU, and a surgical ward. Additional support functions such as central sterile equipment, radiology, lab, and pharmacy are needed. There should be more nurses than physicians (two to three times), sufficient support personnel to move patients, supplies, and perform non-medical tasks. In general, there is at least one non-medical staff member for every medical one. Consider if lab, X-ray, blood bank, or mortuary services will be organic or provided by another entity. When considering deploying with a group, their level of preparation and experience in disaster relief should be considered. A good way to gain personal experience is to deploy with organizations like Operation Smile, Médecins Sans Frontières (MSF, Doctors Without Borders), etc. doing charity work under less stressful (non-disaster) circumstances.

It is critical to know, before leaving, how you will be fed and who is providing logistical support. You must bring with you whatever you will need. The best assumption is that nothing will be available. Even if guaranteed support, it should be expected that you will take the basic means for subsistence along with you. You should not deploy unless you have a reasonable exercise tolerance and no acute or chronic diseases that require specialized support (e.g. orthopedic injuries, diabetes requiring insulin, coronary artery disease requiring medication, obstructive sleep apnea requiring CPAP.) It goes without saying that you should bring an adequate supply of personal medications and hygiene items.

Reconnaissance and Intelligence

Before agreeing to deploy, a detailed country study of the disaster area and adjacent geography must be performed. A Google search is a good place to start, but more specific (and reliable) information can be had from other sources (http://www.country-studies.com/). Trip Advisor (http://www.tripadvisor.com/) and other travel sites like Lonely Planet (http://www.lonelyplanet.com/) can provide general information, but should not be relied upon for disaster situations.

Topics covered should include climate and weather, terrain, transportation infrastructure, economics, customs, culture, religion, demographics, languages, and common foods found in the area. The CIA World Fact Book provides an additional overview (https://www.cia.gov/library/publications/the-world-factbook/geos/vm.html). The US Department of State (http://www.state.gov/p/) provides guidance for US citizens. Maps of the affected area and adjacent, non-affected areas should be obtained and studied. Google Maps, Google Earth, Bing, and Yahoo Maps are reasonable places to start, but often are not up to date. It is wise to download digital maps to carry with you since the Internet is unlikely to be available. Paper maps should also be carried as a backup. ESRI sells a high-end mapping product called ArcGIS® (www.arcgis.com/). While it is expensive software, intended for professional use, they also have a low-cost home license and a free trial. ESRI provides free support to relief organizations, including disaster maps, data, and technical support (http://www.esri.com/services/di saster-response). There is usually a posting of current disaster maps soon after an occurrence.

The World Health Organization (http://www.who.int/countries/en/) and Centers for Disease Control (http://wwwnc.cdc.gov/travel/destinations/list/) provide current disease data. One must understand the pre-disaster burden of medical and surgical disease and the normal level of medical care available to the population. It is wise to consult a tropical medicine text to brush up on endemic diseases in the target country like malaria, schistosomiasis, and helminthiasis. Vaccinations should be up to date for the intended travel itinerary. Visit a travel medicine clinic well before deploying to be sure all immunizations are current.

Attention should be given to the bottom levels of Maslow's hierarchy of needs and essential infrastructure: air, water, shelter, clothing, food, security, sanitation, transportation, communications, energy, and medical care – both for those deploying and for those you intend to serve.

Training: Things to Know and Brush up on

Ideally, anyone thinking of deploying should actively train and study on an ongoing basis. General medical knowledge should include a large dose of family medicine topics required of a general practitioner. That includes the basics of pediatrics, obstetrics, psychiatry, medicine, and surgery. Tropical medicine and wilderness medicine techniques should also be reviewed. We also recommend studying triage, ATLS skills, long bone fixation, wound care, and obstetrical skills. It would be wise to obtain a refresher in how to deliver a baby, both routine and complicated presentations (breech, obstructed), and neonatal resuscitation. Many modern academic departments now have vaginal delivery and cesarian delivery simulators available. Austere anesthesia courses such as the ones run in Australia, UK, Canada, and the US can help reinforce skills.

Insurance

An often-neglected area by those deploying is insurance coverage. Will your health insurance cover you if you become sick or injured? How can you be evacuated back home and who will pay? If you are delayed or become ill, will you get your job back when you return home? For those who deploy as part of the US government (military and National Disaster Medical System) the Uniformed Services Employment and Reemployment Rights Act (USERRA) provides disability insurance and workers compensation insurance coverage. All others should check their current insurance policies. Supplemental travel medical and evacuation insurance can be had through third parties listed on the US Department of State website (https://travel.state.gov/content/travel/en/international-travel/before-you-go/your-health-abroad/insurance-providers-overseas.html).

Malpractice insurance is also essential. Legal liability does not end at your own country's border. It is wise to try to determine how malpractice liability works in the target country. Many policies only cover you at your primary job or in your own specialty. If you are called on to act as a general physician (very likely), coverage is essential. You should first ask your carrier if a supplemental policy can be issued. The deploying agency you are joining is another good source of information.

Family Care

Another neglected planning issue is family care. While you are gone, how will your family get along? Will there be child care or elder care needs? What if your significant other becomes ill? How will the bills be paid? Who will look after your home if you are single? Do you have a reliable communication plan if your family needs to reach you? Do you have living wills, powers of attorney, and an emergency communications plan?

Medication Transport

Unless you are traveling with a well-equipped, professional force, you will need to arrange for transportation of essential medications. A licensed pharmacist can be invaluable at home and on deployment. Bottled oxygen is difficult to move in quantity. Oxygen concentrators are a better choice, although they do require a power source. Intravenous fluids also are bulky to move. Some drugs, like succinylcholine, require refrigeration. A decision to have succinylcholine also requires consideration for dantrolene. Many of the routine anesthetics are heavily regulated in various countries. Importation and possession of sedatives and narcotics in many African, Middle Eastern, and Asian countries is prohibited. Severe penalties for narcotic trafficking (smuggling) can be imposed. Many foreign countries have specific requirements for importation and monitoring. It is best to obtain information and written permission from the embassy or consulate of the target country as well as any countries that you will pass through in transit. Copies of permissions, including appropriate stamps, bearing the name of the permitting official must be carried along with any permitted medications. Since medical supplies are frequently diverted, high-value medications should be carried in the aircraft cabin and secured at all times.

Many foreign countries also restrict personal medications, requiring valid prescriptions and limited supplies for personal use. Check applicable embassy websites.

In addition to foreign laws, US state and federal laws must also be followed. Controlled substances can be exported using US DEA Form 222. It would be wise to contact the DEA far in advance to ensure ability to comply with US Law. (https://apps.deadiversion.usdoj.gov/web forms/orderFormsRequest.jsp)

Equipment

Equipment can be divided into three areas: personal, medical specialty specific, and organizational.

Personal

Essential personal equipment is required for survival and sustainment. A partial list includes:

Rugged waterproof watch	Glow sticks	Multitool/Swiss Army knife
Flashlight(s)	Compass	Collapsible entrenching tool
Headlamp(s)	Pocket knife and sharpener	Small machete (if jungle)
Waterproof solar radio	Personal hygiene items	Personal medications
Water- and oilproof pens and markers	Water purification tablets and straws	Safety glasses
Waterproof notebooks	Face shields	Mosquito nets
Waterproof paper charts	Insect repellant	Leather work gloves
Non-sterile gloves	Waterproof apron	N-95 masks
Ear plugs	Hand sanitizer and wipes	Weather-appropriate clothing for deployment and transit sites

Specialty Equipment

Anesthesia equipment both disposable and durable. Airway, ventilation, drug and fluid administration, ability to clean and sterilize. Drugs and anesthetics.

Organizational Equipment

Power and oxygen generation, fuel, fans/air conditioning, tools for plumbing, electrical, electronics, light construction/repair.

[SEE Appendix 1 on DMAT Gear by Malloch for a more extensive list.]

Principles of Emergency and Trauma Surgery

Christos Giannou and Bruce Paix

Introduction

Natural disasters and armed conflict kill and maim. In the immediate, emergency phase, patients suffering from trauma receive the highest priority. It is only later that the public health effects of destroyed infrastructure, displacement of population, and disorganization of the health system come into play and take precedence. [1-4] However, one major difference between a natural disaster and armed conflict is that the former is a one-off event: most injuries take place at the time of the event, whereas during combat, the injured arrive day after day, every day, until fighting ceases. Thus, during armed conflict, trauma remains a high priority even while the larger public health effects take their toll.

Acute pathologies during a disaster or armed conflict do not take a holiday. Surgical, and obstetric, emergencies continue to occur in any population: appendicitis, cholecystitis, complications of childbearing. However, the extreme event often compromises the capacity of the health system; access to ordinary health care is then decreased. [5] Some surgical pathologies, such as the complications of typhoid fever, can actually increase in those regions where the disease is endemic because of the destruction of basic sanitation infrastructure.

Most evident during major disasters, however, are the "new" circumstances under which trauma and emergency surgery must be undertaken. There are, of course, minor disasters where the hospital system continues to function as before and the extra patient burden is well accommodated. This is often not the case after a major event or in the case of armed conflict. In this chapter, we shall deal with how surgical care should be developed and performed after a major natural disaster or intense armed conflict.

These new circumstances are often described by many surgeons as "primitive" or "austere." In many respects, however, they reflect the normal working conditions in a low-income country. Good, scientifically based surgery is performed every day around the world in simple or austere circumstances, without a disaster having taken place. Techniques are adapted and are appropriate to the working conditions. Poverty does not forcibly result in poor surgery. Working with limited yet appropriate resources is often the most challenging aspect of disaster or war surgery for inexperienced or expatriate surgical personnel. [6]

Epidemiology

Two-thirds, and even more, of injuries suffered after most natural disasters and armed conflicts involve the limbs. [7,8] Although not usually life-threatening in modern surgery, in the disaster setting these injuries represent the major surgical and nursing burden and are often associated with various degrees of long-term disability. Infection, nonetheless, remains a major problem in these dirty and contaminated wounds: tetanus, gas gangrene, and invasive β-streptococcal sepsis.

Life-threatening injuries usually kill within minutes or hours and, unless extraction and evacuation are performed early, relatively few such patients reach hospital in time for surgery to be performed.[i] Even so, only well-functioning local hospitals can intervene in the management of these patients. Outside surgical teams deployed to the scene of a major disaster usually arrive too late to be of help with these patients.[9] In contrast, during armed conflict, casualties may continue to arrive over long periods and a foreign surgical team often has to manage these patients.

Delay in evacuation of the wounded – whether due to a lack of pre-hospital services, destruction of the road infrastructure, or simply distance – is a commonplace event after a major disaster or during armed conflict. This obviously has many follow-on consequences for the types of wounds encountered and the requirements for resuscitation.[10]

Triage of Casualties

It is important for medical personnel to understand the difference between a multiple-casualty incident (where resources can ramp up to deal with the load in the normal manner: surge capacity) and mass casualties (where medical services are overwhelmed and must accept limitations of care) or what has been called a compensated or uncompensated event.[11] In the latter, there exists a category of patients that are best left to die in peace and with dignity. Their management would consume an extraordinary amount of limited resources when faced with the total number of victims, and their survival, in a dependent state, no blessing for them, their families, or their societies.

The pre-hospital organization of triage is essential if the hospital is not to be over-whelmed with patients suffering from minor injuries that can be treated successfully by simple first aid measures. When deployed to the site of a natural disaster the first measure to undertake is the setting up of first aid posts to filter the patients and organize patient flow to the hospitals. For reasons of security, this is usually not the case in situations of armed conflict: pre-hospital care and evacuation become more problematic and take more time to set up. Ultimately, the efficiency of pre-hospital measures depends largely on the pre-existing capacity of the affected country's system of first aid.

Hygiene

A natural disaster or armed conflict severely affects the environment. Infrastructure is devastated, water supplies contaminated or cut off, shelter destroyed (Figure 3.1). One of the consequences is a deterioration in the level of personal hygiene. Scarce water for drinking and cooking is too precious for bathing, and facilities for personal cleanliness are often no longer available. The scene of the event is also in ruins: dust and dirt from rubble after an earthquake or bombardment; mud from a tsunami that infiltrates everything.

A field hospital, or still-functioning structure, should try to organize a facility for showering patients on admission, except obviously for those *in extremis*. Whether this

---

[i] We are speaking here of a civilian context. The military services of industrialized countries have sophisticated capacities for evacuation of the wounded.

(a)

(b)

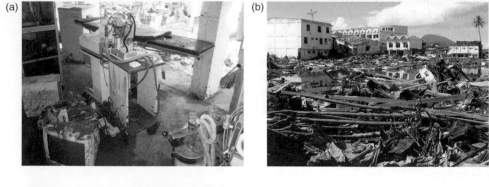

(c)

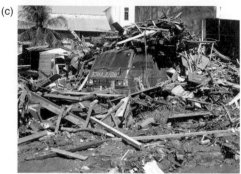

Figure 3.1 Typical environment after a major disaster: Banda Aceh, 2004 (photo credit: B. Paix).

can be improvised or not, or if water supplies are inadequate, in the operating theatre and under anesthesia, a proper scrub of the relevant body part with soap, water, and a brush should be performed. Any excessive hair should be shaved, if necessary. If we have written about basic hygiene here, it is because many surgeons often forget or ignore the obvious: there is no use in putting povidone iodine on top of dirt; it is still dirt. A proper scrub of the body part to be operated on is essential.

Examination and Resuscitation

The initial examination and resuscitation of injured patients proceeds in parallel according to the C-ABCDE algorithm, although most of the injured seen in disasters or armed conflicts will have minor to moderate rather than severe injuries.[12]

Whether due to the large number of patients or constraints of infrastructure, the major clinical problem facing the surgeon will be a lack of diagnostic technologies. Whereas multislice CT scanners are considered essential for first-world management of trauma patients, in a disaster, even a working plain X-ray machine is a great plus! The staff of the emergency reception department must learn (or re-learn) the "eye-ear-nose and ten-finger whole body scan": a proper and complete examination of the patient, from head-to-toe, based primarily on one's clinical skills.

Hypothermia is an especially acute problem for victims trapped under the rubble of collapsed buildings. Pre-hospital intervention in this regard is essential and simply covering the patient with a recovered blanket or sheet is beneficial. It should be noted that a bleeding patient loses body heat even in a tropical climate and environmental measures in the hospital must be undertaken to prevent or correct the condition. Resuscitation rooms and operating theatres should be warmed to around 30°C for trauma patients where possible; an uncomfortable temperature for those unaccustomed.

Quite commonly after natural disasters or during armed conflicts and primarily due to delay in evacuation, many patients in hypovolemic shock have not suffered severe hemorrhage, but rather are dehydrated by the time they arrive at a hospital. Rehydration here equals resuscitation.

Classically, resuscitation is begun with a balanced crystalloid solution (Ringers lactate is preferred) and for a great many patients is adequate, particularly for late arriving patients where hemorrhage has been modest and self-limited. The use of crystalloids in severely injured patients with massive hemorrhage is no longer advised, however.[13] Recent developments in damage control resuscitation for this subpopulation implies limited use of crystalloids and early administration of a balanced composition of blood products, which poses a dilemma in situations of limited blood for transfusion.

Blood Transfusion

The willingness of potential donors to give blood is a function of many social and cultural factors. In some societies it is not a problem at all and the only limiting factor is the setting up of the facilities for collection, screening, and cross-matching. In other societies, however, much discussion and "negotiation" with family and clan members may be required. After many major catastrophes blood is simply not available in the quantities that most doctors would use under normal circumstances. Under these conditions a massive transfusion protocol is irrelevant; a simple transfusion protocol defining the criteria for the administration of blood and the maximum quantity to be administered to an individual patient should be introduced after discussion with all the members of the hospital team.

In these extreme circumstances the resort to "traditional" transfusion practice is the norm: no blood components; whole fresh blood is given, usually with very positive results.[14] It should also be mentioned here that this is standard practice in many low- and medium-income countries. The fractionization/fractionation of blood into components is an expensive procedure and is common only in countries with a certain degree of industrialization.

Autotransfusion – giving shed blood back to the patient – is a time-tested method, especially in situations of limited resources, especially in remote rural hospitals in low-income countries.[15] The hospital should have a protocol for such an event and preparation of the required materials made. Autotransfusion is most often employed in a patient with massive hemothorax, a ruptured spleen, or an ectopic pregnancy.

Antibiotics

Tetanus is an ever-present danger with open and dirty wounds, and immunization coverage around the world is unequal and inconsistant. Knowledge of local vaccination practice and rates is important. A routine protocol of antitetanic serum and toxoid vaccination should be implemented.

For many minor injuries simple wound toilet and antibiotic coverage is sufficient. This is not a call for the misuse of antibiotics, rather a selection of patients to the extent possible based on the experience of the surgeon.[16]

For those patients undergoing surgery, antibiotics are preferably given pre-operatively, or at least intra-operatively, and before the application of any tourniquet.

It is a misuse to give a cocktail of antibiotics in the attempt to prevent all types of post-traumatic infection. Prophylaxis should be targeted: *Clostridia* and β-hemolytic streptococcus are most important in soft tissue wounds. The best antibiotics are thus penicillin or a first-generation cephalosporin. For injuries to the chest, abdomen, or brain, standard protocols involving penicillin, ampicillin, first-generation cephalosporin, gentamycin, metronidazole, and chloramphenicol exist (Table 3.1). These antibiotics are relatively inexpensive and widely available. Their use should not, however, take the place of proper technique and good surgery: the best antibiotic.

Preparation and Anesthesia

Positioning and draping of the patient should allow for exposure of any predictable extension of the surgery: vascular exposure, for example. The use of a pneumatic tourniquet for operations on the limbs should be standard practice in the attempt to conserve the patient's blood.

Provided the surgeon is aware of its limitations, nearly all trauma and emergency surgery can be performed under ketamine anesthesia, with or without muscle relaxation (Figure 3.2); the only exception being surgery on the eye due to the nystagmus. This method has proven safe and effective after disasters and during warfare, particularly where patients are in poor condition due to injury, malnutrition, and pneumonia, and resources are limited.[17] Local, spinal, and intravenous regional anesthesia can be widely used, especially at delayed primary closure of wounds, with the added benefit of providing post-operative analgesia, which may be otherwise unavailable. The logistics of oxygen supply can be daunting and the means of anesthesia used should take this into account. Ketamine anesthesia is usually possible with the patient self-ventilating on room air.

Surgical Decision-Making

The decision to operate, or not, and the sequence of operations, is perhaps the most difficult decision to make in the extreme circumstances of a natural disaster or armed conflict. Supplies are limited, beds are limited, nursing care is limited, and blood for transfusion is limited; these limitations can be very constraining.

The most important factors that define the extent of operations to be performed are post-operative nursing care, the availability of blood, and level of expertise in anesthesia. Not surgical competency: an important lesson for many surgeons.

After many major events the number of surgeons is limited and the individual surgeon is often called upon to perform operations outside his/her speciality. This calls for the approach of a very "general surgeon," not one of subspecialties. Consequently, the operative sequence in a multiply injured patient is of great significance.

Simple measures can have a great effect if the number of patients is overwhelming. The classic triage principle of "the greatest good for the greatest number" must guide the surgeon always. Procedures should be swift and beneficial and, at times, a simple treatment approach based on basic first aid and resuscitation only (fluids, antibiotics, and analgesia) may provide a greater overall benefit than surgery, especially if patients present late.[18]

On the other hand, not all wounds require formal wound excision or debridement (Figure 3.3). Many low-energy wounds can be managed conservatively. A good clinical

Table 3.1 Example of antibiotic protocol for war wounds: ICRC

Injury	Antibiotic	Remarks
Minor soft tissue wounds	Penicillin-V tablets 500 mg QID for five days	
Compound fractures Traumatic amputations Major soft tissue wounds	Penicillin-G 5 MIU iv QID for 48 hours Follow with penicillin-V tablets 500 mg QID until DPC	Continue penicillin-V for five days if closure is performed with a split skin graft.
Compound fractures or major soft tissue wounds with delay of more than 72 hours Antipersonnel land mine injuries of limbs whatever the delay	Penicillin-G 5 MIU iv QID and metronidazole 500 mg iv TID for 48 hours Follow with penicillin-V tablets 500 mg QID and metronidazole tablets 500 mg TID until DPC	If redebridement is performed instead of delayed primary closure (DPC): stop antibiotic unless there are signs of systemic infection or active local inflammation. In this case, add metronidazole 500 mg iv TID and gentamycin 80 mg iv TID.
Hemothorax	Ampicillin 1 g iv QID for 48 hours, followed by amoxicillin tablets 500 mg QID	Total 5 days
Penetrating cranio-cerebral wounds	Penicillin-G 5 MIU iv QID and chloramphenicol 1 g iv TID for at least 72 hours	Continue iv or orally according to patient's condition for a total of 10 days
Brain abscess	Same regime as for cranio-cerebral wounds plus metronidazole 500 mg iv TID	
Penetrating eye injuries	Penicillin-G 5 MIU iv QID and chloramphenicol 1 g iv TID for 48 hours	Continue iv or orally according to patient's condition for a total of 10 days. Local instillation of antibiotic eye drops
Maxillo-facial wounds	Ampicillin 1 g iv QID and metronidazole 500 mg iv TID for 48 hours	Continue iv or orally according to patient's condition for total of 5 days
Abdominal wounds A: Solid organs only: liver, spleen, kidney; and isolated bladder B: Stomach, small intestines C: Colon, rectum, anus	A: Penicillin-G 5 MIU iv QID B: Ampicillin 1 g iv QID and metronidazole 500 mg iv TID C: Ampicillin 1 g iv QID and metronidazole 500 mg iv TID and gentamycin 80 mg iv TID	Continue for 3 days depending on drainage

Anti-tetanus measures for all patients.
Penicillin-G may be replaced by ampicillin or a first-generation cephalosporin according to availability.
Allergy to β-lactam antibiotics: replace with known standards (erythromycin, clindamycin etc.)

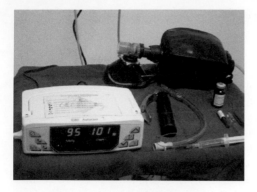

Figure 3.2 Standard anesthesia equipment and supplies necessary after a natural disaster or during armed conflict: ketamine, muscle relaxants, diazepam and analgesics (credit: ICRC *War Surgery: Working with Limited Resources in Armed Conflict and Other Situations of Violence*, Volume 1, ICRC, 2009).

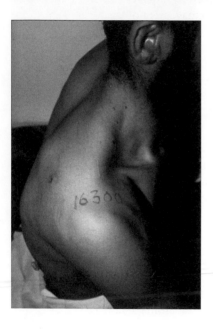

Figure 3.3 Palpation reveals no hematoma, no edema, and a soft pliable muscle. At the most, excision of the skin wounds under local anesthesia is all that is required (credit: R. Coupland/ICRC *War Surgery: Working with Limited Resources in Armed Conflict and Other Situations of Violence*, Volume 1).

examination of the affected body part determines if there has been significant tissue damage or not and, therefore, whether the body's natural defenses are sufficient to deal with the trauma.[16]

Even some abdominal wounds, usually if patients present late or are due to low-energy fragments mimicking a stab wound, can be managed conservatively. Nonetheless, the non-operative management of abdominal wounds requires time, diagnostic means, and the capacity to re-examine the patient regularly; not always the case.

Damage Control Surgery

The practice of staged management of the severely injured patient has become standard today. In the extreme circumstances under discussion, several questions must be asked: Will the surgeon see the patient a second time? What level of nursing care is available? Is there a functioning ICU? Usually, ward care is limited, mechanical ventilation is scarce or nonexistent, and often, the patient's post-operative care and rehabilitation will be largely carried out by family members as "volunteers."

Surgical Technique

The techniques for emergency surgery follow standard procedures and protocols; the only compromise being due to the availability or not of technology, the capacity for sterilization, and the adequacy of logistic supply. As a result, laparoscopic and other minimally invasive surgery is usually contraindicated. "Old-fashioned" invasive surgery should be the standard.

The great difference in surgical technique is to be found in the management of trauma, especially open wounds, and, above all, those with fractures. The wounds of disasters and armed conflict are dirty and contaminated and the rules of septic surgery apply: wound excision or debridement; no unnecessary change of dressings; delayed primary closure of the wounds four to seven days later; and conservative management of fractures (Table 3.2). Even for closed fractures, the conditions of sterility in the operating theatre and the difficulties of logistic supply (having enough plates, screws, and nails of the appropriate size, and their re-supply after use) usually mean that conservative orthopedic measures are called for: splinting, traction, plaster-of-Paris and external fixation.[15]

The technique of wound excision is a classical lesson of surgery that every new generation of surgeons must re-learn.

Initial Wound Excision

Wound excision or debridement is best performed layer by anatomic layer: from the skin through the soft tissues down to the periosteum and bone.

Skin is elastic, has a good blood supply, and will be necessary for later closure. Conservative debridement of skin wounds is the rule. The wound track is laid open through generous skin incisions in the long axis of the extremity (Figure 3.4). Subcutaneous fat has a poor blood supply and contaminants readily stick to it; excision should be generous, all around the original wound. Deep fascia should be divided throughout the length of the skin incision to allow adequate exposure and decompression of the tissues.

Wearing two pairs of gloves and being careful of sharp fractured bone ends, the surgeon should now explore the wound cavity, usually filled with hematoma, damaged muscle, bone fragments, and foreign material.

Muscles are debrided according to the classical four Cs: color, consistency, contractility (on pinching), and circulation (bleeds when cut) – all foreign material is removed (Figure 3.5). Gas gangrene is a myositis and muscle excision should be

Table 3.2 Basic principles in the management of disaster and war wounds

- Wound incision for drainage
- Excision of devitalized and necrotic tissues, layer by anatomic layer
- Copious irrigation: normal saline or potable water
- Hemostasis
- Leave the wound open for drainage: no sutures
- Large bulky, absorbent dressing
- No unnecessary change of dressings
- Delayed primary closure (DPC)

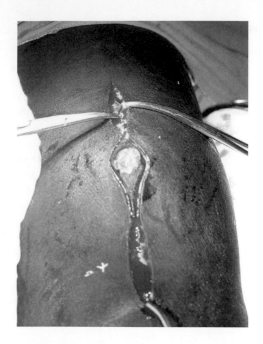

Figure 3.4 Excision of the entry wound and extension incision of the skin to give access to the depths of the wound (credit: F. Jamet/ICRC *War Surgery: Working with Limited Resources in Armed Conflict and Other Situations of Violence*, Volume 2, ICRC, 2013).

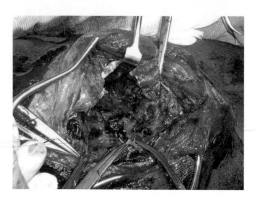

Figure 3.5 The wound cavity debrided, hemostasis is ensured. The wound is now copiously irrigated with normal saline or potable water, depending on availability (credit: F. Jamet/ICRC *War Surgery: Working with Limited Resources in Armed Conflict and Other Situations of Violence*, Volume 2).

adequate, but not excessive in removing viable tissue that would result in unnecessary disability.

Periosteum has a good blood supply and is necessary for fracture healing; excision should be conservative. Bone, on the other hand, has a very poor blood supply. Unattached fragments of cortical bone should be discarded and the fracture properly aligned.

A major blood vessel should be repaired, shunted, or ligated. Severed nerves or tendons should not be repaired primarily. The cut ends are tagged with a colored non-absorbable suture and fixed to a nearby muscle to prevent retraction. Repair is a delayed procedure once all inflammation has subsided.

Foreign bodies such as bullets or metallic fragments are removed if found during wound excision, but otherwise should not be sought out. The indications for removal of such foreign bodies at the initial operation are few: jeopardy to a major vessel or nerve;

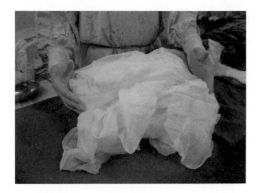

Figure 3.6 Large, bulky, absorbent dressing (credit: ICRC *War Surgery: Working with Limited Resources in Armed Conflict and Other Situations of Violence*, Volume 1).

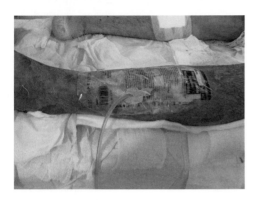

Figure 3.7 Improvised vacuum-assisted dressing (credit: ICRC *War Surgery: Working with Limited Resources in Armed Conflict and Other Situations of Violence*, Volume 2).

intra-articular; a very small fragment in the anterior chamber of the eye. Most fragments or bullets requiring removal – superficial causing pain on movement or over pressure points, or causing an abscess – can be dealt with at a later date.

The tourniquet is now removed and hemostasis confirmed. All compartments should be checked for proper decompression. A fasciotomy may be required.

The wound is copiously irrigated – up to 8–10 liters for a large wound – using normal saline or simple potable water, depending on availability. Any fracture is stabilized by an initial method of bone immobilization. Even without a fracture, the limb may be favorably immobilized by means of a splint to reduce pain and edema.

The wound is then left open to drain, not sutured primarily or packed tightly, and a bulky dressing of loose, fluffed dry gauze and absorbent cotton wool applied (Figure 3.6). This cannot be overemphasized: the wound should not be sutured closed, but left open. The use of vacuum-assisted wound closure (VAC; Figure 3.7) is a positive development, but commercially available devices are prohibitively expensive and the constant low-flow suction apparatus rarely available under the circumstances. Low-cost alternatives have been improvised and may be used if conditions permit.[19,20]

The limb is kept elevated and physiotherapy commenced immediately the day after wound debridement. The limb should be observed for any compromise of circulation denoting an incipient compartment syndrome. Signs of hemorrhage or acute infection require a return to theatre for re-exploration, not a change of dressings on the ward. A soaked dressing should be overdressed with more cotton and a bandage. Otherwise, the original dressing is left intact until return to theatre for delayed primary closure.

Second Operation: Delayed Primary Closure

Delayed primary closure (DPC) – suturing the wound after a period of four to seven days – results in healing by primary intention, just like immediate closure of a wound, but without the risk of enclosing an infective process causing greater tissue destruction and possible invasive sepsis. This is a time-tested procedure for dirty, contaminated, or late-presenting wounds. The delay also allows for soft-tissue edema to be largely absorbed. A clean and healthy wound ready for DPC has a distinct presentation: after removal of the dressing, the last gauze compress covering the wound adheres to the raw surface. Upon its removal, the muscle contracts and bleeds.

In addition, most open wounds and amputation stumps have a particular ammoniac odor. In the parlance of ICRC surgeons, this is called the "good bad odor," and results from the normal products of serum protein degradation. It should not be confused with the "bad bad odour" of an infective process. In addition, wounds are sometimes covered by a yellowish fibrin film, to be differentiated from pus. DPC must never be performed over pus; the presence of fibrin will not adversely affect healing.

The skin is closed with large, widely spaced interrupted sutures; the muscular tissues collapse into place. A drain should be placed if there is any dead space. Sutures should not be placed under tension. If this is the case, then skin grafting and/or a local rotation skin flap should be used.

If at the second operation the wound is found to be infected or necrotic tissue has become apparent, it should be re-excised and left open again, not re-excised and sutured. The patient returns to theatre for attempted DPC four to five days later. There is no need to re-visit the wound every day or so. This only increases trauma to the wound, delays healing, and exposes the patient to nosocomial infection.

The second operation is the best occasion to decide on the best method for the definitive fixation of fractures.

The Exceptions

As in all of medicine, there are exceptions to this general rule of leaving the wound open and some wounds can and should be closed immediately. Wounds of the scalp, face, and neck, and genitals can be closed primarily after debridement. The relatively small amount of soft tissue, easily but carefully excised, and excellent blood supply allow for immediate suturing. Closure of the dura, if possible, is recommended in penetrating cranio-cerebral injuries. After debridement of an open pneumothorax (sucking chest wound), the innermost muscle layers and the pleura are sutured closed in order to recreate a functional pleural cavity; the same applies to open abdominal wounds, to prevent herniation of the intestines. The skin and subcutaneous tissues are left open for DPC. In addition, at least the capsule if not the synovial membrane of joints should be closed; blood vessels require a muscle flap if repaired primarily to prevent desiccation and secondary hemorrhage, and tendons and nerves of the hand covered by means of a rotation flap.

Another exception is the patient who requires serial debridement because of the large extent of the wound and where the surgeon is unsure of the viability of the remaining tissues and further excision would result in greater disability. Here, the surgeon takes a conscious decision to stop the operation and revisit the wound 48 hours later, to allow a line of demarcation to form, should this be the case. Any newly necrotic tissue is excised, and the standard protocol for DPC then followed (Figure 3.8).

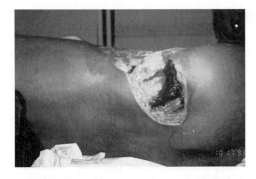

Figure 3.8 Serial debridement of a large wound with questionable viability of the tissues at the first debridement; the second look reveals an area of necrotic tissue (credit: ICRC *War Surgery: Working with Limited Resources in Armed Conflict and Other Situations of Violence*, Volume 1).

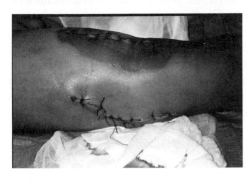

Figure 3.9 Mismanaged wound: the wound has been sutured with little or no debridement: fever, edema, and incipient gas gangrene (credit: D. Cooke/ICRC *War Surgery: Working with Limited Resources in Armed Conflict and Other Situations of Violence*, Volume 2).

Neglected and Mismanaged Wounds

Many patients present very late after a natural disaster or during an armed conflict due to difficulties in evacuation and transport. Their wounds are often grossly infected; amputations are common but should not be considered a universal response. Many limbs can be saved through repeated debridements to remove all sequestra and other necrotic tissues, and honey or sugar dressings.

Often, someone has sutured a wound closed, usually with little or no debridement. The sutures should be immediately removed. These mismanaged wounds are usually full of pus (Figure 3.9).

Definitive Post-Operative Care

Resources permitting, the general principles for nursing care, nutrition, patient hygiene, and physiotherapy continue as before. Mobilization on crutches – unless skeletal traction is used – and exercises to maintain muscle mass and joint mobility are important. Often, other family members will be responsible for the patients ongoing wound care, nutrition, and hygiene, and may need instruction in this.

Drains should be removed as soon as possible, usually within 24–48 hours. A clean, dry wound requires no change of dressing until removal of sutures as per routine.

A large wound cavity not amenable to flaps or grafting should be left to granulate until skin grafting or a rotation flap can be performed. Dressings with honey or sugar are traditional methods that have been found to enhance the formation of granulation tissue and combat infection.[21,22] Superficial *Pseudomonas aeruginosa* infection is common and can be easily treated with dressings of acetic acid (diluted vinegar).[23]

Reconstructive Surgery of the Limbs

Limb salvage following disaster and war wounds often requires major reconstructive surgery to obtain a reasonable functional result. Limited hospital facilities and time constraints generally argue against performing such surgery during the emergency phase after a major event. Whereas early amputation is often the only option given the resources available, there are occasions when appropriate reconstructive surgery can and should be performed as part of the basic management of the wound.[24]

Exposed major blood vessels of the limbs – repaired or not – should be covered by a mobilized skin or muscle flap; this qualifies as primary emergency reconstruction performed as part of the initial surgery. Reconstruction performed at the time of DPC follows significant soft-tissue loss preventing approximation of the wound edges without tension or a large dead space making direct suture inappropriate; skin grafts or flaps are required. If an external fixator is applied at DPC, simultaneous soft-tissue reconstruction can be performed and the pins placed so as not to interfere with the flap. Myoepithelial flaps incorporating skin, fascia, and muscle are preferred.

Late elective reconstruction procedures such as scar revision, burn contractures, or tendon transfer for nerve lesions are usually undertaken three to six months after complete soft-tissue healing. Special expertise, proper hospital facilities, and available time implying a reduced patient load are essential.

Physiotherapy and Patient Rehabilitation

Disasters and war result in many amputees and other disabilities. Re-education and physical rehabilitation are essential for socio-economic re-integration of wounded patients. Psychological support is also important if one considers the terror suffered by many survivors of an earthquake, tsunami, or armed conflict that has cost thousands of lives.

Summary

The surgery of conflict and disaster is often conducted under challenging conditions, with large numbers of patients, scarce resources, damaged infrastructure, and uncertain security. Provided appropriate attention is paid to the limitations imposed, classic triage principles applied, procedures appropriately chosen, and sound surgical principles followed, much good can be done, even under precarious circumstances.

References

1. Aboutanos MB, Baker SP. Wartime civilian injuries: epidemiology and intervention strategies. *J Trauma* 1997;**43**:719–726.

2. Horton R. Croatia and Bosnia: the imprints of war – 1. Consequences. *Lancet* 1999;**353**:2139–2144.

3. Salama P, Spiegel P, Talley L, Waldman R. Lessons learned from complex emergencies over past decade. *Lancet* 2004;**364**:1801–1813.

4. Spiegel PB, Checchi F, Colombo S, Paik E. Health-care needs of people affected by conflict: future trends and changing frameworks. *Lancet* 2010;**375**:341–345.

5. Korver AJH. Outcome of war-injured patients treated at first aid posts of the International Committee of the Red Cross. *Injury* 1994;**25**:25–30.

6. Wong EG, Razek T, Elsharkawi H, et al. Promoting quality of care in disaster response: a survey of core surgical competencies. *Surgery* 2015;**158**:78–84.

7. Giannou C, Baldan M. *War Surgery : Working with Limited Resources in Armed Conflict and Other Situations of Violence,* Vol. 1. Geneva: ICRC, 2009.

8. Mohebbi HA, Mehrvarz S, Saghafinia M, et al. Earthquake related injuries: assessment of 854 victims of the 2003 Bam disaster transported to tertiary referral hospitals. *Prehosp Disast Med* 2008;**23**:510–515.

9. von Schreeb J, Riddez L, Samnegard H, Rosling H. Foreign field hospitals in the recent sudden-onset disasters in Iran, Haiti, Indonesia, and Pakistan. *Prehosp Disast Med* 2008;**23**:144–153.

10. Bhatnagar MK, Smith GS. Trauma in the Afghan guerrilla war: effects of lack of access to care. *Surgery* 1989;**105**:699–705.

11. Lennquist S (ed). *Medical Response to Major Incidents and Disasters: A Practical Guide for All Medical Staff*. Berlin: Springer, 2012.

12. Bellamy RF. Combat trauma overview. In: Sajtchuk R, Grande CM, eds. *Textbook of Military Medicine, Anesthesia and Perioperative Care of the Combat Casualty*. Falls Church, VA: Office of the Surgeon General, United States Army; 1995:1–42.

13. Holcomb JB, Jenkins D, Rhee P, et al. Damage control resuscitation: directly addressing the early coagulopathy of trauma. *J Trauma* 2007;**62**:307–310.

14. Rhee P, Koustova E, Alam HB. Searching for the optimal resuscitation method: recommendations for the initial fluid resuscitation of combat casualties. *J Trauma* 2003;**54**(Suppl.):S52–S62.

15. Giannou C, Baldan M, Molde Å. *War Surgery: Working with Limited Resources in Armed Conflict and Other Situations of Violence,* Vol. 2. Geneva: ICRC, 2013.

16. Bowyer GW. Management of small fragment wounds: experience from the Afghan border. *J Trauma* 1996;**40**(3 Suppl.):S170–S172.

17. Paix BR, Capps R, Neumeister G, Semple T. Anaesthesia in a disaster zone: a report on the experience of an Australian medical team in Banda Aceh following the "Boxing Day tsunami". *Anaesth Intensive Care* 2005;**33**:629–634.

18. Coupland RM. Epidemiological approach to surgical management of the casualties of war. *BMJ* 1994;**308**:1693–1696.

19. Andreassen GS, Madsen JE. A simple and cheap method for vacuum-assisted wound closure. *Acta Orthop* 2006;**77**:820–824.

20. Bui TD, Huerta S, Gordon IL. Negative pressure wound therapy with off-the-shelf components. *Am J Surg* 2006;**192**:235–237.

21. Lee DS, Sinno S, Khachemoune A. Honey and wound healing: an overview. *Am J Clin Dermatol* 2011;**12**:181–190.

22. Mphande ANG, Killowe C, Phalira S, Wynn Jones H, Harrison WJ. Effects of honey and sugar dressings on wound healing. *J Wound Care* 2007;**16**:317–319.

23. Nagoba B, Wadher B, Kulkarni P, Kolhe S. Acetic acid treatment of pseudomonal wound infections. *Eur J Gen Med* 2008;**5**:104–106.

24. Coupland RM. The role of reconstructive surgery in the management of war wounds. *Ann R Coll Surg Engl* 1991;**73**:21–25.

Total Intravenous Anesthesia in Disaster Medicine

4

Phillip Blum and Martin Graves

As Admiral Gordon-Taylor of the British Navy has so aptly said, "Spinal anaesthesia is the ideal form of euthanasia in war surgery" – then let it be said that intravenous anesthesia is also an ideal method of euthanasia"

FJ Halford, MD, FACS, Critique of Intravenous Anesthesia in War Surgery[1]

The above famous critique of intravenous anesthesia occurred following the bombing of Pearl Harbor, where anesthesia folklore tells us more Americans died from the use of thiopental than from the Japanese attack. However, in the same journal that published Halford's statement there appeared a case study of the use of thiopental in a shocked patient with a gunshot wound to her chest and upper abdomen.[2] In this case the anesthetist administered a more modest bolus of thiopental (25 mg compared to the 500 mg boluses used at Pearl Harbor), supplemented anesthesia with nitrous oxide, secured the airway with endotracheal intubation, and allowed the patient to breathe spontaneously.

The austere environment of disaster medicine provides the anesthetist with a number of challenges. including:

1. Logistics of supply and re-supply of drugs and equipment
2. Prolonged evacuation times
3. Reduced specialist support
4. Limited and unreliable power and medical gas supply
5. Exposure to extremes of temperature and dust.

While high fidelity and complex anesthetic machines have allowed the First-World anesthetist to handle sicker and more complex patients, they are unlikely to function in the above environment. In this setting total intravenous anesthesia can offer the anesthetist many advantages over volatile anesthesia. Volatile anesthetics are affected by temperature and can be a logistical burden as large volumes are required. Volatile anesthetics are also classed as dangerous cargos by airlines and are unable to be transported in passenger baggage.

Disadvantages of Volatile Anesthesia

- Logistics of supply
- Volatiles are "dangerous cargo"
- Requirement for scavenging
- Storage issues (temp requirement of large volumes)
- Varied performance at extremes of temperature
- Agents are very costly due to large flows
- Many anesthetists are unfamiliar with draw-over vaporizers.

Total intravenous anesthesia (TIVA) is a technique for providing general anesthesia using only intravenous agents. In the First World it is normally performed by syringe drivers controlled by complex pharmacodynamic formula,[3] but in a resource-poor situation it can be performed using a simple ml/h syringe driver, a gravity-fed intravenous infusion set, or, in its simplest form, by intermittent boluses.

Propofol

Due to its favorable pharmacokinetics the most common agent used for TIVA in hospital-based anesthesia is propofol.[4] The simplest regimen delivers a bolus followed by infusion at a reducing rate as fat stores become saturated. This is known as the Bristol method, which produces a plasma propofol concentration of 3 to 3.5 µg/ml by delivery of a 1 mg/kg bolus followed by an infusion that decreases from 10 to 8 to 6 mg/kg/h every 10 minutes.[5]

Following an intravenous injection the drug is lost from the plasma by redistribution into the tissues, metabolism, and pulmonary and renal clearance. A graph of plasma concentration vs time reveals that the plasma concentration falls in a triexponential manner, with the pharmacokinetics best being described by a three compartment model.[6] In order to maintain a steady-state plasma concentration the lost drug needs to be replaced by a stepwise decreasing infusion. Depth of anesthesia can be increased by a bolus followed by an increase in the infusion rate. Anesthesia depth is decreased by pausing the infusion for a short period before re-starting it at a lower rate.

Whilst propofol has many advantages as an agent for TIVA, in the situation of disaster and austere medicine it has some drawbacks. Its pharmacokinetics and dynamics are adversely affected by hemorrhagic shock[7] such that compartmental clearances are reduced and volume of distribution is increased, leading to an increased plasma concentration of propofol. This effect is compounded by an increase in patient sensitivity to the drug leading to a two and a half times reduction in the plasma concentration required to achieve anesthesia. Whilst the effect of hemorrhagic shock on propofol pharmacokinetics is reversed by volume resuscitation, pharmacodynamic effects of hemorrhage are unchanged.[8] Propofol is also affected by storage temperature, and has adverse effects on respiration, requiring a high level of monitoring and vigilance in order to ensure an adequate safety profile.

Ketamine

Ketamine is the most widely used intravenous anesthetic in disaster medicine. It has a number of advantages for its use in this situation, including a very wide safety profile.[9] Ketamine is a dissociative anesthetic. Its mechanism of action is through competitive antagonism of the excitatory neurotransmitter glutamate at the N-methyl-D-aspartate receptor Ca^{2+} channel, thus disconnecting the thalamus from the neocortex.[10] It is prepared as a racemic mixture in an acidic solution. It is commonly presented as the ketamine hydrochloride salt in 200 mg per 2 ml and 500 mg per 10 ml ampoules. It is soluble in water and is able to be mixed with other acidic drugs such as midazolam, propofol, fentanyl, morphine, and vecuronium.

Advantages of Ketamine

- Wide safety profile
- Available in high concentrations allowing easy carriage

- Provides good analgesia, allowing it to be used as a sole anesthetic agent
- Safer in hemorrhagic shock
- Respiration and airway reflexes relatively maintained
- Can be given orally, IM or IV
- Doesn't trigger MH.

Disadvantages of Ketamine

- Emergence delirium
- Salivation
- Increased muscle tone and semi-purposeful movement
- First-World anesthetists less familiar with its use.

Ketamine Pharmacokinetics

Ketamine is metabolized in the liver by hydroxylation and demethylation to norketamine which is excreted in the urine. When given intravenously it has an onset of action of 30 seconds, a distribution half life of 10 minutes, and an elimination half life of 2 to 3 hours. Unlike propofol, its pharmacokinetics are best described by a two-compartment model.[11] Ketamine is also well absorbed when given intramuscularly, having a bioavailability of 90 to 95%. When given via this route a 6 to 8 mg/kg dose has an onset of 3 to 5 minutes and duration of up to 25 minutes.

Ketamine Pharmacodynamics

Ketamine's pharmacodynamics have been well described in the literature.[12] The dissociative anesthetic state it produces is quite different to other anesthetic agents. There is no loss of corneal reflex such as occurs with other induction agents and it often produces a slow nystagmus, with dilation of the pupils. Its use is often associated with non-purposeful movements, which can be of concern to anesthetists and surgeons not familiar with its use.

Cardiovascular Effects

Ketamine produces favorable hemodynamics as a result of inhibition of re-uptake of norepinephrine.[13] This often results in an increase in heart rate, systemic vascular resistance, and blood pressure. These affects make ketamine anesthesia a particularly good choice in hypovolemic and unstable patients, but can be blunted by the co-administration of midazolam or opiates.[14] Of note, however, is that ketamine has direct cardiac inhibitory affects which are unmasked when the sympathetic nervous system is exhausted, resulting in a fall in blood pressure.[15]

Respiratory Effects

The effects of ketamine on the respiratory center are also of advantage to the anesthetist involved in disaster surgery. Ketamine causes bronchodilation which is of benefit to patients with exposure to toxic gases, as might occur in a disaster situation. Ketamine also maintains respiratory drive much more than other anesthetic agents, improving its safety profile and lessening the risk of airway loss and the requirement to ventilate a patient under anesthetic. Ventilation perfusion mismatch is less with ketamine compared to other anesthetic agents.[16] These properties can result in a lower inspired oxygen concentration requirement, in some cases being able to provide anesthesia without any added oxygen.[17] This relieves a large burden to the anesthetist operating in an austere environment with limited gas supplies.

Salivation is increased with ketamine, which could possibly cause laryngospasm or upper airway obstruction. Secretions can be reduced by pre-medication with either atropine or glycopyrolate; however, care is needed in tropical environments as the concurrent decrease in sweating caused by these agents may lead to hyperthermia. Although swallowing and gag reflexes are maintained with this anesthetic more than with other IV agents, aspiration is still possible and so care is needed when the patient is unfasted, which is likely in a disaster situation.

Many anesthetists in the past have avoided ketamine in patients where pulmonary hypertension may be present as it had been reported to increase pulmonary vascular resistance; however, this action does not occur when hypercapnia is controlled by mechanical ventilation.[18,19]

Central Nervous System Effects

In the past the use of ketamine in head injury has been controversial as there were case reports of increase intracranial pressure during ketamine anesthesia.[20,21] Review of these case reports reveals that end-tidal CO_2 was not controlled. A recent review article has challenged previous doctrine and suggests that ketamine is safe in the setting of head injury, if attention is paid to avoidance of secondary injury caused by hypotension, hypoxia, and hypercapnia.[22] In view of its favorable cardiac effects, ketamine may be a better choice than propofol in the hemodynamically compromised trauma patient with a co-existing head injury.

One of the most disturbing side effects of ketamine is that of emergence phenomenon. This can take the form of alterations in mood, vivid dreaming, and visual hallucinations to frank delirium. The incidence is of the order of 3 to 30%, increases with age and is more common in females. Pre-medication with benzodiazepams such as midazolam (0.05–0.1 mg/kg) or diazepam (0.1–0.2 mg/kg)[23] reduce the incidence of this, as does co-administration with propofol. In the pediatric population the incidence and severity of delirium is significantly less; midazolam has not proved to decrease the incidence in children and is avoided, since its use may increase unwanted side effects such as respiratory depression.[24] In a disaster situation, injured patients requiring surgery risk developing PTSD. It is reasonable to question whether ketamine anesthesia is implicated in the etiology of PTSD. However, a study involving US military personnel compared the incidence of PTSD between a group receiving ketamine infusion and a control group receiving only morphine analgesia for burns surgery. The incidence of PTSD was lower in the ketamine group.[25] Research has recently been commenced investigating ketamine as a treatment for PTSD.[26]

Other Effects

Ketamine causes an increase in muscle tone. This may cause difficulties in reduction of joint dislocation or fractures, and in laparotomy requiring abdominal muscle relaxation for surgical access. The use of a muscle relaxant such as vecuronium negates this issue, at the cost of a more complex anesthetic, necessitating endotracheal intubation, ventilation, and the increased monitoring that is required with muscle paralysis.

Ketamine also increases smooth muscle tone. A study on pregnant females by Oats et al. found that uterine tone during the first and second trimesters of pregnancy was increased with ketamine to the same extent as ergotamine, but there was no increase in uterine tone in the third trimester.[27] There are no studies on teratogenicity of ketamine and the FDA has listed ketamine as a category B medication. Except in cases of eclampsia and pre-eclampsia, the World Health Organization recommend ketamine as a suitable anesthetic for cesarean sections.[28]

Ketamine Anesthetic Practicalities

A number of ketamine anesthetic techniques have been described. The following are options the anesthetist can use depending upon patient assessment and available resources.

Ketamine Co-administered with Propofol using Sophisticated Syringe Drivers[29]

This technique relies on power to drive syringe pumps and oxygen to enhance the inspiratory concentration, as well as the logistical requirement of servicing equipment.

Equipment
1. Syringe driver – may be either simple ml/h, or able to be run as mg/kg/min
2. Oxygen in the form of a tank or oxygen concentrator
3. 200 mg/2 ml or 500 mg/10 ml ampoules of ketamine
4. 50 or 20 ml syringes
5. Low volume extension set
6. IV access and infusion set preferably with an antireflux line
7. Monitoring of pulse and blood pressure, oxygen saturations, and end-tidal capnography, if available
8. Airway equipment
9. Ability to ventilate the patient with a t-piece or self-inflating bag.

Ketamine may be mixed with propofol and loaded in the same syringe to create a ketamine 10 mg/ml and propofol 10 mg/ml solution. This reduces the amount of equipment required; however, it prevents the flexibility of adjusting infusions of the two agents independently.

The advantage with co-administration of propofol is reduced emergence phenomenon, and reduction of tachycardia and hypertension; however, this compromises the safety profile of the ketamine by loss of protective airway reflexes and respiratory drive. A ketamine-only technique is preferred in hemodynamically unstable patients.

Following pre-medication with 0.07 mg/kg of midazolam and pre-oxygenation, the patient is induced with a combined dose of propofol 1.0 mg/kg and ketamine 1.0 mg/kg. When using the agents in the same syringe as above this equates to a volume of 0.1 ml/kg.

Maintenance is obtained with an infusion of propofol at 1 to 2 mg/kg/h and ketamine 1 to 2 mg/kg/h. When combined this is a rate of 0.1 to 0.2 ml/kg/h.

If the patient appears light, a bolus dose of 0.1 mg/kg (0.01 to 0.02 ml/kg) of both drugs is given, followed by an increase in the infusion rate of 0.1 mg/kg/h. If anesthesia appears too deep it can be lightened by pausing the infusion for a short period. The infusion is then recommenced at a rate reduced by 0.1 mg/kg/h of both drugs.

The infusion should be ceased 5 to 7 minutes prior to the anticipated end of surgery.

Ketamine Infusion[30]

This technique may be performed using a mechanical infusion pump, or by adjusting the rate using a manual drip calculation method. When using a drip calculation method the use of a 60 drop per ml microdrip set will aid in the accuracy of delivery. Depending upon patient factors and surgical requirements the patient can be allowed to spontaneously ventilate using a Hudson mask, or be paralyzed, intubated, and ventilated.

Equipment:
1. Infusion pump or IV infusion set with drip chamber
2. 200 mg/2 ml or 500 mg/10 ml ampoules of ketamine
3. 500 or 1000 ml bag of normal saline
4. Intravenous access equipment
5. Airway equipment
6. Pulse, blood pressure, respiration, oxygen saturation, and capnography monitoring, as available
7. Oxygen in the form of a tank or oxygen concentrator
8. Airway equipment and self-inflating bag if using muscle paralysis.

500 mg to 1000 mg ketamine is added to the saline bag to make up a 1 mg/ml solution for maintenance. For shorter surgery 250 ml N/S bags may be more practical if available. A syringe containing 200 mg of ketamine in 20 ml is used for induction.

Following pre-oxygenation and pre-medication with 0.05–0.1 mg/kg midazolam, anesthesia is induced with an IV bolus of 1 to 2 mg/kg of ketamine.

Anesthesia is then maintained with a ketamine infusion at the rate of 1.5–3.0 mg/kg/h. If practical it is best for the ketamine infusion to run in an independent cannula separate to the maintenance or resuscitation line. Using the above solution of 1 mg/ml and a 10 drop per ml infusion set this ends up being 5 to 10 drops per min for a 20 kg child, 10 to 30 drops per minute for a 60 kg adult and 15 to 40 drops per min for an 80 kg adult.

If a drop per ml micro drip set is available, a more concentrated solution should be used by diluting 400 mg of ketamine in a 100 ml bag of normal saline to produce a 4 mg/ml solution. To achieve a maintenance rate of 2 mg/kg/h will require a drip rate of 0.5 drops/kg/min (half the patients weight in drops per min).

To increase the depth of anesthesia a bolus of 0.1 mg/kg should be given, followed by an increase in the rate of the infusion. To decrease anesthetic depth the infusion should be ceased for 10 to 20 seconds followed by resumption at a slower rate. The infusion should be ceased 5 to 7 minutes prior to the anticipated end of surgery.

Ketamine Intermittent Boluses[31]

This technique requires the least amount of equipment, giving it significant advantages over the others in an extremely austere environment; however, it is a less smooth technique given the larger variation in plasma drug concentration caused by intermittent boluses.

Equipment:
1. 200 mg/ml or 500 mg/10 ml ampoule of ketamine
2. Intravenous injection equipment
3. Intravenous cannulation equipment
4. Oxygen if available
5. Monitoring of pulse, respiration, BP, saturation, and capnography, if available.

A 10 mg/ml solution of ketamine is drawn up in a 20 ml syringe. An induction dose of 1 to 2 mg/kg is given intravenously. As the patient becomes light further intravenous boluses of 0.5 mg/kg are given. Boluses are likely to be required every 5 to 10 minutes.

If due to environmental situations it is impossible to obtain IV access (e.g. entrapment situations), a 4 to 6 mg/kg dose can be given by deep intramuscular injection. This will have an onset of 3 to 5 minutes and duration of 20 to 30 minutes. Further IM boluses, if required, should be half the original dose.

Special Scenarios

Hypovolemic Shock

The anesthetist in a disaster situation must assume that a significant number of their patients will be suffering from some amount of blood loss on top of dehydration and possible sepsis. In addition with the logistical limitations of the austere environment it is likely that the anesthetist has only very limited access to blood products and inotrope infusions. The pharmacokinetics and dynamics of ketamine are particularly suited to these critically ill patients.

In uncorrected hemorrhage, ketamine has reduced central compartment clearance as well as a decrease in the size of the central compartment, resulting in a higher plasma concentration following an intravenous bolus. However, the changes in pharmacokinetics of ketamine are much less compared to propofol in hypovolemia, this may be related to ketamine's low plasma protein binding of 12% compared with 95 to 99% in propofol.[32] Ketamine's pharmacodynamic effects are relatively unchanged by hemorrhage. This results in a reduction of induction dose to 0.5 mg/kg, but requires minimal alteration to maintenance dosing.[33] The addition of midazolam to the ketamine mixture, however, may adversely affect hemodynamics in an under-resuscitated patient.

Pediatrics

A significant amount of work during disaster relief missions involves pediatric patients. Ketamine has been extensively used in the pediatric population for both sedation and induction of anesthesia.

Ketamine has been shown to have a similar central compartment volume in the pediatric population, meaning that the induction dose is the same as in adult patients (1–2 mg/kg). Clearances, however, increase with decreasing age, meaning that the pediatric population will require an increased infusion rate to maintain depth of anesthesia compared with adults.

Dallimore et al. recommend a decreasing infusion rate similar to the Bristol methods 10–8–6 rule for patients weighing between 12 and 40 kg where a loading dose of 2 mg/kg is followed by an infusion of 11 mg/kg/h for the first 20 minutes, 7 mg/kg/h for the next 20 minutes, 5 mg/kg/h for the next 20 minutes, 4 mg/kg/h for the following hour, and 3.5 mg/kg/h thereafter.[34] Whilst this regimen is possible when using a syringe driver it may prove impractical when using a gravity drop infusion set. In this situation simplifying the infusion by starting with a rate of 7 mg/kg/h that is reduced to 5 mg/kg/h after 30 mins and the use of boluses of 0.2 mg/kg if the patient appears light may reduce the risk of drug error. Similar regimes have been used with success.[35]

As noted earlier, emergence phenomenon are much less common and less severe in the pediatric population, lessening the requirement for co-administration of midazolam or diazepam.[24] Excess salivation in the pediatric population may result in more laryngospasm, requiring a higher level of vigilance.

Of concern in the pediatric population is recent evidence of ketamine-induced apoptosis of immature neurones.[36] Whilst this may prompt a change of agent in your home practice it is worth remembering that studies in humans have not shown differences in learning in children having undergone ketamine sedation and so in the disaster situation the advantages may outweigh the risks.

Future Issues

Whilst ketamine has proved itself to be invaluable in the field of disaster, Third-World, and trauma anesthesia, there has been a move by member nations of the UN to have the Commission on Narcotic Drugs place ketamine in Schedule 1 of the 1971 Convention.[37] This would restrict the supply and carriage of this medication and could possibly make it unavailable for use in disaster situations. So far the WHO has voted against this occurring, but international anesthetists need to maintain vigilance against moves to have this valuable drug removed from our armamentarium.

References

1. Halford FJ. Critique of intravenous anesthesia in war surgery. *Anesthesiology* 1943;4:67–69.

2. Adams RC, Gray HK. Intravenous anesthesia with pentothal sodium in the case of gunshot wound associated with accompanying severe traumatic shock and loss of blood: report of a case. *Anesthesiology* 1943;4:70–73.

3. Miller DR. Intravenous infusion anesthesia and delivery devices. *Can J of Anaesth* 1994; 41(7):639–652.

4. Morgan DJ, Campbell GA, Crankshaw DP. Pharmacokinetics of propofol when given by intravenous infusion. *Br J Clin Pharmacol.* 1990;30(1):144–148.

5. Roberts FL, Dixon J, Lewis GT, Tackley RM, Prys-Roberts C. Induction and maintenance of propofol anaesthesia: a manual infusion scheme. *Anaesthesia* 1988;43(Suppl):14–17.

6. Absalom AR, Mani V, De Smet T, Struys MMRF. Pharmacokinetic models for propofol: defining and illuminating the devil in the detail. *BJA* 2009;103 (1):26–37.

7. Johnson KB, Egan TD, Kern SE, et al. The influence of haemorrhagic shock on propofol: a pharmacokinetic and pharmacodynamic analysis. *Anesthesiology* 2003;99(2):409–420.

8. Jonson KB, Egan TD, Kern SE, et al. Influence of hemorrhagic shock followed by crystalloid resuscitation on propofol: a pharmacokinetic and pharmacodynamic analysis. *Anesthesiology* 2004;101 (3):647–658.

9. Green SM, Clem KJ, Rothrock SG. Ketamine safety profile in the developing world: survey of practitioners. *Acad Emerg Med* 1996;3(6):598–604.

10. Mion G, Villevielle T. Ketamine pharmacology: an update (pharmacodynamics and molecular aspects, recent findings). *CNS Neurosci Ther* 2013;19:370–380.

11. Clements JA, Nimmo WS, Grant IS. Bioavailability, pharmacokinetics and analgesic activity of ketamine in humans. *J Pharmaceutical Sci* 1981;71 (5):539–542.

12. Pai A, Heining M. Ketamine. *CEACCP* 2007;7(2):59–63.

13. Lundy PM, Lockwood PA, Thompson G, Frew R. Differential effects of ketamine isomers on neuronal and extraneuronal catcholamine uptake mechanisms. *Anesthesiology* 1986;64:359–363.

14. Svenson JE, Abernathy MK. Ketamine for prehospital use: new look at an old drug. *Am J Em Med* 2007;**25**:977–980.

15. Saegusa K, Furukawa Y, Ogiwara Y, Chiba S. Pharmacologic analysis of ketamine induced cardiac actions in isolated, blood-perfused canine atria. *J Cardiovasc Pharmacol* 1986;**8**:414–419.

16. Tokics L, Strandberg A, Brismar B, Lundquist H, Hedenstierna G. Computerised tomography of the chest and gas exchange measurements during ketamine anaesthesia. *Acta Anaesthesiol Scand* 1987;**31**:684–692.

17. Pesonen P. Pulse oximetry during ketamine anaesthesia in war conditions. *Can J Anaesth* 1991;**38**(5):592–594.

18. Balfors E, Haggmark S, Nyhman H, Rydvall A, Reiz S. Droperidol inhibits the effects of intravenous ketamine on central hemodynamics and myocardial oxygen consumption in patients with generalized atherosclerotic disease. *Anesth Analg* 1983;**62**:183–187.

19. Williams GD, Philip BM, Chu LF, et al. Ketamine does not increase pulmonary vascular resistance in children with pulmonary hypertension undergoing sevoflurane anaesthesia and spontaneous ventilation. *Anesth Analg* 2007;**105**(6):1578–1584.

20. Shapiro HM, Whyte SR, Harris AB. Ketamine anaesthesia in patients with intracranial pathology. *Br J Anaesth* 1972;**44**:1200–1204.

21. Gibbs JM. The effect of intravenous ketamine on cerebrospinal fluid pressure. *Br J Anaesth* 1972;**44**:1298–1302.

22. Cohen L, Athaide V, Wickham ME, et al. The effect of ketamine on intracranial and cerebral perfusion pressure and health outcomes: a systematic review. *Ann Em Med* 2015;**65**(1):43–51.

23. Cartwright PD, Pingel SM. Midazolam and diazepam in ketamine anaesthesia. *Anaesthesia* 1984;**39**:439–442.

24. Wathen JE, Roback MG, MacKenzie T, Bothner JP. Does midazolam alter the clinical effects of intravenous ketamine sedation in children? A double-blind, randomized, controlled, emergency department trial. *Ann Em Med* 2000;**36**(6):579–588.

25. McGhee LL, Maani CV, Garza TH, Gaylord KM, Black IH. The correlation between ketamine and post traumatic stress disorder in burned service members. *J Trauma* 2008;**64**(2):195–199.

26. Feder A, Parides MK, Murrough JW, et al. Efficacy of intravenous ketamine for treatment of chronic posttraumatic stress disorder: a randomized clinical trial. *JAMA Psychiatry* 2014;**71**(6):681–688.

27. Oats JN, Vasey MB, Waldron BA. Effects of ketamine on the pregnant uterus. *BJA* 1979;**51**(12):1163–1166.

28. *WHO Model Prescribing Information: Drugs Used in Anaesthesia*. Geneva: WHO 1989.

29. Bajwa SJS, Bajwa SK, Kaur J. Comparison of two drug combinations in total intravenous anesthesia: propofol–ketamine and propofol–fentanyl. *Saudi J Anaesth* 2010;**4**(2):72–79.

30. Ketcham DW. Where there is no anaesthesiologist: the many uses of ketamine. *Tropical Doctor* 1990;**20**:163–166.

31. Cottingham R, Thomson K. Use of ketamine in prolonged entrapment. *J Accid Emerg Med* 1994;**11**:189–191.

32. Black IH, Grathwohl KW, Terrazas IB, Martini WZ, Johnson KB. The influence of hemorrhagic shock on ketamine: a pharmacokinetic analysis. *Anesthesiology* 2006;**105**:A203.

33. Weiskopf RB, Bogetz MS. Haemorrhage decreases the anaesthetic requirement for ketamine and thiopentone in the pig. *Br J Anaesth* 1985;**57**:1022–1025.

34. Dallimore D, Anderson BJ, Short TG, Herd DW. Ketamine anesthesia in children: exploring infusion regimens. *Pediatr Anesth* 2008;**18**:708–714.

35. Tugrul M, Camci E, Pembeci K, et al. Ketamine infusion versus isoflurane for

the maintenance of anesthesia in the prebypass period in children with tetralogy of Fallot. *J Cardiothorac Vasc Anesth* 2000;**14**:557–561.

36. Liu F, Paule MG, Ali S, Wang C. Ketamine induced neurotoxicity and changes in gene expression in the developing rat brain. *Curr Neuropharmacol* 2011;**9**:256–261.

37. UN Commission on Narcotic Drugs uno dc.org/unodc/en/commissions/CND/Ma ndate_Functions/Mandate-and-Functions_index.html (accessed September 2019).

Inhaled Anesthetics and Draw-Over Devices in Disaster Response

Carlton Brown

Inhaled anesthetics remain the primary pharmacologic agents for administering general anesthesia in current surgical practices. Anesthesia providers enjoy familiarity and extensive experience with these inhaled agents in the context of modern anesthesia delivery equipment. In providing anesthetic care during disasters, providers will often have access to the same technically sophisticated anesthetic vaporization and monitoring systems typical of modern, brick-and-mortar hospital facilities. For example, anesthetic care rendered after a focal mass casualty event in an urban area would likely be done with a reliable supply of pharmaceutical agents, modern anesthetic machines, modern monitors, and reliable electricity. Even in rare circumstances of regional natural disasters where local healthcare facilities have lost electricity, water, or other infrastructure support, it is still often possible to transfer patients to facilities in adjacent geographic areas where these services remain intact. In this context, the use of inhaled anesthetics in disaster response is likely to be simply a direct extension of our daily practices. "No one gets smarter in a disaster," and our use of familiar equipment, familiar agents, in familiar settings, and with familiar patient flow patterns yields the highest probability of successful anesthetic outcomes. In the anesthetic care of patients in disaster settings, it is incumbent that providers not augment the misery and mortality of the actual disaster with any additional morbidity or mortality from their anesthetic care. As disaster triage directs patients into surgical care, the availability of the most sophisticated anesthetic care – familiar anesthetic equipment, agents, resources, and providers – should be part of that decision-making process.

In those rare circumstances where surgical care must be undertaken in very austere conditions, providers should carefully consider the advantages and disadvantages of delivering inhaled anesthetics and the concomitant need of airway manipulation and ventilation that generally accompanies them. Even for extensive surgical procedures, there are often alternatives to inhaled anesthetics. Total intravenous anesthesia (TIVA), intravenous or intramuscular ketamine, or regional anesthetic techniques may offer safer and more efficient resource utilization for austere surgical care. TIVA, typically with propofol, can be administered if necessary with only gravity fed IV and a mini-dripper. Ketamine, either IV or IM, can allow the completion of remarkably extensive surgical procedures while maintaining spontaneous ventilation and hemodynamic stability. Regional anesthetics often avoid airway issues and offer extremely efficient use of pharmaceutical resources. By example, a 30 ml vial of preservative-free 0.75% bupivacaine may yield as many as 15 isobaric spinal anesthetics. For procedures on the lower extremities or even into the abdomen up to the diaphragm, spinal anesthesia is a reasonable alternative to inhaled general anesthesia. Procedures on the upper extremities can be done with modest amounts of local anesthetic in regional plexus blocks. Trauma involving extremity injuries as seen in natural disasters is often amenable to regional anesthetics. Before anesthesia providers commit themselves and their patients to unfamiliar inhaled anesthetics delivered through unfamiliar equipment, a careful risk–benefit analysis should be considered given these alternative techniques for supporting surgical care.

Absent global apocalypse, modern anesthesia disaster resources and equipment are often delivered within a day or two of the primary event, even into extremely remote areas. These resources include readily transportable, scaled-down versions of commercial anesthesia machines that have many of the modern safety features appropriate for inhaled anesthetic delivery. These "field anesthesia machines" combine a small footprint, minimal logistic demands, and some intrinsic monitoring capabilities to provide safe inhaled anesthetic delivery. The US military currently issues and supports the Draeger Fabius Tiro "M" model for deployable use. This is only one of many such compact "field machines" available worldwide. Many of these machines are capable of providing PEEP, triggered and controlled ventilation, air dilution, and other features now considered part of normal contemporary anesthetic practice. As the care of trauma patients often involves penetrating wounds, crush injuries, and thoraco-abdominal surgery, these ventilator modes are most useful. The ability of these portable anesthesia machines to measure exhaled carbon dioxide is particularly important for assessing adequacy of ventilation and persistence of cardiac output. End-tidal inhaled anesthetic agent measurement is very helpful both in avoiding over-dosage and optimally timing emergence. Combined with a small portable monitor, these "field anesthesia machines" allow safe inhaled anesthetic delivery outside of a traditional hospital setting. Whenever possible, providers involved in disaster relief should become familiar with the machines with which they will practice prior to deployment. Both carefully reading the operator's manual and some prior clinical experience are highly recommended, as some of these devices may have limited capabilities or unique characteristics (hidden on–off switches). Patient safety dictates familiarity with these machines *before* use in a high-stress disaster setting. Although comparable in safety to hospital equipment, these machines require reliable compressed gas supplies and electricity, and their vaporizers are typically agent-specific. These resources may be problematic in the most austere of locations. The decision to deliver inhaled anesthetics should consider availability of these machines, provider familiarity (or time available to learn their proper use), availability and reliability of infrastructure resources, and availability of inhaled anesthetic agents compatible with agent-specific vaporizers.

Disaster anesthesia often involves care of trauma patients, and most anesthesia providers are familiar with the relative advantages and disadvantages of inhaled anesthetics in this population (Box 5.1). The hemodynamic effects of inhaled anesthetics as sole agents may be clinically limiting. Modern fluoro-methyl ether anesthetics are vaso-depressant largely through decreases in systemic vascular resistance. This can be offset in part by using nitrous oxide in lieu of higher doses of these ethers. In field anesthesia, however, nitrous oxide may be either unavailable or inappropriate at altitude. The use of intravenous narcotics such as fentanyl may also allow reduced doses of inhaled drugs, but the availability of controlled substances in field settings may be problematic for both logistical and regulatory reasons. The absence of nitrous oxide or readily available intravenous narcotics may be a substantial change in practice for many anesthesia providers.

Box 5.1 Advantages of Inhaled Anesthetics

Modern inhaled anesthetics do have *potential advantages* in disaster response planning. These include:

- Low relative cost (isoflurane in particular)
- Easily shipped – small size and weight
- Long shelf-life storage
- No refrigeration required
- Provider familiarity
- Predictable administration with appropriate equipment
- Rapid titration
- Rapid onset
- Rapid recovery
- Allows spontaneous ventilation
- Muscle relaxant properties without neuromuscular blockade
- Minimal long-term toxicity
- Possible cyto-protection through pre-conditioning.

Disadvantages of inhalational anesthetic agents include:

- Some issues with shipping (hazardous materials regulations)
- Cost in Third-World countries
- Logistics of primary and re-supply
- May be agent-specific for vaporizers
- Abusable substances
- Theft for profit or abuse
- Require complex delivery devices (anesthesia machines)
- Hemodynamic depression – dose dependent
- Risk of malignant hyperthermia
- Atmospheric contamination
- Older agents (halothane, enflurane) myocardial depressants.

In all, disaster relief planning should include an integrated approach to the logistics of pharmaceutical supply, patient monitoring, and anesthetic delivery devices *if* inhalational anesthetics are to be used.

Draw-Over Vaporizer

To paraphrase Antony in *Julius Caesar*, "Friends, Romans, countrymen, lend me your ears. I come to bury Caesar, not to praise him. The evil that men do lives after them; the good is oft interred with their bones. So let it be with [*the draw-over vaporizer.*]"

The "draw-over vaporizer" is a device that, much like Caesar, is and should remain a part of history. The tradition of inhaled anesthesia since the nineteenth century has involved devices that take a liquid anesthetic and convert it into a vapor, often in haphazard, unreliable, or even dangerous concentrations. Morton used ether delivered through his inhaler – in effect, a draw-over vaporizer – in the first public demonstration of inhaled anesthesia in 1846. Current "draw-over vaporizers" follow in that tradition. Attempts at creating "simple" disaster response vaporizers have been described for more than 50 years.[1] The "draw-over vaporizer" was suddenly re-discovered and enjoyed near-mythical status

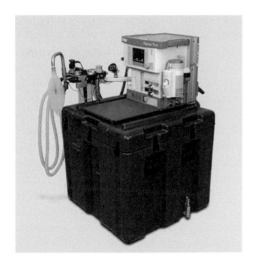

Figure 5.1 Draeger Fabius Tiro Model "M" – current US deployable anesthesia machine.

after being employed by British forces during the Falklands/Malvinas War in 1982. Shortly thereafter, the US military placed draw-over devices into its medical inventory. The US Army and Navy still issue the Ohmeda Universal Portable Anesthesia Complete (UPAC) draw-over device[2] to some forward-deployed units. However, changes in anesthetic practice over the last 25 years have nearly obviated the need for such devices. TIVA, ketamine, and regional anesthesia often offer superior anesthetic care to the draw-over device in austere settings. Simply because any device is issued by the US military does not necessarily commend its use. When one of the authors (CQB) was deployed on an aircraft carrier in 1983, the Navy still had "open drop ether" (Yankauer) masks in its Authorized Medical Allowance List (AMAL). While anesthesia machines have been designed to deliver volatile anesthetics more safely over the last 30 years, the design of the draw-over vaporizer has steadfastly avoided any of these important patient safety features.

The general premise of the draw-over vaporizer is that of an ultra-austere device, requiring no electricity, no compressed gas, and capable of converting any anesthetic liquid into a vapor. While this simplicity may be appealing, the draw-over device lacks even the most rudimentary safety features for the delivery of inhaled anesthetics. In fact, it does not meet the current United States Food and Drug Administration's safety requirements for the administration of inhaled anesthetics. By simple example, there is no in-circuit oxygen analyzer. The device is pictured in Figure 5.1. Part of its mythical attractiveness is that it packages into a small box that is readily transportable. The standard issue components can be seen in the picture.

In its standard form, the draw-over vaporizer relies on the inspiratory efforts of a patient to "draw over vapor" by entraining room air into the vaporizer, saturating a fraction of that air with anesthetic vapor, and then delivering that vapor to the patient. This is similar in general design to modern proportional flow vaporizers, with the significant difference that modern anesthesia machine vaporizers require compressed gas to pick up and deliver the vapor. Calibration cards allow the anesthesia provider to convert the dial setting into approximate concentrations of the various inhaled anesthetics. Corrections for temperature and atmospheric pressure are additionally required. Manual assistance of patient ventilation requires a self-inflating bag, absent a compressed gas supply. Supplemental oxygen may be added to the circuit, but is not required for operation of the vaporizer.

There are several obvious limitations to this device. In its most basic form, there are no accommodations for mechanical ventilation or supplemental oxygenation. There is no oxygen analyzer. There is no deliberate re-breathing within the anesthesia circuit, resulting in high anesthetic vapor consumption, loss of heat, and loss of humidity. The absence of an anesthetic agent-specific interlock on the filling port permits the introduction of any agent into the device, along with the uncertainty and safety issues accompanying such easy substitutions. It unfortunately also allows for inadvertent agent mixing of two agents within the device. If one chooses to use this device, *there should never be a mixture of agents* in the vaporizer. Absent an azeotropic mixture, each anesthetic agent will volatilize independently and a massive anesthetic over-dosage may result. There is no alarm or indicator to identify this mixed agent condition. The device is not fully "tip resistant," and if not maintained in a vertical position with liquid agent in the vaporizer, it can deliver lethal anesthetic concentrations. In all, the draw-over device is potentially very hazardous.

There have been several attempts at modifying the draw-over vaporizer to accommodate some of these limitations. Figures 5.2 and 5.3 below shows the Gegel–Mercado modifications[3] that measure circuit-inspired concentration of oxygen (FiO_2) and provide

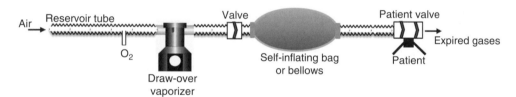

Figure 5.2 Basic draw-over setup.

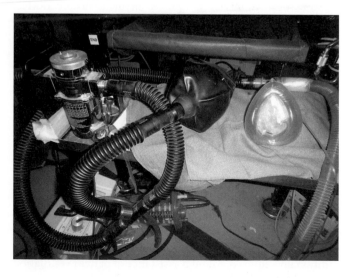

Figure 5.3 Added tubing and monitors for ventilator support.

for mechanical ventilation. As mechanical ventilation is added to this device, however, a basic safety premise is compromised: in its original design, anesthetic over-dose is avoided in this device when the increasing levels of anesthesia resulted in decreasing respiratory efforts by the patient. With mechanical ventilation, this feedback loop is lost and over-dosage can easily result. Additionally, the use of a mechanical ventilator adds one-way valves, additional connections, and other sources of potential failure into the breathing circuit. Further, the addition of an electrically powered ventilator and an electrical FiO_2 measurement device increase the complexity of the overall circuit and require, at a minimum, battery power. At some point, any claim of "elegant simplicity" is lost.

Although these devices are currently issued by the US military, one might draw an inference of caution from a requirement within a military manual regarding them: the Navy Bureau of Medicine and Surgery Notice (BUMEDNOTE) 1520 (29SEP2014) still suggests utility in training personnel with draw-over vaporizers. However, also in September 2014, the Surgeon General of the Navy issued an extensive set of training requirements before Navy personnel are allowed to use a draw-over vaporizer (NAVMED 1520/30 (09/2014)). This training includes a practicum for equipment setup, required didactic and training materials, a minimum number of clinical cases, and final signatory permission before Navy personnel are allowed to use this device. (As the draw-over device does not meet minimum FDA safety standards for clinical anesthesia delivery devices, it raises an interesting ethical question about obtaining clinical experience.) As general advice to disaster anesthesia response personnel who have not previously used the draw-over device, it is hazardous to your patients to learn in an "on-the-job" disaster setting. In all, passing historical familiarity with the draw-over device may be all that is needed for most disaster response anesthesia personnel.

References

1. Coursey JW, Wilson RD. A new draw-over halothane vaporizer. *Anesth Analg* 1965;4:147–157.

2. Ohmeda *Ohmeda Universal Portable Anesthesia Complete Manual*. Madison, WI: Ohmeda, 1990.

3. Gegel BT. Field-expedient Ohmeda universal portable anesthesia complete draw-over vaporizer setup. *AANA J* 2008;76:185–187.

Chapter 6

Airway Management

Michael J. Murray

Introduction

There is a great deal of information about the management of the airway during many different scenarios, but very little of that information addresses the management of the airway during a mass casualty event following a disaster. There are guidelines for managing a difficult airway,[1] for managing a failed intubation,[2] and for managing the airway of a patient who has sustained trauma,[3] but one can find very little information about how to manage the airway during a mass casualty event (MCE). In 2015 two journals devoted entire issues to airway management but neither journal has any information about airway management following a disaster,[4,5] when a health care facility may have a multitude of patients who require emergent airway management to minimize morbidity and mortality. The lack of such information is surprising because following a major disaster that results in an MCE, health care providers consistently state that better preparedness would have resulted in decreased morbidity and mortality.[6] One interpretation of this lack of information is that mass casualty events that generate a multitude of patients that require emergency airway management are so rare that there is no way that health care providers can prepare for, and anticipate, such events. However, if one performs a hazard-analysis risk-management assessment, although the chances of such events occurring are quite low, when they do occur, the resulting morbidity and mortality are incredible.[7] For example, the worst disaster in the past 100 years was the 1918 Spanish influenza pandemic, during which 20% of the world's population was infected with the virus, which killed one of every 40 people in the world; the mortality rate was in the thousands per 100 000. The numbers of patients requiring respiratory care was enormous. Likewise, the polio epidemic in the 1950s resulted in so many patients requiring mechanical ventilation that patients were housed in hospital auditoriums. In more recent times the SARS[8] and H5N1[9] epidemics had the potential to create equally large numbers of patients requiring respiratory care. In addition to natural biologic events, there is always the potential for rogue nations and terrorists to use biologic agents or chemical agents that would result in a large number of patients requiring emergency airway management. For example, the recent use of chlorine gas by Syria against Kurdish fighters in March of 2015,[10] and the use of sarin by the Aum Shinrikyo cult in the subway system of Tokyo in 1994[11] underscore the fact that such agents could be used again in the future. Finally, one cannot discount the possibility of an industrial disaster that would precipitate an MCE in which the majority of patients would require emergency airway management, e.g. the isocyanate gas leak in Bhopal, India that affected tens of thousands of individuals.[12]

This chapter focuses therefore, not on how one would manage several patients who might require emergent airway management (a mass casualty incident), but potentially hundreds of patients (a mass casualty event) who might require emergency airway management.

Disaster Management

Prevention/Mitigation

While there is little that we as health care providers can do to prevent or mitigate disasters that would result in a large number of patients who might require emergent respiratory care following a disaster, one should at least be aware of what resources are available should the unthinkable occur. Aside from the need for surge capacity, a need that would be addressed by the community's emergency response plan, as occurred in Paris following the terrorist attacks of November 13, 2015,[13] the greatest need in terms of equipment would be for ventilators. The Center for Disease Control and Prevention's (CDC) Strategic National Stockpile is a repository of ventilators that would be used to supplement the supply currently in use by the nation's acute care facilities. These ventilators can be requested and allocated to areas of need and could be delivered within several hours (~12 h) to a facility that required them.[14]

Preparedness

Preparing for an MCE that would require the emergency airway management of dozens if not hundreds of patients is difficult. Anesthesia departments' emergency response plans typically do not contain guidance for this scenario. The primary reason for "emergency preparedness," the second component of an over-all disaster response plan, is to prepare for different scenarios, especially one that though unlikely, would result in considerable morbidity and mortality. Therefore, it might behoove a hospital when planning its biannual emergency response drill, as required by The Joint Commission (TJC), to plan a "disaster drill" that would include a large number of patients coming to the hospital in respiratory distress. Anesthesia providers – anesthesiologists, CRNAs, and anesthesia assistants – would have the requisite skills to provide assistance in managing the airway in most mass casualty situations. However, these individuals probably have little or no experience managing an airway while wearing personal protective equipment (PPE). Ambulatory patients coming to a hospital following exposure to a chemical agent such as sarin, would be asked to disrobe and undergo decontamination before being seen by a health care provider. However, those patients with significant nerve agent poisoning may have acute respiratory failure requiring emergency airway management by an individual wearing a hazardous materials (HAZMAT) suit. Once the life threatening condition is treated, then patients' clothing is removed and the patient decontaminated.[15]

HAZMAT PPE presents several challenges. The suits are not insulated and external temperatures can significantly impede performance. The gloves are usually constructed from Teflon, polyvinyl chloride or rubber, and polyethylene and although they are impermeable to most chemical agents, they significantly decrease manual dexterity. Similarly, the face hoods or masks may impair visual acuity. Prior training wearing these suits is recommended to improve performance during an actual mass casualty event. As will be discussed later, consideration should be given to securing the airway with a supraglottic airway (SGA) device, disrobing and decontaminating the patient, and placing a tracheal tube at a later time under better circumstances.[15]

There is more to emergency preparedness though, than just practicing airway management while wearing PPE. The anesthesiologist in charge of a department's disaster management plan should incorporate a section that addresses the airway management issues that might arise in an MCE following a disaster. Issues that should be addressed include personnel, equipment and supplies, human factors, training, and diagnosis-management paradigms.

Personnel

In order to mount an adequate response to an MCE in which there are scores of patients with respiratory compromise, it is probably most important that a facility or an emergency response system have an adequate number of well-trained individuals. In one study of pre-hospital airway management in emergency and trauma patients, there was no deficiency of equipment, but a majority of the emergency response personnel had inadequate training in airway management.[16]

Equipment and Supplies

The hospital must have the ability to establish a triage site outside the emergency department that has the capacity to evaluate, decontaminate, and treat patients before they are allowed to enter the facility. Obviously, in order to respond to a mass casualty event, defined as an event that overwhelms the hospital's ability to provide the usual standard of care, there must be an adequate supply of 100% oxygen (pressurized outlets or cylinders) along with tubing, facemasks, equipment for mask ventilation etc.[17] In an MCE the use of supraglottic airways (SGAs) may be lifesaving in that more patients can have a definitive airway device placed and ventilated with 100% oxygen. One might argue that the same could be achieved with bag-mask ventilation but only about one-third of novice providers are able to do so effectively. Even with additional training success rates increase to only 80–90%.[18]

There are several different SGAs that potentially could be used in an MCE, but the number of choices should be limited. The Supreme LMA® and the I-gel LMA® have been found to be superior to other LMAs when placed by novice operators.[19] They have the additional advantage that they can be placed in the dark if need be, e.g. if facilities lose electrical power and lighting is suboptimal.[20]

Human Factors

The psychological stress that health care providers will experience when responding to a disaster will impair performance.[21] Therefore, any plan should attenuate, if not eliminate, any additional stressors. The plan should be as simple as possible – an algorithm that offers a multitude of management pathways, or airway devices that one could use, creates a "paradox of choice" and may delay an appropriate response.[22] A similar factor that should also be taken into account when designing the plan is "analysis paralysis."[22] An anesthesiologist may over-analyze the situation to try to find an ideal management strategy, one that will save the life of every casualty that arrives at the hospital. However, in a true mass casualty situation one cannot act as one would act in one's normal everyday practice. If one focuses on trying to save every patient, and spends too much time with a single patient, many more patients' lives are put at risk. The goal in disaster management is to save as many lives as possible, recognizing that not all lives can be saved. Although an individual caring for a single patient may focus on securing the airway by placing a tracheal tube or SGA, the team leader must have more "situational awareness." He or she must allocate resources so that the maximum number of patients will undergo appropriate airway management with maintenance of oxygenation and ventilation by whatever available means.

Training

Aircraft pilots undergo periodic training in a flight simulator so that they maintain familiarity with the appropriate response to uncommon mechanical failures that could potentially result in an airplane crash. Because these events are so rare and for which one cannot train in a real-world scenario, the training must be obtained in a flight simulator. In addition, because recall of the correct pilot response to mechanical failure deteriorates with time, the training must be repeated on a regular basis. The same is true for disaster management skills and this is the reason that TJC requires hospitals to have biannual disaster management drills. The same is also true for airway management skills of individuals who may infrequently use those skills. Currently, most health care providers must undergo basic life support (BLS) (and advanced cardiac life support) training every two years. There is evidence however, that retraining in BLS every six months helps individuals better maintain their basic skills e.g. jaw-thrust, assisted ventilation etc.[23]

Diagnosis-Management Paradigms

The anesthesiologist in charge of this periodic training should have a disaster management plan that is focused and with an easily understood algorithm. All members of the team must be educated on what the priorities are, the most fundamental of which is having the correct diagnosis-management paradigm.[22] The best-trained individuals with adequate supplies and equipment will have poor outcomes if they have the wrong paradigm. For example, when authorities ended the hostage crisis in the Moscow Dubrovka Theater in 2002, it is presumed that they immobilized everyone with a potent aerosolized opioid,[24] most likely carfentanyl. This information was not communicated to emergency response personnel so that when the hostages and their captors arrived at local hospitals, physicians interpreted their meiosis and respiratory difficulty as manifestations of nerve agent poisoning. They managed patients' airways appropriately, but because they used an anticholinergic to treat patients and not an opioid antagonist, more than 130 hostages died. The physician in charge of this mass casualty event had the wrong disease-management paradigm; more situational awareness may have improved patients' outcome.

Additional Personnel

In most MCEs hospitals would have an adequate number of individuals with the necessary airway management skills to manage patients with respiratory compromise. However, depending on the number of patients, additional personnel may be required. There are lessons that individuals and facilities can learn from the military, an organization whose health care teams have as one of their primary foci, the management of mass casualties. All medics carry nasopharyngeal airways to be placed when indicated in the field. These medics, and combat lifesavers and nurses also may have attended a basic airway skills course that includes training in mask ventilation, insertion of oral and nasopharyngeal airways, SGA devices, tracheal intubation, and even cricothyroidotomy. However, in training such individuals, one must be careful not to overwhelm novice providers with too complicated an airway management algorithm or too many choices of equipment.[22] In providing pre-hospital care or care in a triage area outside the hospital, placement of an SGA in an unconscious patient may be the most effective means to manage airway and respiratory compromise.[25] Individuals who may be called upon to assist in airway management in a mass casualty event should receive training in the anesthesia department in placement of SGA devices.[18]

Response

If a hospital is notified that there has been a disaster and that a large number of patients with respiratory difficulties are being transported to the facility, the institution should immediately activate its emergency response plan; time is of the essence. The Aum Shinrikyo terrorist group released sarin into the Tokyo subway system at 07:55 on March 20, 1995. St. Luke's hospital was notified at 08:16 and the first patient arrived at 08:28. The first patient arrived by ambulance at 08:43, and within an hour the hospital was trying to manage over 500 patients.

Depending on the scope of the disaster, and the precipitating cause of the respiratory distress, e.g. use of chlorine or phosgene by a terrorist group, consideration should be given to accessing ventilators in the Strategic National Stockpile. A triage and decontamination site must be quickly established outside the emergency department. Personnel with training in airway management wearing PPE should be assigned to the decontamination area. The number of casualties and the etiology of the respiratory distress will dictate the scope of the hospital's response, but independent of that, a very simple algorithm for managing equipment and scenarios should be followed (Box 6.1) Unconscious and apneic patients should have a definitive airway established and should be ventilated with 100% oxygen. Conscious patients with respiratory distress should be supplied 100% oxygen via a mask while additional evaluation and treatment is undertaken in the emergency department. Patients who require mechanical ventilation should be admitted to an ICU following treatment in the emergency department.

Box 6.1 Algorithm for Selection of Airway Devices for Use During a Mass Casualty Event

1. Oxygenation is the priority, and then ventilation.
2. Choose devices and equipment that can be used by the least experienced personnel with an approximately 100% success rate.
3. Devices and equipment must be clinically reliable – not just in routine use, but in emergency situations as well.
4. Devices should be tested in a number of circumstances over a period of time by a cross-section of personnel.
5. Extubation procedures should similarly be managed by a protocol, with a plan for reintubation should end-points not be maintained.
6. Sufficient staff should be trained to manage not only oxygenation and ventilation in mass casualty events, but of all forms of respiratory therapy.

Recovery

Following the incident there must to be an evaluation of the adequacy of the response, and again depending on the size and severity of the MCE, counseling should be made available to all providers who participated in the response.

Conclusion

Hopefully, none of us will be involved in a MCE in which there are scores of patients requiring emergency airway management, but the best way to anticipate a successful response to such an event is to begin to prepare for it now, and to develop a plan that is as straightforward as possible.

References

1. Apfelbaum JL, Hagberg CA, Caplan RA, et al. Practice guidelines for management of the difficult airway: an updated report by the American Society of Anesthesiologists Task Force on Management of the Difficult Airway. *Anesthesiology*, 2013;**118**:251–270.

2. Frerk C, Mitchell VS, McNarry AF, et al. Difficult Airway Society 2015 guidelines for management of unanticipated difficult intubation in adults. *Br J Anaesth* 2015;**115**:847–848.

3. Jain U, McCunn M, Smith CE, Pittet JF. Management of the traumatized airway. *Anesthesiology* 2016;**124**:199–206.

4. Fleisher LA. Airway management. *Anesthesiol Clin* 2015;**33**:viii–xiv.

5. Gaszynski T, Toker K, Carassiti M, Chalkias A, Carlson JN. Advances in airway management and ventilation strategies in emergency medicine. *Biomed Res Int* 2015;**2015**:425715.

6. Ciraulo DL. A survey assessment of the level of preparedness for domestic terrorism and mass casualty incidents among Eastern Association for the Surgery of Trauma members. *J Trauma* 2004;**56**:1033–1041.

7. Arnold J. Disaster medicine in the 21st century: future hazards, vulnerabilities, and risk. *Prehosp Disaster Med* 2002;**17**:3–11.

8. Zhong N, Zeng G. What we have learnt from SARS epidemics in China. *BMJ* 2006;**333**:389–391.

9. Oner AF, Bay A, Arslan S et al. Avian influenza A (H5N1) infection in eastern Turkey in 2006. *N Engl J Med* 2006;**355**:2179–2185.

10. Abdulrahim R. Six die from alleged chlorine-gas bomb attack in northwest Syria. *Wall Street Journal*, March 17, 2015:3.

11. Okumura T, Takasu N, Ishimatsu S et al. Report on 640 victims of the Tokyo subway sarin attack. *Ann Emerg Med* 1996;**28**:129–135.

12. Das J. The Bhopal tragedy. *J Indian Med Assoc* 1985;**83**:72–74.

13. Hirsch M, Carli P, Nizard R et al. The medical response to multisite terrorist attacks in Paris. *Lancet* 2015;**386**:2535–2538.

14. Malatino E. Strategic national stockpile: overview and ventilator assets. *Respir Care* 2008;**53**:91–95.

15. Murray M. Emergency preparedness for, and disaster management of, casualties from natural disasters and chemical, biologic, radiologic, nuclear and high-yield explosive (CBRNE) events. In Barash P, Cullen BF, Stoelting RK et al. (eds.) *Clinical Anesthesia*, 7th edn. Philadelphia, PA: Lippincott, Williams & Wilkins, 2013:1535–1554.

16. Ismail S, Zia N, Samad K, et al. Prehospital airway management in emergency and trauma patients: a cross-sectional study of ambulance service providers and staff in a low- and middle-income country. *Prehosp Disaster Med* 2015;**30**:1–7.

17. Becker D, Rosenberg MB, Phero JC. Essentials of airway management, oxygenation, and ventilation. *Anesth Prog* 2014;**61**:78–83.

18. Soleimanpour H, Gholipouri C, Panahi JR, et al. Role of anesthesiology curriculum in improving bag-mask ventilation and intubation success rates of emergency medicine residents: a prospective descriptive study. *BMC Emerg Med* 2011;**11**:8–14.

19. Henlin T, Sotak M, Kovaricek P, et al. Comparison of five 2nd-generation supraglottic airway devices for airway management performed by novice military operators. *Biomed Res Int* 2015;**2015**:20189.

20. Ohchi F, Komasawa N, Imagawa K, Okamoto K, Minami T. Evaluation of the efficacy of six supraglottic devices for airway management in dark conditions: a crossover randomized simulation trial. *J Anesth* 2015;**29**:887–892.

21. Donchin Y, Gopher D, Olin M, et al. A look into the nature and causes of human errors in the intensive care unit. *Crit Care Med* 1995;**23**:294–300.

22. Greenland K. Art of airway management: the concept of 'Ma'. *BJA* 2015;**115**:809–812.

23. Nishiyamaa C, Iwami T, Murakami Y, et al. Effectiveness of simplified 15-min refresher BLS training program: a randomized controlled trial. *Resuscitation* 2015;**90**:56–60.

24. Anonymous. Russia Names Moscow Siege Gas. 2002. Retrieved from BBC News: http://news.bbc.co.uk/2/hi/eur ope/2377563.stm (accessed September 2019).

25. Khosravan S, Alami A, Hamzei A, Borna J. Comparing the effectiveness of airway management devices in pre-hospital emergency care: a randomized clinical trial. *Pak J Med Sci* 2015;**31**:946–949.

Vascular Access, Hydration, and Fluids

Michael J. Murray

Introduction

Following a major disaster from which a large number of casualties result, a community's ability to rescue, triage, transport, evaluate, and treat these casualties quickly and effectively leads to the best possible outcome. The best outcomes occur if treatment is judiciously applied within the "golden hour," the 60 minutes following the injury to the patient.[1] However, the golden hour rule most commonly applies to individuals who have sustained traumatic injury and not to mass casualty events during which tens if not hundreds or thousands of patients must be treated, in which case the first 24 hours become critical.[2] Medical care provided during such events is quite different from that provided during one's regular civilian medical practice.[3] However, independent of the number of casualties, at some point in time, depending on the severity of the injuries, those patients who are moderately to severely injured will require primary and secondary surveys with special attention to the ABCs and, with respect to "circulation," these patients will need vascular access established and fluid resuscitation. This chapter will focus on those issues common to all patients who have sustained traumatic injury and require fluid resuscitation, and on the requirements for those patients who are victims of earthquakes, thermal injury, explosions, and infectious agents.

General Principles

Mass casualty events are situations in which a hospital's facilities are overwhelmed by the number of casualties arriving at the hospital's emergency department (ED), either because of the absolute number of casualties or because the facility's capability is degraded, e.g. from damage to the physical plant from an earthquake or tornado or from loss of electrical power because of a hurricane or flood. Therefore, an anesthesiologist or other health care provider must be prepared to function in an austere environment, one that may be quite chaotic, one in which even blood pressure cuffs and stethoscopes are not available or are not practical. Or the anesthesiologist may be called upon to treat a patient trapped in the rubble of a collapsed building following an earthquake, tornado, or explosion.

Fluids

A patient with a respiratory rate of ≥30 breaths per minute, or a pulse of greater than 100 beats per minute or one that has a barely palpable pulse will require placement of an intravenous cannula and administration of intravenous fluids. Isotonic saline is commonly recommended initially for most patients,[4] whereas Ringer's lactate is recommended for patients who have sustained thermal injury.[5] The goal is to maintain intravascular volume, cardiac output, and tissue perfusion until further evaluation and treatment can be undertaken. The disadvantage of isotonic saline is that it has a relatively large amount of chloride compared to that contained in Ringer's lactate, which may worsen a pre-existing metabolic acidosis. The disadvantage of Ringer's lactate, on the other hand, is that the small amount of K^+ it contains may cause fatal hyperkalemia, even in patients with a crush injury sustained in an earthquake or explosion who do not have acute kidney injury (AKI).[6] The goal during fluid resuscitation is to maintain blood pressure and urine output. However, excessive fluid administration can create as many problems as under-resuscitation, including abdominal compartment syndrome, which may worsen AKI.

Route of Administration

Those who practice in high-income countries are accustomed to resuscitating patients with intravenous fluids. However, following a disaster, in an austere environment intravenous cannulas and sterilized intravenous fluids may not be readily available. In 1950, the Surgical Study Section of the National Institutes of Health recommended that "the use of an oral saline solution is adopted as standard procedure in the treatment of shock due to burns and other serious injuries in the event of a large scale civilian catastrophe."[7] The solution that was recommended was Myers solution: a hypotonic (160 mOsm) solution containing 85 mEq of Na^+ that is buffered with either bicarbonate or citrate. These recommendations are relatively easy to implement in a timely fashion and their application may result in improved outcome, at least from AKI in patients who have sustained crush injury[8] or thermal injury.[9]

Other alternatives to intravenous resuscitation must be considered, e.g. when dealing with patients with highly contagious and lethal (Class A bioweapon) infectious diseases. In the 2014–2016 Ebola viral disease (EVD) pandemic, treatment was largely supportive and quite basic. Because of EVD's effects on the gastrointestinal system, enteral resuscitation was not an option, and the placement of intravenous cannulas by personnel wearing PPE (personal protective equipment) in patients whose extremities were edematous presented a major challenge. In such circumstances the placement of intraosseous cannulas for fluid resuscitation is more readily achieved and can be lifesaving.[10]

Specific Considerations

Crush Injuries

In the December 1988 earthquake in Armenia there were 25 000 fatalities; there were more than 900 severely injured patients of whom 900 had AKI, one-third of whom required dialysis.[11] AKI is the leading cause of delayed mortality following an earthquake (the majority of patients die acutely from head or thoracic crush injury in collapsed buildings at the time of the event). AKI and death can be avoided by the timely administration of fluid.[12] Saline is recommended as it is efficacious and associated with few side effects. Sodium bicarbonate added to 0.5 N saline attenuates the deposition of uric acid and myoglobin in the renal tubules, decreases the incidence of hyperkalemia, and corrects metabolic acidosis, but may not be available in an austere environment.[4] As discussed previously, solutions containing even small amounts of K^+ should be avoided. The administration of mannitol to treat the rhabdomyolysis associated with crush injury is somewhat controversial. Mannitol is believed to be therapeutic because of its diuretic, vasodilating, and antioxidant properties. Mannitol increases intravascular volume, prevents deposition of myoglobin and uric acid in renal tubules, decreases intercompartmental pressures and muscle edema, and decreases the incidence of compartment syndrome. Mannitol is not without risk though, as it may worsen congestive heart failure in at-risk patients, and is associated with nephrotoxicity *per se*. The decision to use mannitol, if available, must be made on a case-by-case basis, under close supervision with appropriate monitoring, which may be difficult, depending on the extent and severity of the mass casualty event. If mannitol is used, a small dose is recommended initially and continued only if there is a satisfactory diuretic response.

Thermal Injury

The care of patients with thermal injuries was significantly improved when it was recognized that they require a large amount of fluid, an amount that was dependent on the extent and severity of the burn, and the patient's body weight. The standard of care for patients who sustain thermal injury is the administration of intravenous fluid, and the sooner the fluid is administered the better the outcome. Administration of fluid either intravenously or enterally in a timely fashion to patients with ≥20% TBSA (total body surface area) third-degree burns significantly decreases the incidence of hypovolemic shock and AKI. There is, however, some controversy as to the best formula for the type and amount of fluid that patients should receive. In the United States the modified Parkland and modified Brooke formulae are the most widely used. Both formulae list the administration of crystalloid during the first 24 hours following a burn, adding colloid during the second 24-hour period. Protein-based colloids (albumin/plasma) are used by most centers. For less serious injuries, <20% TBSA, or for situations in which the number of casualties overwhelms the healthcare system, e.g. following a nuclear blast, administration of oral rehydration fluid may be lifesaving.

Explosions

The explosions in the warehouses along the docks in Tianjen, China in August 2015 destroyed >17 000 homes, killed 777 people and injured more than 2000 others. IEDs (improvised explosive devices) are being used with increased frequency by terrorists the world over. Health care providers therefore, independent of where they practice, must be prepared to render assistance either at the site of the explosion, or in the healthcare facility where they work. The most vital actions at the scene are assessment and establishment of an airway, ventilatory assistance if necessary, and stopping any bleeding immediately, e.g. application of a tourniquet to a bleeding extremity. At the health care facility damage control resuscitation (stopping internal bleeding as soon as possible) is associated with the best outcomes. Unfortunately, depending on the number of patients, less seriously injured patients may have surgery delayed and will require intravenous fluid therapy. In such a situation, hypotensive resuscitation initially, until bleeding is under control, is increasingly advocated.[13] The only exception would be in patients with traumatic brain injury, in whom mean arterial pressures of less than 90 mmHg are associated with worse neurologic outcomes.

Epidemics

The Ebola virus disease (EVD) epidemic of 2014–2016 underscored how ill-prepared the civilized world is to prevent and treat such infectious outbreaks, and how much panic occurs in the general population when such an infectious outbreak occurs. In an illness such as a viral hemorrhagic fever like EVD in which there is widespread third spacing of fluids and extensive gastrointestinal losses of blood and intravascular fluid, fluid resuscitation is literally lifesaving. Providing this treatment in the austere environment found in West Africa was a considerable challenge. Wearing PPE for extended periods of time in an extremely warm hospital tent was one such challenge, as was the placement of intravenous cannulas in edematous extremities for administration of fluids (oral rehydration was not a realistic option because of the gastrointestinal side effects of the disease) while wearing PPE. If these difficulties could be overcome, the chances of survival were considerably improved, but nonetheless, the overall mortality rates in West Africa during the EVD pandemic was approximately 80%. The few patients with EVD who were treated in resource-rich countries had much better outcomes, underscoring what was discussed previously about the difference in providing care to a few patients vs hundreds of patients with either traumatic injury or a debilitating infectious process during a mass casualty event.

Conclusion

For a multitude of reasons, the world in which we live is experiencing more disasters, whether natural or man-made, than ever has occurred in the past. Physicians and other healthcare providers must educate themselves so that they're prepared to deal with the number of casualties that might arise from a disaster in their locality in the future. Part of the preparedness is the ability to work under austere conditions, and the ability to triage patients – those with less severe injuries can be delayed or even rendered at home with enteral fluids. Those with more severe injuries must be managed immediately – stopping the bleeding from any source – with the administration of 0.9% saline for crush victims, Ringer's lactated fluid for burn victims, hypotensive resuscitation initially for victims of blast injury, and the establishment of intravenous or intraosseous access in patients with infectious illnesses, while wearing PPE.

References

1. Rady MY. Triage and resuscitation of critically ill patients in the emergency department: current concepts and practice. *Eur J Emerg Med* 1994;**1**(4):175–189.

2. Blow O, Magliore L, Claridge JA, Butler K, Young JS. The golden hour and the silver day: detection and correction of occult hypoperfusion within 24 hours improves outcome from major trauma. *J Trauma* 1999;**47**(5):964–969.

3. Holcomb JB. Fluid resuscitation in modern combat casualty care: lessons learned from Somalia. *J Trauma* 2003;**54**(5 Suppl): S46–S51.

4. Sever MS, Vanholder R. Management of crush victims in mass disasters: highlights from recently published recommendations. *Clin J Am Soc Nephrol* 2013;**8**(2):328–335.

5. Fodor L, Fodor A, Ramon Y, et al. Controversies in fluid resuscitation for burn management: literature review and our experience. *Injury* 2006;**37**(5):374–379.

6. Sever MS, Erek E, Vanholder R, et al. Serum potassium in the crush syndrome victims of the Marmara disaster. *Clin Nephrol* 2003;**59**(5):326–333.

7. [No Authors Listed] Saline solution in treatment of burn shock. *Public Health Rep* 1950;**65**(41):1317–1320.

8. Cancio LC, Kramer GC, Hoskins SL. Gastrointestinal fluid resuscitation of thermally injured patients. *J Burn Care Res* 2006;**27**(5):561–569.

9. Michell MW, Oliveira HM, Kinsky MP, et al. Enteral resuscitation of burn shock using

World Health Organization oral
rehydration solution: a potential solution
for mass casualty care. *J Burn Care Res*
2006;**27**(6):819–825.

10. Ben-Abraham R, Gur I, Vater Y,
Weinbroum AA. Intraosseous emergency
access by physicians wearing full
protective gear. *Acad Emerg Med* 2003;**10**
(12):1407–1410.

11. Collins AJ, Burzstein S. Renal failure in
disasters. *Crit Care Clin* 1991;**7**(2):421–435.

12. Better OS, Stein JH. Early management of
shock and prophylaxis of acute renal
failure in traumatic rhabdomyolysis.
N Engl J Med 1990;**322**(12):825–829.

13. Kirkman E, Watts S, Cooper G. Blast
injury research models. *Philos Trans R Soc
Lond B Biol Sci* 2011;**366**(1562):144–159.

Critical Care Delivery for Disasters in Austere Environments

Liza Weavind

Natural disasters (Japan tsunami 2011), terrorism attacks (Boston marathon bombing 2013) and industrial accidents (Bhopal disaster 1984) create mass casualty situations, with large numbers of critically ill or injured patients. These mass casualties create a surge in resource utilization (space, people, and equipment), which places stresses on the most resilient, well-resourced, and integrated healthcare systems.[1,2]

One hundred million people are injured every year, of which 5 million will succumb to these injuries, and 90% of this mortality occurs in low- and middle-income countries (LMICs).[3] Critical care needs following disasters occurring in austere and remote settings quickly outstrip the local resources available and can lead to preventable loss of life, increasing morbidity and disability for survivors. This increase in the number of disability-adjusted life years burdens entire communities. The demand for critical care services may not arise directly from the violence or disaster itself, but from chronic medical disorders following the breakdown of public health infrastructure (e.g. clean water resulting in cholera, waste removal in the recent Ebola crisis) or interruption in the ability to get medications.[4]

This chapter outlines best practices and key points in planning for and delivering critical care following a disaster in austere environments:

- Planning
- Logistics
- Systems planning
- Ethical considerations
- Sustainability after the disaster
- Data and research.

Planning

Pre-disaster planning by LMICs improves their ability to utilize international aid when a disaster occurs and decreases the time to rescue efforts being initiated to limit life loss associated with these events.[5] Foreign medical teams, even if deployed immediately, often fail to arrive in time to provide emergency trauma interventions in the immediate aftermath of an event. This task falls to the local medical or surgical providers, who, in the chaos directly following the disaster, lack a coordinated response and are unable to access needed medical supplies, transportation, and hospitalization for the victims. The more robust the public health infrastructure (primary care, emergency care, and medical transport) prior to a disaster, the more effective the local disaster responders can be in the rescue of the initial victims.[6] The time required to mobilize disaster medical teams and the fact that these teams can only deploy to the affected areas at the invitation of the host nation lead to prolonged delays before these teams become effective. Strategic relationships with world bodies such as the World Health Organization (WHO), United Nations, Non-Government Organizations (NGOs), and governments as well as academic or professional organizations from developed countries can limit this delay and allow disaster teams to mobilize efficaciously. Professional critical care societies in developed countries should invest in critical care education (resuscitation, evacuation, and transport of critically ill patients) and protocol development to be utilized in these LMICs in a disaster, prior to the arrival of international medical responders.

Disaster Medical Responders

Who should provide critical care services in a disaster?

1. Skilled and experienced adult and pediatric trained critical care providers, preferably with previous training/expertise in disaster response.[5] Skills required to be an effective provider:
   - Leadership skills, but also a team player
   - Flexibility/self sufficiency to work in a variety of non-traditional critical care arenas
   - Experience/training in mass casualty incidents with diverse medical equipment and with specific training in the unique injury patterns that may be encountered
   - Ability to communicate and coordinate workflows across multidisciplinary and multicultural teams
   - An understanding of the political and cultural background contributing to the disaster
2. Providers aligned with groups who provide this type of care (Médecins Sans Frontières, Red Cross, military responders, NGOs, etc.)

Who shouldn't provide critical care services in a disaster? Well-intentioned, but poorly prepared, inexperienced or untrained disaster responders, who may be unable to adapt their skills in austere environments and thus hinder the process rather than help.[5]

Disaster Logistics

Critical care delivery is resource intensive and is challenging when barriers such as a poor economy, lack of infrastructure, and lack of trained staff are exacerbated by crisis and disaster. Successful delivery of care in this environment depends on meticulous planning, fastidious management of resources, and having the right people on the team (local and foreign). Disaster responders should engage with the local medical staff and stakeholders, preferably giving them strategic and leadership roles in managing the disaster victims.[7] This integration will allow teams to garner locally available resources and technologies, as well as get buy-in to facilitate care of the victims. These relationships with also allow for a smooth disengagement in the post-disaster period.[9]

1. Leadership and supervisory systems to support care – a critical care team leader (CCTL) is appointed to lead the unit/team. The CCTL should be a competent, disaster trained, and respected clinician, as well as an effective communicator, a flexible leader, and a consummate professional. The intensivist in this role will be responsible for patient triage in conjunction with surgical teams, resource allocation, medical direction, and

oversight of the other providers. The CCTL should have final decision-making authority regarding who receives and does not receive critical care services.

2. Clinical staff shortages – a 1:2 nurse-to-patient ratio may not be feasible with shortages and should rather be determined by provider experience and clinical demands. To remove variability and allow less skilled providers to safely care for critically ill patients, safety checklists, nurse-driven care guidelines, and protocols can be utilized. The use of adaptive staffing models with innovative shift structures can maximize care delivery without causing staff burnout.[4]

3. Biomedical engineers (for repairs and to keep equipment in working order), translators and research personnel are key non-clinical team members to facilitate workflow.

4. Supply chain – an administrative director (this may be a role shared by the nursing and physician leader of the ICU) is helpful to take care of the supply chain while the clinical team focuses on the medical needs of the patients. Some issues that the administrator will need to address are as follows:

   a. Security for staff in insecure environments, which will require high-level situational awareness, communication with military or other groups in the disaster area, along with contingency and evacuation plans (for staff and patients) should an unsafe environment deteriorate

   b. Support services for staff such as food, housing, and transport

   c. Equipment, which should be appropriate for the local environment, affordable, portable, multiuse and simple to operate. A list of essential emergency equipment can be found at: www.who.int/surgery/publications/EEEGenericListFormatted%20 06, but include ICU specific additions:

      i. Beds/stretchers

      ii. Ventilators – both adult and pediatric with flexible electric/battery power with the ability to run on low-flow oxygen without a high-pressure gas source. These ventilators need to be easy to operate and repair

      iii. Cardiopulmonary monitors and point-of-care (POC) testing devices for blood work, which are simple to calibrate and maintain

      iv. Arterial and central venous lines

   d. Essential medications (narcotics, antibiotics, inotropes, and vasopressors) to provide comfort and supportive care for critically ill patients

   e. Intravenous fluids (crystalloids and colloids) available on hand and a stable supply chain, as the initial amount that can be transported may be limited

   f. Oxygen (tanks or a concentrator) – tanks are robust, but transport and refilling of tanks is expensive and unreliable

   g. Personal protective equipment for staff to maintain universal precautions for the duration of the relief effort.

Systems Planning

Resource-poor nations struggle with access to fundamental resources such as a consistent supply of electricity, access to fuel, and clean water, and this may be exacerbated during the disaster. These constraints force ingenuity and flexibility when disaster teams are tasked with providing critical care services in this environment. A focus on the following issues facilitate care:

1. Power – an independent supply of electricity from a portable energy source (batteries, generators, or solar devices) to power equipment is essential as the national grid for the country may be unreliable. If generators are being used as a fuel source a consistent supply will need to be identified. Consider the implication that electricity may not always be available and have a contingency plan in place to best manage the scenario.

2. Water – clean and continuous water supply as ICU patients require about 40–60 liters/day, but can be as high as 100–300 liters/day per patient undergoing a surgical intervention.[10]

3. Sanitation and disposal of waste – the WHO guideline on the management of healthcare-associated waste should be followed.[11]

4. Blood and blood product availability – this is a scarce and high-risk resource. The reliance on donation of whole blood by volunteers (living donor blood bank) with limited ability to screen for endemic diseases, viral diseases, or even cross-matching makes the unintended consequences of utilizing this resource fraught with danger. Disaster-specific transfusion guidelines are required with the ability to recognize and treat transfusion-related complications.[7,8]

5. Diagnostic technology – such as X-rays, ultrasound and ECGs to facilitate early diagnosis and intervention for life-threatening conditions is only valuable if it can be maintained and repaired.

Ethics

Rationing of critical care is a reality in a disaster scenario with many considerations, other than population-level short-term survival, being taken into account. Rationing should be fair and just, to maximize the benefits to the population being served, and should be based on objective factors (physiologic criteria, likelihood of survival, need for long-term reliance on scare resources) applied consistently to all patients.[12]

Strict triage practices must be instituted early to minimize utilizing scarce resources on patients who are unlikely to survive or who will require ongoing care (dialysis, prolonged mechanical ventilation) which will be unavailable following withdrawal of the disaster medical teams. Chronically critically ill patients or those with an increase in the number of disability-adjusted life years burden entire communities and the impact of providing life prolonging support services for them should be weighed against the benefit to the community. Long-term chronic care is not available in most LMICs and this, coupled with socio-cultural, religious norms, and expectations which impact the ability to withdraw life support once it has been initiated, should be taken into consideration before initiating lifesaving supportive care.[12] Ethically there is no difference between withholding or withdrawing life support, but it may be impossible to do so without losing the trust of the people and patients you are here to serve.[13,14]

The legal ramifications of applying a triage algorithm to ration scare resources in a disaster are untested in the international arena, but when applied consistently, in good faith and with transparency, the provider should be protected. This remains an area of research.[15,16]

Triage Principles in a Disaster[14]

1. The triage officer (usually the senior surgeon in a trauma situation), who has ultimate triage authority on site, should consult with both surgical and critical care teams about

which patients are appropriate to undergo surgical intervention and subsequent admission to the ICU, as this leads to optimized utilization of resources and smooth patient flow from the operating room to the ICU.[5] ICU admission criteria and knowledge of critical care resource constraints can facilitate this discussion.

2. Critical care will be rationed only after all attempts to augment services or transfer patients elsewhere have been exhausted.

3. Limitations on critical care will be proportional to actual limitations of resources.

4. Rationing will be transparent, will occur uniformly, and abide by objective criteria laid down in triage protocols/algorithms rather than by clinical judgment and will be communicated to patients and families on admission to the hospital.

5. Rationing will apply equally to withholding and withdrawing life support with frequent patient re-evaluation for appropriateness of ongoing critical care support.

6. Patients not eligible for critical care will still be provided with comfort care and transitioned to palliation, not with the intent of hastening death, but relieving suffering.

7. These decisions should be documented in the medical record with the data to support the decisions for transparency and consistency.

Post-Disaster Hand-Off and Long-Term Provision of Services

What happens after the disaster? In many LMICs the existing medical infrastructure, facilities and expertise are inadequate prior to the disaster and remain so afterward. The disengagement of surge resources and reintegration of these services into the medical delivery model of the community will require coordination between the disaster teams and the pre-existing healthcare stakeholders (local government officials, health care providers, hospitals, and national public health care officials). The lack of baseline emergency and critical care services prior to the disaster makes the constitution of these services after a disaster challenging and must be done in conjunction with, and not at the expense of, preventative and primary care programs. A focus on improving patient care through the use of routines, checklists, and protocols can result in better outcomes for all patients and a more efficient use of resources than a large financial or technological investment by disaster teams.[17] Education and curricula development by foreign medical teams may have more value than leaving behind equipment that health care providers cannot use once the disaster teams have withdrawn.

Data Collection and Quality Improvement Factors

1. In a disaster, research and data collection are not top priorities, but are vital to improve mass casualty response and resource utilization at the time of a disaster. The clinical and cost-effectiveness of the interventions by disaster teams as well as the long-term economic impact on host countries needs to be tracked and reported out to optimize the response for the next disaster.

2. Standardized data collection tools should be deployed to facilitate education and provide data to local authorities, increase accountability of care, and facilitate review of the event later to improve response in future.

3. Data should be collected in crisis and non-crisis situations to evaluate structure, process, and outcomes, as it will drive improved design of critical networks of care, unit staffing, and use of intensive care beds.[12]

Conclusion

Disasters, both natural and man-made, create injury and compound the complexities of chronic illness, requiring the need for critical care and lifesaving interventions. Providing high-quality and exceptional critical care in these austere environments requires comprehensive planning, training, and education to prepare medical personnel responding to disaster, transporting equipment and supplies to the affected areas, and careful management of resources once in place. It can be done and continues to be done by a varied group of exceptional civilian and military providers.

References

1. Emergency preparedness and response. Centers for Disease Control and Prevention website. http://emergency .cdc.gov/ (accessed September 2019).

2. Emergency preparedness: preparing hospital for disasters. California Hospital Association website. www .calhospitalprepare.org/ (accessed September 2019).

3. *The Injury Chart Book: A Graphical Overview of the Global Burden of Injuries.* Geneva: World Health Organization, 2002.

4. Adhikari NKJ, Fowler RA, Bhagwanjee S, Rubenfeld GD. Critical care and the global burden of critical illness in adults. *Lancet* 2010;**375**:1339–1346.

5. Task Force for Mass Critical Care. Care of the critically ill and injured during pandemics and disasters: CHEST consensus statement *Chest* 2014;**146**(4 Suppl):8S–34S.

6. Alexander D. Disaster and emergency planning for preparedness, response, and recovery. 2015 https://oxfordre.com/natur alhazardscience/view/10.1093/acrefore/978 0199389407.001.0001/acrefore-978019938 9407-e-12 (accessed September 2019).

7. Chackungal S, Nickerson JW, Knowlton LM, et al. Best practice guidelines on surgical response in disasters and humanitarian emergencies: report of the 2011 Humanitarian Action Summit Working Group on Surgical Issues within the Humanitarian Space. *Prehosp Disaster Med* 2011;**26**(6):1–8.

8. Schmidt PJ. Blood and disaster: supply and demand. *N Engl J Med* 2002;**346** (8):617–620.

9. McQueen K, Parmar P, Kene M, et al. Burden of surgical disease: strategies to manage an existing public health emergency. *Prehosp Disaster Med* 2009;**24** (4):s228–s231.

10. Pruss A, Giroult E, Rushbrook P. *Safe Management of Wastes from Health Care Activities.* Geneva: WHO, 1999.

11. Prin M, Wunsch H. International comparisons of intensive care: informing outcomes and improving standards. *Curr Opin Crit Care* 2012; **18**(6):700–706.

12. Evans TW, Nava S, Mata GV, et al. Critical care rationing: international comparisons. *Chest* 2011;**140**(6):1618–1624.

13. Devereaux AV, Dichter JR, Christian MD, et al. Definitive care for the critically ill during a disaster: a framework for allocation of scarce resources in mass critical care. *Chest* 2008;**133**:51S–66S.

14. Gostin L, Bayer R, Fairchild A. Ethical and legal challenges posed by severe acute respiratory syndrome: implications for the control of severe infectious disease threats. *JAMA* 2003;**290**:3229–3237.

15. Center for Law and the Public's Health. Model State Emergency Health Powers Act. www.aapsonline.org/legis/msehpa2 .pdf (accessed September 2019).

16. Waters D, Wilson I, Leaver RJ, et al. *Care of the Critically Ill Patient in the Tropics.* Oxford: Macmillan, 2004.

17. Rhodes A, Moreno RP, Azoulay E, et al. Prospectively defined indicators to improve safety and quality of care for critically ill patients. *Intensive Care Med* 2012;**38**:598–605.

Chapter 9

Children in Disasters

Simon Hendel

Introduction

Children are amongst the most vulnerable members of society. In disasters that vulnerability is magnified, especially for the very young and those children who are unaccompanied or have pre-existing medical needs.

The intention of this chapter is to serve as a useful and pragmatic guide to the occasional pediatric practitioner or for the health worker who is in or preparing for a disaster.

There are a number of key differences between the management of children and adults in disasters. These differences will form the basis of the discussion in this chapter. There are also many differences in the availability of expertise and resources to prepare for and manage disasters when they occur. This changes how different jurisdictions may be able to realistically respond, but not the key principles of how to respond.

Children are not little adults and so the key differences in their physiology and development will be examined, as will the different equipment, drugs, and fluids used to treat children in disasters. Responding to disasters involving children is emotionally challenging and psychologically draining. This may have significant effects on health workers and emergency personnel.

There is an enormous difference in development and independence between a newborn through to a 16-year-old young person. This difference is reflected in the broad range of issues that can affect children in disasters. For example, the risk of environmental extremes is significantly greater in a newborn than a teenager. Conversely, the risk of emotional trauma or post-traumatic stress disorder is greater in the teenager exposed to a disaster.

Preparing for, responding to, and recovering from any disaster requires complex systems and multi-agency collaboration. Doing so with children in mind needs all the same responses in addition to an approach that addresses children's unique needs and special vulnerabilities.

The general principles for disaster preparedness and specific responses in a disaster have been discussed in previous chapters and so they will not be repeated in detail here, except where they are necessary for making the point about caring for children.

Preparing for a Disaster

A disaster involving children may overwhelm a non-pediatric hospital, or the emergency medical services response more rapidly than an equivalent event not involving children.

In a disaster, it is highly likely that organisations and individuals who do not usually manage pediatric patients will need to have the capacity to respond outside their normal scope of practice.

The World Association of Disaster Emergency Medicine defines a disaster as:

"A situation or event that overwhelms local capacity, necessitating a request to national or international level for external assistance, or an unforeseen and often sudden event that causes great damage, destruction and human suffering."

Disasters are then further described in terms of natural or man-made. When managing involved children the specific type of disaster will present slightly different issues and challenges for planning and response. More distinctly defined are mass casualty incidents. These events are distinct from larger scale disasters in that they may not effect the community-at-large, despite nonetheless overwhelming local capacity for effective response. It is also important to distinguish these from multiple casualty incidents. By definition, these do not overwhelm local resources or capacity to respond.

This definition is useful in terms of understanding the types of events that are likely to be "disasters." It is important to note that disasters are not contingent only on a significant number of affected individuals but on the overwhelming of local capacity. This is an important consideration for organizations as they prepare for dealing with children involved in a disaster.

Responding to disasters is stressful. For responders it is physically and emotionally draining work. When children are involved the added degree of emotional and psychological stress may make the risk of exhaustion and burnout amongst responding health staff greater. This risk should be discussed in the preparation phase and, as best possible, plans made to mitigate this risk.

From previous chapters, we know that disasters can and do take many forms. Both natural and man-made disasters occur in a variety of contexts and settings, from Paris to small mountaintop villages in Nepal and everywhere in between. Children are also affected by context; however, specific plans for how best to respond to a particular disaster in a particular place are beyond the scope of this chapter. The intent of this chapter is to provide general information and structures that can be adapted and applied to local planning needs and practices.

A structured, multi-agency approach to disaster management forms the basis of the preparedness and response when it comes to dealing with children in disasters as it does for dealing with disasters in general.

Planning at the local level will inevitably involve discussions with key local stakeholders. Pediatric specialists should be identified and involved early in the planning process. At a minimum, experts in pediatric pre-hospital care, pediatric emergency medicine, childhood mental health experts, and pediatric critical care experts should be involved in planning for disaster response. Ideally this planning process should be integrated with broader disaster plans to enable a response for pediatric care in disasters that dovetails with other emergency response plans.

Wherever and however disaster strikes, prior preparation and planning will enable a more coordinated and effective response to coping with and managing children involved. During the early stages of planning and preparedness, consideration of which groups of children will likely be at more risk than baseline or those children with likely the highest risk may help to focus efforts to benefit the whole community.

Understanding the ways in which children differ from adults in disasters is a first step in preparing effectively.

Amongst other medical concerns in a disaster event, children are particularly vulnerable to clinical problems like diarrheal illness, respiratory compromise, effects of environmental extremes, trauma, and burns (see Table 9.1).

Planning for Communication During the Disaster Response

Clear communication between authorities and the population-at-large is an important part of maintaining free flow of information and in managing presentations to care centers. Children and young people may or may not be accompanied by adult guardians following a disaster event and so means of communicating information about the event must be pitched at a basic level and across platforms. Communication about issues relating to children in disasters must be "simple, poignant, accessible and timely," according to the American Academy of Pediatrics, Pediatric Preparedness Resource Kit.

The method of communication most likely to be successful in reaching the population needs to be considered early in the planning phase. It is likely that a cross-platform approach including radio, television, mobile phone networks, and social media will be utilized by disaster management agencies. The success of this communication will depend on the pre-existing capacity of communications infrastructure and the degree to which that infrastructure has been interrupted by the disaster event.

While mass communications will form a part of the disaster response in general, it is important that specific thought be given to how information relevant to childhood risks will be communicated to parents and guardians, and also to children themselves.

Responding to a Disaster

The medical response to a disaster involving children is likely to involve multiple groups of health personnel. While it is beyond the scope of this chapter to set out rigid doctrine in relation to methods of scene command and control or to delve into the inner workings of major incident management, effective command and control is essential and is discussed elsewhere.

It is also beyond the scope of this book to dictate fundamental clinical skills such as in the management of pediatric trauma or burns. There are many easily accessible online resources for in-depth approaches to clinical management of the pediatric patient in the pre-hospital or austere environment. These will be linked at the end of this chapter.

Many of the pre-hospital and in-hospital response teams will have some experience managing pediatric clinical problems. As such, much of the discussion below will be revision. The intention is for the following paragraphs to provide a few useful pieces of practical guidance to adapt familiar practice or function as an aide memoire rather than as an exhaustive coverage of the topic.

There are no major differences in the operational command and control of disasters simply because children are involved, and so instead the next few paragraphs will focus on the practical points of difference between responding to any disaster and responding to one involving children.

Triage

Triage is the process by which severity of presenting cases are assessed and prioritized and available resources are allocated to address those priorities. There are key differences between the objectives of triage in normal circumstances and in disasters.

Table 9.1 Pediatric risks in disasters

Illness/injury	Pediatric risk	Example of disaster event	Potential mitigation
Diarrheal illness	Age-dependent susceptibility (influenced by hygiene, crowding, water and sanitation) More susceptible to effects of dehydration More specialised knowledge and skills required for intravenous rehydration Infants and young children much more susceptible to hypoglycemia and malnutrition	Natural: any that disrupts routine sanitation and/or displaces populations into areas of high density (e.g. Nepal earthquake, Cyclone Winston in Fiji) Man-made: war (e.g. Syrian refugee crisis)	Caches and ready supply of oral rehydration solution (ORS) Access to and supply of infant formula Intravenous and nasogastric rehydration capability
Respiratory infection/ compromise	Higher minute ventilation Greater susceptibility to infectious agents Many chemical agents settle low to ground closer to children's breathing level Smaller, narrower airways more susceptible to inflammation or inhalational agents	Natural: fires, pandemic influenza Man-made: fires, terrcrist attack, nuclear accidents	Established relationships with regional pediatric centers for advice and training Oxygen supplies Specific chemical and radiological antidotes if available
Trauma	Smaller circulating volume and therefore less total volume loss required before onset of shock Inexperience in most centers dealing with pediatric trauma Pain management difficulties	Natural: floods, earthquake, major storm event Man-made: war, terrorism, major transport incident	Structured approach to pediatric trauma following APLS/ ATLS guidelines Early pharmacologic management of pain (see Table 9.3)

Table 9.1 (cont.)

Illness/injury	Pediatric risk	Example of disaster event	Potential mitigation
Burns[a]	More susceptible to effects of fluid shifts in major burns Inexperience of most practitioners	Natural: fires, earthquakes Man-made: fires, war	Accuracy in estimating total body surface area (TBSA) burned using either "rule of nines" (see Figure 9.2) or other validated approach. Early initiation of fluid resuscitation based on modified Parkland's formula[a] or aiming for urine output of 1 ml/kg/h
Environmental extremes	Greater risk of hypothermia and heat illness (especially the very young)	Natural: flooding, storms Man-made: war	Early priority to dry, cover, and shelter young children
Developmental	Less capacity for independent survival High risk of impaired childhood development if displacement/trauma prolonged	All	
Emotional	Less mature coping strategies Less able to process events High chance of separation from family	All	See Chapter 13

[a] Modified Parkland's formula for calculating 1st 24 h of fluid resus in burns: 3–4 ml × wt in kg × %TBSA over 24 h 1st half given in the 1st 8 h since time of burn and next half in remaining 16 h.

These have been addressed in detail elsewhere, but the major difference is that allocating resources to treat the sickest or most severely injured patients may not be the wisest application of available resources and may ultimately place other patients at risk.

This may mean that, in a disaster, children who would survive in other circumstances may die. This is a difficult and distressing concept in any circumstance for health providers to prepare for and ultimately implement if needed, making planning and forethought even more crucial.

Having an accepted system for triage is an important part of ensuring that decisions around health resource allocation are made in as objective and reproducible a way as possible.

There are a number of accepted pediatric triage tools that have been applied to disasters. None of these systems is foolproof and none is widely accepted across the world. There is variation across and within jurisdictions as to which pediatric triage tool is used. The specifics of the tool are less important than the adoption of an easy to use system that is decided upon early in the preparation phase and practiced by disaster response teams prior to implementation in an actual disaster event.

All triage systems are susceptible to under- and over-triage. Under-triage is the inappropriate under-estimation of casualty severity. Under-triage rates should ideally not be more than 5%. Over-triage is the inappropriate over-estimation of casualty severity and is less likely to lead to adverse morbidity or mortality. Accepted rates are around 50%.

One effective method of triaging pediatric patients in a disaster or mass casualty incident is utilizing SALT – Sort, Assess, Life-saving interventions, Transport – combined with the Pediatric Assessment Triangle (PAT). This approach is used by a number of emergency medical services in the USA and around the world. The advantage of combining the PAT into the triage of pediatric disasters is that it is familiar to many pre-hospital providers, simple to use, and does not require sophisticated equipment.

Triage Step 1: Sort

The triage process begins with sorting patients into three groups:

- Priority 1: Obvious threat to life or unresponsive
- Priority 2: Purposeful movement
- Priority 3: Walking

Triage Step 2: Assess

Using the PAT to rapidly assess children provides a valid starting point for initial reception and clinical reassessment of injured children. Under most circumstances, those children allocated priority 1 should be assessed first.

The PAT has three components – represented by sides of a triangle (see Figure 9.1). These components are appearance, work of breathing, and circulation. It is analogous to a rapid pre-primary survey with the ABC approach familiar to most emergency personnel.

The PAT is not an exhaustive head to toe examination and should not take more than a minute to complete.

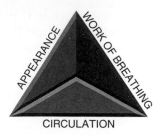

Figure 9.1 The Pediatric Assessment Tool (source: emedicine.com).

Appearance is an "end-of-the-bed" assessment of body position, activity, and tone, and a general view of whether this child is sick or not. Is the child crying or not? Are they alert and aware of your assessment or are they indifferent?

Assessing work of breathing rapidly requires an assessment of respiratory rate and the nature of breathing. Are accessory muscles being used? Is there nasal flaring or noisy breathing? If a pulse oximeter is available, measuring oxygen saturation at this stage provides some objective data to reference reassessment and confirm overall impression.

Circulation is assessed by capillary refill time (>2 s is abnormal), color, and managing any obvious sources of hemorrhage. Blood pressure, while useful in older children, is not a reliable measure of shock in the very young and therefore has limited utility at this stage of the assessment.

Triage Step 3: Life-Saving Interventions

Once the children have been allocated either priority 1, 2 or 3, and priority 1 patients have been assessed using the PAT, lifesaving interventions should be initiated.

This is where the familiar full primary survey (ABCDE) occurs and interventions within the practitioner's scope of practice should be initiated.

The question as to whether cardiopulmonary resuscitation should occur in the disaster or mass casualty incident remains contentious. As we have discussed, disasters and mass casualty incidents are not homogeneous events. As such, judgment must be shown as to what is most appropriate in a particular circumstance. The decision as to whether CPR and other critical care interventions should be instituted will rely heavily on local knowledge and whether time and resources invested in saving one life will endanger many others or will be futile in any event.

In many circumstances, however, it will be completely appropriate to initiate advanced critical care treatments to injured or unwell children in a disaster. Clinical response to the very seriously injured or unwell child in a disaster or mass casualty incident will be greatly improved with clear planning and early interaction and training with first responders by those tasked with establishing local disaster response protocols.

Triage Step 4: Transport

The priority at this stage of the disaster triage process is to further allocate patients in increasing order of urgency in order to remove them from the immediate disaster or major incident site.

Table 9.2 Transport priorities based on triage assessment

Color	Meaning	Comments
Green	Minimal	Minor injuries. Can tolerate delay without increased morbidity or mortality
Red	Immediate	Patients who do not obey commands (age appropriate), are in respiratory distress, do not have a peripheral pulse, or have uncontrolled major hemorrhage
Gray	Expectant	Those patients whose injuries or condition are not compatible with life, given available resources. There is controversy in utilizing this category. Ideally the most senior health worker on scene or in the triage area should be involved in the decision to categorize someone as "expectant" – especially with children
Black	Dead	Patients who are not breathing after initiating lifesaving interventions are classified as dead
Yellow	Delayed	Patients who do not fit into any other category. These patients are essentially the second priority for transport

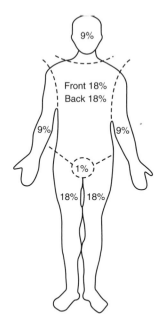

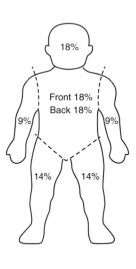

Figure 9.2 Pediatric "rule of nines." For each year after age 1 up to age 10, 1% is taken from the head and 0.5% is added to each lower limb. From age 10, adult proportions are used.

The easiest and most widely accepted method for doing this is to allocate color-coded tags to patients based on clinical assessment (Table 9.2). It is the same system used in adult disaster management If specialized tags are not available, colored pens, tape, or paper are more than adequate.

Equipment, Fluids, and Medications for Pediatric Disaster Response

Many institutions and pre-hospital providers will have their own pediatric equipment lists. Availability of equipment and skill sets to be able to use certain pieces of equipment will vary across the globe.

Most equipment required for pediatric emergency use will mirror that of adult emergency use, but will be obviously smaller in size and assessment of appropriate size is often weight based. Accurate estimation of weight is therefore important. There are several available aids to assist the occasional pediatric provider in making this assessment as accurate as possible, such as the Broselow tape.

Fluid management and rehydration is an important part of minimizing morbidity and mortality amongst children in disasters. There is enormous variation in practices in this area across the world. The particular brand of fluid used is less important than the principles involved in rehydration.

As a rule, oral or nasogastric rehydration is cheaper, safer, more effective, and less labor intensive than intravenous therapy. Resuscitation and rehydration for severe dehydration or shock will need to be intravenous.

Broadly, intravenous therapy consists of replacement of losses (e.g. hemorrhage, diarrhea, vomiting) and maintenance. Losses should be replaced with isotonic crystalloid (normal saline, lactated Ringers/Hartman's solution, plasmalyte, or equivalent). Maintenance should also be isotonic but in most circumstances it should also contain 5% or 10% dextrose solution, especially in the very young. Ultimately local experience and practices will dominate fluid therapy; however, the key point is that hypotonic solutions and maintenance fluids without dextrose should be avoided, especially in infants, due to the increased risk of cerebral edema and hypoglycemia.

Pediatric Analgesia

Table 9.3 Pediatric analgesia drug doses

Drug (generic name)	Dose	Interval	Max dose
Paracetamol/ Acetominophen	15 mg/kg	6hrs	1000 mg
Ibuprofen	10 mg/kg	8hrs	400 mg
Codeine	0.5–1 mg/kg	4hrs	60 mg
Morphine	0.1–0.2 mg/kg	2hrs	20 mg
Fentanyl	1-2mcg/kg	30 mins	300mcg

Useful Links

1. www.nyc.gov/html/doh/downloads/pdf/bhpp/hepp-peds-childrenindisasters-010709.pdf
2. www.nationaltraumacentre.nt.gov.au
3. www.nationaltraumacentre.nt.gov.au/sites/default/files/PDFs/AUSMAT/2011/web.pdf
4. www.ceep.ca/publications/PaedDisasterPreparedness.pdf

Special Populations: Children

Proshad Efune and Mohammed Iqbal Ahmed

Introduction

Anesthesiologists are likely to face pediatric disaster victims both in the developed world and in developing countries, as children are a significant percentage of the global population. Although many challenges in taking care of children in disasters, especially in resource-poor countries, are like the ones described elsewhere in this book, pediatric disaster preparedness involves some unique considerations. The following provides a brief overview of essential equipment, training, and resuscitation as applicable to the anesthesiologist caring for a child in a disaster.

Pre-Operative Evaluation

As most pediatric drugs are weight based, obtaining an accurate weight prior to surgery is important. In the event a measurement is not available (due to absence of scales or presence of injury), there are multiple strategies for estimating weight:

- *Broselow tape:* Color-coded tape measure that estimates a child's weight based on length. The tape measure also lists medication doses and equipment sizes.
- *Best Guess:* Australian formula that estimates weight:
  - infants 1–11 months: weight (kg) = (age in months+9)/2
  - children 1–4 years: weight (kg) = 2 × (age +5)
  - children 5–14 years: weight (kg) = 4 × age
- *The advanced pediatric life support (APLS) formula*:
  - infants 0–12 months: weight (kg) = (0.5 × age in months) + 4
  - children 1–5 years: weight (kg) = (2 × age in years) + 8
  - children 6–12 years: weight (kg) = (3 × age in years) + 7.

For children < 1 year old, the Broselow tape is the most accurate, whereas Best Guess is most accurate for ages 1–5 years and 11–14 years and the APLS formula is most accurate for ages 6–10.[1]

Pediatric patients may present for a variety of procedures during disasters. In addition to immediate post-disaster trauma surgeries such as exploratory laparotomy for control of blunt abdominal trauma or craniotomy for hematoma evacuation, pediatric patients may present in the more sub-acute phase for reduction of long-bone fractures, or for surgery unrelated to the disaster, such as appendectomy. Even the most emergent of surgeries allow for at least a brief pre-operative evaluation:

1. Assessment of the airway including determination of structural derangements or bleeding which may make intubation difficult or impossible. The obtunded child at risk for aspiration requires immediate intubation even prior to surgery.
2. Assessment of circulatory volume: vital signs such as heart rate and blood pressure, as well as physical exam findings such as the strength of the peripheral pulse, duration of capillary refill, skin turgor, fullness of the anterior fontanelle, and mentation are invaluable in the assessment of volume status and shock. Signs and symptoms of shock include hypotension, rapid and weak pulse, restlessness, tachypnea, and diaphoresis. Internal hemorrhage is often more difficult to recognize than external hemorrhage.

The pre-operative evaluation prior to non-emergent surgery should include a thorough history and physical exam including:

1. Birth and postnatal history
2. Assessment of problems with prior anesthetics
3. Family history of problems with anesthesia
4. Drug allergies
5. Recent upper respiratory tract infection symptoms
6. Loose teeth
7. History of easy bruising or bleeding.

The child should be examined for mouth opening and neck extension, as well as a basic heart, lung, and neurologic exam. Depending on the nature of the surgery and the severity of the patient's underlying illness, and pending available resources, laboratory evaluation and imaging studies may be necessary prior to surgery.

The recent or current upper respiratory tract infection in children presenting for elective surgery poses a dilemma for many anesthesiologists caring for children. On one hand, a recent viral infection places the child at increased risk of peri-operative respiratory complications; on the other hand, recent viral infections are frequently common in children, and an attempt to wait for recovery may be thwarted by recurrent infections. The presence of fever, purulent secretions, or active respiratory symptoms such as wheezing need to be factored prior to deciding whether to proceed. If the decision is made to proceed, the family should be counseled on the risks.

Whenever possible, parental consent should be obtained prior to surgery and anesthesia. For the unaccompanied child and in urgent or emergent situations, appropriate medical care should not be withheld. Non-urgent treatment may prove more difficult. Policies, whether on an institutional or national level, should be in place prior to deployment to disaster settings to address these issues and reduce confusion.

Pre-Operative Preparation of the Child

Pre-operative fasting guidelines are as follows in children:

1. Two hours for clears
2. Four hours for breast milk
3. Six hours for formula or a light meal
4. Eight hours for a heavy meal.

The anesthesiologist caring for children should be cautioned about the possibility of incomplete or inaccurate disclosure of fasting times by parents and information lost in translation. Appropriate precautions should be undertaken in these situations.

In non-disaster settings, surgery and anesthesia are very stressful experiences for children and their parents. This stress is undoubtedly amplified in the disaster setting. Young children between the ages of 1 and 5 tend to be at highest risk for developing significant pre-operative anxiety. Even in a disaster, steps should be taken to reduce or abolish this stress response through behavioral interventions and distraction techniques:

1. Distraction techniques are generally more effective than encouraging or consoling remarks.
2. Pre-operative anxiolysis with IV or PO benzodiazepines such as midazolam can be very effective.
3. Small doses of an anesthetic such as ketamine can be efficacious in the pre-operative period.
4. Opioids given alone as a pre-medication do not tend to allay anxiety, however, they should not be spared in the pediatric patient who has significant pain prior to surgery.

To the extent possible, during evacuation or transport, children should not be separated from their families or caregivers in the disaster environment. Should separation occur, reunification should be attempted as quickly as possible. The anesthesiologist caring for children in a disaster should be aware of such reunification resources.

Monitoring

The American Society of Anesthesiologists (ASA) standards for basic monitoring apply also to pediatric patients and should be adhered to even in resource-poor settings. Occasionally, deviation from these standards may be necessary to provide essential care in a timely fashion. These decisions should be a shared responsibility of the team where urgency, locally applicable guidelines, and alternative facilities with better resources form part of the risk/benefit calculation. The experience of the anesthesiologist in low-resource settings becomes very important in guiding these difficult decisions.

Oxygenation

When an anesthesia machine is used to deliver general anesthesia, an oxygen analyzer should be used to measure the concentration of delivered oxygen in the patient breathing system. Blood oxygenation should be measured via continuous pulse oximetry.[2] In resource-poor or devastated areas, pulse oximetry may be unavailable or unreliable. The Lifebox[TM] project is a non-governmental organization that has delivered pulse oximeters to more than 100 countries to address this need. The aim is to make surgery safer by eliminating the need to conduct any anesthetic without pulse oximetry.

Circulation

Arterial blood pressure and heart rate should be determined at least every 5 minutes. Additionally, circulatory function should be continually evaluated by one of the following:

1. Palpation of a pulse
2. Auscultation of heart sounds

3. Monitoring of intra-arterial pressure tracing
4. Pulse oximetry.[2]

Automated oscillometric blood pressure cuffs are preferred, but manual sphygmoman-ometer measurements suffice if unavailable.

Electrocardiogram

Every patient receiving general anesthesia should have the electrocardiogram displaying continuously from the beginning of anesthesia until preparing to leave the anesthetizing location.[2]

Ventilation

All patients under moderate or deep sedation or general anesthesia should have continual monitoring for the presence of expired carbon dioxide. When an endotra-cheal tube or laryngeal mask airway is used to support ventilation, quantitative monitoring of expired carbon dioxide is recommended.[2] In the disaster setting, this technology may have limited availability, and one expired carbon dioxide monitor may need to be shared by more than one operating room for critical parts of the case, such as during airway placement.

The Precordial Stethoscope

A precordial stethoscope will allow for continuous assessment of heart sounds, as well as breath sounds, complementing other monitors. It becomes especially useful if other mon-itoring modalities are unavailable. Every anesthesia provider traveling to a disaster area is advised to invest in a customized earpiece (approximate cost $50) that makes using the precordial stethoscope comfortable and practical for long periods. Endobronchial intuba-tion, unintended extubation, apnea, bronchospasm, and circuit disconnections can be instantly diagnosed in addition to significant drops in cardiac output by change in heart sounds or heart rate. The patient end of the system is easily fashioned with intravenous tubing and stethoscope chest pieces, though pediatric and infant-designed chest pieces are readily available. More expensive modern iterations are Bluetooth wireless-based technol-ogies that require battery power.

Temperature

Every child receiving anesthesia should have temperature monitored when clinically sig-nificant changes in body temperature are intended, anticipated, or suspected.[2] Skin tem-perature monitoring suffices if other monitoring modalities are not available. Neonates and infants are particularly at risk of hypothermia during surgery and anesthesia due to their thinner skin and large surface area relative to body mass. A variety of warming strategies are effective, including warming the operating room, overhead warming lights, forced air warmers, fluid warmers, covering exposed skin with plastic wrap, and warming mattresses.

Foley Catheter

Monitoring of urine output is invaluable in the management of the patient in or at risk of shock due to hypovolemia or hemorrhage. Foley catheters as small as 6 Fr may be necessary in neonates or infants. The minimal acceptable urine output in pediatric patients is 1 ml/kg/h.

Access

Peripheral Access

Peripheral access in infants can be particularly difficult as the amount and distribution of subcutaneous fat makes visualization difficult. The saphenous vein is often more easily accessible, and IVs can be placed when the vein is not visible. The IV catheter is inserted into the skin at a 10–20° angle just anterior to the medial malleolus and directed toward the back of the knee. Butterfly needles inserted into small veins are not adequate for infusions during surgery as they easily dislodge, but can be used for induction. Local infiltration with buffered lidocaine can be helpful prior to awake IV placements, even in young children. In particular, the smaller gauge needles (26 G or 27 G) are well tolerated. The following IV catheter sizes are typically utilized:

1. Neonates and small infants: 24 G. Larger catheters may run the risk of rupturing the vessel. 22 G catheters can be used in the saphenous vein.
2. Toddlers and small children: 22 G.
3. Older children and adolescents: 18 or 20 G.

Intraosseous Line

Consider intraosseous (IO) placement if IV access cannot be obtained after two attempts. Consult the specific IO device instructions for proper utilization of the device. The insertion site of choice in infants and children is the proximal tibia. Alternative sites include the distal femur or distal tibia. Any medication or resuscitation fluid can be delivered through an IO, including blood products. A vigorous flush of 10 ml of normal saline is required before the catheter will flow. An IO is typically not maintained for longer than 24 hours.

Central Venous Access

Central venous lines (CVLs) suitable for pediatric patients come in multiple sizes and lengths. The femoral, subclavian, and internal jugular veins may be accessed. The internal jugular is typically larger than the femoral, but access is often impeded due to the presence of a cervical collar in trauma patients. The subclavian has a higher rate of requiring multiple attempts, unintended arterial puncture, and higher rates of pneumothorax as compared to the internal jugular vein.[3] For internal jugular catheterization, the catheter tip should ideally be at the superior vena cava–right atrial junction, just outside the heart. Typical CVL sizes and insertion depths for internal jugular catheterization are presented in the Table 10.1.

Tools to Improve the Success of Venous Catheterization

Ultrasound guidance improves vascular access success rates in children.[4] However, these may be unavailable in the disaster setting. Portable and handheld machines are becoming more readily available and economical, and disaster teams should strongly consider having at least one of these devices. Portable infrared-based vein finding technology is useful in

Table 10.1 Typical CVL sizes and insertion depths for internal jugular catheterization

	CVL size	Insertion depth
Neonates and infants	4 Fr	5 cm
Toddlers and small children	5 Fr	8 cm
Older children and adolescents	7 Fr	10–12 cm

small children. Warm packs are helpful in patients with decreased perfusion to the distal extremities.

Airway Management

Mask

Cushion seal facemasks of various sizes should be available for every anesthetic. A properly sized mask covers the nose and mouth without overlying the eyes or extending beyond the chin. The use of proper technique is important.

1. Avoid depressing the submental soft tissues of small children during a chin lift. This maneuver often closes the mouth in neonates and infants which can sometimes, but not always, be relieved by extending the neck.
2. In difficult mask ventilation situations in infants, perform temporomandibular subluxation by placing the 5th digit in the retromandibular notch and pulling the condyles in an upward direction. This anteriorly translocates the jaw and rotates the temporomandibular joint, which opens the mouth and pulls the tongue off the posterior pharyngeal wall.

Airway Adjuncts

Oral and nasopharyngeal airways of various pediatric sizes should be available for every anesthetic.

1. Estimate oral airway size by measuring the distance from the teeth to the base of the tongue. Too small an oral airway may push the tongue into the glottic opening, whereas too large an oral airway may push the epiglottis into the glottic opening, worsening airway obstruction.
2. Nasopharyngeal airways must be lubricated and inserted gently to avoid traumatizing the turbinates or adenoids. Estimate the proper length by measuring the distance between the patient's auditory meatus and the tip of the nose.

Endotracheal Tubes

Endotracheal tube (ETT) sizing in the pediatric patient is typically based on age. The most frequently used formula is:

ETT size = age (in years)/4 + 4

Subtract 0.5 mm for a cuffed ETT

Neonates and infants – 3.0 to 3.5 ETT

Premature infants may require ETTs as small as 2.0

Depth of insertion (cm) = ETT size × 3

Cuffed ETTs have several advantages over uncuffed ETTs:

1. Fewer repeat intubations typically required as inflation or deflation of the cuff often will allow for an appropriate leak
2. Less contamination of the airway in patients at risk for aspiration
3. More precisely controlled ventilation is allowed
4. Improved ventilation in patients with poor lung compliance is allowed.

A variety of ETTs are available for special needs. Pre-formed oral or nasotracheal tubes may not be available in an austere setting. Double lumen tubes may also be unavailable for one-lung ventilation. The anesthesiologist may have to rely upon selective lung ventilation using a single lumen tube, or occlusion of a main stem bronchus with a 5 Fr Fogarty type balloon-tipped catheter.

Early intubation should be considered for burn patients at risk for inhalation injury. Signs and symptoms of inhalational injury include difficulty breathing or swallowing, hoarseness, stridor, wheezing, or singed nasal hairs, but history of smoke inhalation should prompt vigilance and early intervention.

Laryngoscopes

Standard straight and curved laryngoscope blades should be available for every anesthetic. The laryngeal opening in infants tends to be more cephalad and anterior, and so it is common to use a Miller 0 or 1, or a Phillips 1 to intubate the trachea of infants and small children. A Macintosh blade, with its curvature and wider spatula, may be more advantageous to control the tongue when intubating an older child. Multiple laryngoscope handles and backup batteries should always be available.

Care should be taken to keep the cervical spine immobilized during laryngoscopy in all trauma patients. Video laryngoscopes allow for visualization of the laryngeal opening with minimal, if any, neck extension. They are unlikely to be available in the austere disaster setting, however.

It should be noted that infants and young children desaturate quickly in the face of apnea due to several factors such as a low functional residual capacity (FRC), a closing volume of small airways that is often higher than their FRC, and their higher oxygen consumption as compared to adults. Airway considerations also differ from adults. Neonates and infants have:

1. A proportionately larger head and tongue
2. An anterior and cephalad larynx
3. An omega-shaped epiglottis.

These features must be considered during placement of an advanced airway. Shoulder rolls can prove to be a useful adjunct to help align the airway axes, but they can also result in hyperextension of the neck, making the direct laryngoscopic view more difficult.

Laryngeal Mask Airway

Pediatric-sized laryngeal mask airways (LMAs) should be available during every anesthetic. The smallest LMA is a size 1, and should be suitable for most neonates and infants. LMA sizing is available on most LMA packaging. The contraindications to LMA use are like those in adults.

Difficult Airway Equipment

The anesthesiologist providing care to children in disaster settings should be adept at rescuing the pediatric airway. Arguably the ability to effectively mask ventilate is the most important skill to master prior to taking on the responsibility of providing anesthesia to children. If a difficult airway is anticipated, the corollary to the "awake intubation" in the adult is the technique of maintaining spontaneous ventilation throughout induction. This is most safely accomplished using agents that do not suppress breathing, such as ketamine, dexmedetomidine, and volatile agents. It is extremely important to avoid neuromuscular blocking agents in the anticipated difficult intubation until the airway is secured. In the event of an unanticipated cannot intubate/cannot ventilate situation, the ASA difficult airway algorithm can be applied to children.[5]

A variety of portable video laryngoscopes are available and may serve as an important rescue device in the disaster setting. LMAs can also be used as a conduit for ETT placement in the difficult airway. This is most easily facilitated with flexible fiberoptic scope use, but understandably, this equipment may not be available in the disaster setting. The Airtraq™ (Prodol Meditec S.A., Vizcaya, Spain) is a disposable fiberoptic intubation device that can be used in difficult airway situations. Some anesthesiologists have successfully reused the disposable device after disinfection, making it a particularly attractive option for use in the resource-poor setting. The smallest blade is a size 0, which is suitable for neonates and fits as small as a 2.5 ETT.

Breathing Systems

In the event an anesthesia machine is unavailable, or one with a circle system is unavailable, Mapleson circuits can be utilized:

1. Mapleson A circuit:
   a. Preferred for spontaneously breathing children
   b. Only results in no rebreathing during spontaneous ventilation when the fresh gas flow is more than 75% of the minute ventilation
2. Mapleson D circuit:
   a. Preferred for assisted ventilation
   b. Requires slightly higher fresh gas flow rates than the Mapleson A during spontaneous ventilation
   c. Despite the need for a higher fresh gas flow rate during spontaneous ventilation, considering both spontaneous and controlled ventilation, the Mapleson D requires the lowest fresh gas flow rates among all Mapleson circuits, which may be an important consideration in the resource-poor setting.

It is important to ensure that pediatric-sized flow or self-inflating bags are available and sized appropriately for each patient.

If oxygen tanks are used, they should consistently be checked to ensure they are not empty. Most healthy children without lung injury can tolerate an anesthetic without supplemental oxygen. If an oxygen source is unavailable, room air with a self-inflating, i.e. Ambu®, bag may be acceptable. The primary goal remains supporting the child's ventilation with adequate minute ventilation. Oxygen concentrators can also be of great value in the resource-limited setting.

Ventilatory Modes

The child without lung injury can tolerate brief anesthetics while spontaneously breathing without the development of severe atelectasis. Longer anesthetics can still be performed with the child breathing spontaneously, however an assist mode such as pressure support with continuous positive end-expiratory pressure (CPAP), or CPAP alone should be employed to prevent atelectasis.

Pressure control and volume control ventilation are the two most common modes employed for controlled ventilation in the pediatric patient in the OR. Pressure control is often favored in neonates and infants due to the inability of most anesthesia machines to be able to deliver precise tidal volumes during volume control ventilation. Pressure control is also useful in cases of large air leaks around uncuffed ETTs. The neonate has less than 10% the number of alveoli as the older child. As such, they are prone to both barotrauma and volutrauma, and ventilatory parameters must be monitored very closely during anesthesia. Tidal volumes should be limited to less than 8 ml/kg in most pediatric patients.

Fluid Management

Infants and children have a smaller circulatory volume and fluid reserve, which puts them at risk for hypovolemic shock.

Choice of Intravenous Fluid

The first step in the resuscitation of shock includes volume resuscitation. The initial fluid bolus should consist of an isotonic fluid such as 0.9% saline or lactated Ringer's solution. Hypotonic fluids should not be used as the sole resuscitative fluid due to the risk of acute hyponatremia and subsequent organ injury. Resuscitation typically begins with 20 ml/kg aliquots with frequent assessment of response and/or adverse effects due to fluid overload, as evidenced by crackles/rales on lung exam or a palpable liver. A reasonable strategy is to transition to colloid (i.e. 5% albumin) boluses for management of ongoing losses and hypotension after 25–30 ml/kg of crystalloid is administered.

Maintenance fluid rates are calculated using the following (Holliday and Segar) formula based on weight:

1. <10 kg = 4 ml/kg/h
2. 10–20 kg = 40 ml/h + 2 ml/kg/h for every kg above 10 kg
3. >20 kg = 60 ml/h + 1 ml/kg/h for every kg above 20 kg (add 40 to the patient's weight to quickly calculate maintenance needs).

Neonates should receive dextrose-containing maintenance fluids to avoid hypoglycemia.

Blood Transfusion

Blood Conservation

In the austere disaster setting where blood is a precious resource, blood conservation techniques can help reduce utilization of blood in the peri-operative environment. Strategies include:

1. Peri-operative erythropoietin
2. Iron supplementation
3. Pre-operative autologous blood donation
4. Acute normovolemic hemodilution
5. Cell-saver techniques.

Apart from erythropoietin and iron supplementation, these techniques are challenging in the management of the pediatric patient. Additionally, it is unlikely cell-saver devices will be available in the disaster setting. Antifibrinolytic drugs such as tranexamic acid and aminocaproic acid can be useful in limiting blood loss and ultimately the need for blood transfusions in certain pediatric surgical procedures.

Blood Sources

In countries without a well-developed health care system, the national response to blood management in disasters is often insufficient. The actual shortage of blood in disasters is usually overshadowed by the massive disruption of the delivery system that often occurs in these countries. There is often an influx of voluntary donors in disaster situations, and blood centers should be prepared to manage volunteers and donors. Relatives of victims may also volunteer to donate to their family member. These donations should be entertained if time permits for safe collection and processing.

Warming Systems

It is imperative that blood products that are administered rapidly be warmed prior to administration to prevent hypothermia. Neonates and infants are particularly at risk of severe hypothermia for the reasons mentioned above. Hypothermia can propagate bleeding in trauma patients due to cold-induced platelet dysfunction. The Hotline® is the fluid warmer most typically used, but in resource-poor disaster settings, immersion of blood products in a water bath prior to transfusion is a safe alternative.[6]

Massive Transfusion

Massive transfusion is typically defined as the need to transfuse more than 1 blood volume in a 24-hour period. Trauma patients appear to benefit from early administration of plasma and platelets. The exact ratio is unknown in children. Ideally laboratory data would guide replacement of coagulation factors, but even in resource-rich settings, these values are frequently unavailable in a timely fashion rendering them unhelpful in the patient with rapid blood loss. The principles of massive transfusion apply to the bleeding non-trauma pediatric surgical patient as well, such as proportionate packed red blood cells (PRBCs), coagulation factor and platelet replacement. However, it is even less clear when to give these and how much to give. Fresh whole blood transfusion should be considered as an alternative, if available. Hypocalcemia and hyperkalemia should be anticipated and appropriately treated during massive transfusion.

Drugs

Induction Agents

IV Agents

Ketamine at a dose of 2 mg/kg produces a catatonic-like state in children in 1–2 minutes. Potential adverse effects include:

1. Sialorrhea (5 µg/kg intravenous glycopyrrolate given 5 minutes prior to ketamine administration may prevent sialorrhea)
2. Laryngospasm
3. Tachycardia
4. Hypertension
5. Emergence delirium (midazolam given prior to ketamine may prevent emergence delirium).

Propofol is the most commonly used IV induction agent in pediatric anesthesia practice. The considerations for its use are like that in adults. It should be avoided in cases of hemodynamic instability. It should be noted that larger doses are often needed to induce a state of general anesthesia in infants and children (i.e. 2–3 mg/kg) due to their larger central compartment and higher clearance rates as compared to adults.

Etomidate is an alternative induction agent that is safe and effective in pediatric patients. It is particularly appealing for induction of the brain-injured child, as it has cerebro-protective effects without producing hypotension which could negatively impact cerebral perfusion. Despite extensive study, there remain concerns about the adrenal suppression that occurs following even a single dose of etomidate, and so care should be taken when using this agent in patients with sepsis.

Inhaled Agents

Inhalational inductions are faster in infants and children due to their higher alveolar ventilation to FRC ratio:

1. Inhalation inductions can be achieved with the child in any position.
2. IV access can be obtained once the child is safely asleep, allowing for a pain-free induction.
3. Care should be taken to avoid force during the induction process, especially for patients who will return to the OR for repeat procedures, as significant anxiety and rejection of the anesthesia mask may occur with repeat visits.
4. As much as possible, the child should be walked through the induction process, and the mask should not be applied without warning.
5. Distraction techniques can be very helpful, as can disguising the odor of the volatile agent with a candy flavor in the mask (i.e. application of a flavored lip balm to the inside of the mask).
6. Sevoflurane is the ideal inhalation agent for induction due to its low solubility and rapid induction.
7. Nitrous oxide speeds induction even further when added to sevoflurane. It is less noxious than desflurane, leading to less coughing and laryngospasm during inhaled inductions.

The anesthesiologist should be prepared to handle upper airway obstruction following inhaled induction:

1. Neck extension, mouth opening, jaw thrust, and gentle CPAP can be effective.
2. If an oral airway is inserted, care should be taken that the patient is deep enough that laryngospasm does not ensue.
3. A well-lubricated nasopharyngeal airway is an alternative.
4. The IV should not be inserted until the patient is unconscious.
5. If nitrous oxide is used during induction, the patient should be transitioned to 100% FiO_2 once unconsciousness is achieved to help delay oxygen desaturation if laryngospasm does develop.

If the above maneuvers do not relieve the upper airway obstruction, the patient may have laryngospasm. The aspiration of saliva often initiates laryngospasm, and so patients with excessive secretions are particularly at risk. Vigorous positive pressure ventilation may worsen the situation, as secretions are pushed further back into the larynx, and due to the closure of the glottis, much of the air is shunted to the stomach, causing gaseous distention, and increasing the risk for aspiration. Moderate CPAP can be maintained with intermittent positive pressure ventilation and the technique of temporomandibular subluxation is often effective. If these techniques fail, and the patient does not have IV access, 4 mg/kg IM succinylcholine and 20 µg/kg IM atropine can be administered. If an IV is in place, a small dose of IV anesthetic can be administered (e.g. 0.5 mg/kg propofol).

Anesthesia providers should be prepared to use inhalational agents other than the ones they normally use, when working in remote areas. Induction techniques with enflurane, halothane, and isoflurane are somewhat different from sevoflurane and require more care and skill. This need can be obviated by placing an IV first, possible and perhaps necessary even in small children.

Maintenance of Anesthesia

Total intravenous anesthesia, particularly a regimen that allows the patient to breathe spontaneously with a natural airway, should be considered when access to technology is compromised secondary to either a lack of electricity or lack of access to necessary equipment. Ketamine is a particularly attractive agent for this purpose. Care should be taken to titrate carefully. A ketamine anesthetic is a reasonable "fall back" method of anesthesia if an anesthesia machine fails or is unavailable, or if the gas supply fails. It is also an excellent anesthetic if one is necessary at the scene of injury.

Volatile agents, when available, are excellent maintenance anesthetics in children. The same considerations apply to children as to adults when using these agents. The minimum alveolar concentration of most inhaled agents tends to be a little higher in children than adults. Children are at higher risk of malignant hyperthermia due to the fact many of them have not been previously exposed and so susceptibility is unknown. Malignant hyperthermia requires a high degree of suspicion. The most common presenting signs are:

1. Sinus tachycardia
2. Hypercarbia
3. Jaw rigidity.

Other symptoms include total body rigidity, arrhythmias, and hyperthermia. The most important initial steps in the management of a suspected episode of malignant hyperthermia include:

1. Stopping the offending agent
2. Administering 100% FiO_2 at high fresh gas flow rates
3. Administering dantrolene at a dose of 2.5 mg/kg.

Even in the austere disaster setting, dantrolene should be stocked and available, given the lifesaving nature of the drug. Repeated doses can be given as clinically indicated. Dantrolene requires large quantities of sterile water for dilution and can be labor intensive. Additional therapies include:

1. Administration of sodium bicarbonate 1–2 mEq/kg to correct metabolic acidosis
2. Additional mannitol (there is 150 mg of mannitol per milligram of dantrolene in the vial)
3. Furosemide 0.5–1 mg/kg to ensure a urine output of at least 2 ml/kg
4. Cooling measures
5. Treatment of hyperkalemia and arrhythmias as appropriate.

Draw-over systems can also be a valuable tool in resource-poor settings or in field anesthesia. Draw-over systems refer to those breathing systems in which an inhalation anesthetic is vaporized by the patient's breathing. The simplest form consists of two reservoir tubes, a vaporizer, and a non-rebreathing valve. The patient inspires and expires via the non-rebreathing valve. Air enters the system from the atmosphere and may be supplemented with oxygen if available. The tubes provide reservoirs of anesthetic-containing gases. A self-inflating bag can be incorporated into the system to assist or control ventilation if necessary, as respiratory depression is a risk with this technique.

Analgesics

Non-Opioid Analgesics
Rectal acetaminophen at a dose of 20 mg/kg can be given after induction or before emergence and can aid in the analgesic management of children. IV non-steroidal anti-inflammatory agents such as ketorolac (0.5 mg/kg) can reduce opioid requirements.

Opioids
A variety of IV opioids can be used for analgesia during and after surgery in pediatric patients. The respiratory depressant effect of opioids can be very unpredictable in neonates, and great care should be taken when administering them to this age group. Premature neonates less than 50–60 weeks corrected gestational age and term neonates less than 44 weeks corrected are at risk for post-operative apnea and should be carefully monitored for at least 24 hours after surgery. Risk factors include a low gestational age at birth, a low corrected gestational age, and anemia. Short-acting opioids such as fentanyl may be more suitable in neonates to avoid over-narcotization.

Neuromuscular Blocking Agents
Neonates and infants tend to have a higher sensitivity for most non-depolarizing neuromuscular blocking agents. In contrast, they require larger doses of

succinylcholine (2–3 mg/kg) than older children and adults due to their relatively larger volume of distribution. The contraindications of succinylcholine are like that in adults. However, it should be noted that there may be a more frequent incidence of neuromuscular diseases that predispose to hyperkalemia and rhabdomyolysis following succinylcholine administration in children, and the anesthesiologist caring for children should be prepared to handle the complication.

Neostigmine is the neuromuscular blocking reversal agent of choice. Infants typically require 50 µg/kg, but if possible, the dose should be based on peripheral nerve stimulator monitoring. Glycopyrrolate is given concomitantly to avoid excessive cholinergic activity leading to bradycardia.

Antibiotics

The prevention of infection starts with standard barriers, including gloves for every patient contact and washing hands with soap and water or alcohol-based cleaners before and after each encounter. Traumatic wounds will often require antibiotic administration. It is important to verify drug allergy status prior to admission. Most reactions of "rash" to penicillin-based agents do not necessarily contraindicate cephalosporin administration. Vancomycin should always be administered at a slow infusion rate due to the risk of severe red man's syndrome and/or hypotension. Surgical site prophylaxis with antibiotics is not necessary for every pediatric procedure, and in the resource-poor disaster setting, should be used judiciously and after careful assessment of the risks and benefits.

Rescue Drugs

The following rescue drugs should be readily available: epinephrine, atropine, calcium gluconate or chloride, and sodium bicarbonate.

Pediatric Dosing

Table 10.2 Pediatric dosing for commonly used peri-operative medications

Acetaminophen	PO	10–15 mg/kg
	IV	10–15 mg/kg
	PR	10–20 mg/kg
Adenosine	IV	Initial: 0.1 mg/kg (max 6 mg) If not effective, increase to: 0.2 mg/kg (max 12 mg)
Albuterol	INH	2.5–5 mg
Atropine	IV	10–20 µg/kg
Calcium gluconate	IV	10–30 mg/kg
Dantrolene	IV	2.5 mg/kg

Table 10.2 (cont.)

Dexamethasone	IV	0.1–0.5 mg/kg
Diphenhydramine	IV	0.5–1 mg/kg
	PO	0.5–1 mg/kg
Dopamine	IV	2–20 µg/kg/min
Epinephrine	IV	1–10 µg/kg bolus 0.01–0.3 µg/kg/min
Ephedrine	IV	0.02–0.2 mg/kg
Furosemide	IV	1 mg/kg
Fentanyl	IV	0.5–5 µg/kg
Glycopyrrolate	IV	5–15 µg/kg
Hydromorphone	IV	10–20 µg/kg
Ibuprofen	PO	10 mg/kg
Ketamine	IV	1–2 mg/kg
	IM	3–10 mg/kg
Ketorolac	IV	0.5–1 mg/kg
Lidocaine	IV	1–2 mg/kg
Mannitol	IV	0.5–1 g/kg
Midazolam	IV	0.1 mg/kg
	PO	0.5 mg/kg
Morphine	IV	0.05–0.1 mg/kg
Naloxone	IV	1–10 µg/kg
Neostigmine	IV	0.02–0.07 mg/kg
Ondansetron	IV	0.1–0.15 mg/kg
Phenylephrine	IV	1–10 µg/kg
Propofol	IV	2–4 mg/kg
Rocuronium	IV	0.6–1.2 mg/kg
Succinylcholine	IV	1–2 mg/kg
	IM	3–5 mg/kg
Vecuronium	IV	0.1 mg/kg

Regional Anesthetics

Regional anesthesia may prove to be the safest anesthetic technique for the cooperative child in a resource-limited disaster setting. Even a local infiltrative technique may be sufficient in certain situations. Local infiltration of a surgical wound should be encouraged whenever possible, even if general anesthesia and systemic analgesia are planned. It is important to keep in mind that however strong the indications may seem for using a technique, the best anesthetic technique remains the one the anesthesiologist is most experienced and confident in.

Caudal Epidural

A commonly employed regional block in pediatric practice is the caudal epidural. It is overall a very safe and simple technique, and can be used for any surgery performed on the lower abdomen or lower extremities. It is most commonly administered as a single shot. Absolute contraindications include myelomeningocoele and meningitis. The procedure is as follows:

1. The child is placed in the lateral position with the hips flexed
2. An equilateral triangle is formed with the fingertips from the bilateral posterior superior iliac spine to the needle insertion at the sacral hiatus. The sacral hiatus is felt as a depression immediately inferior to the sacral cornua and in the midline.
3. The needle is placed at $\leq$45° angle to the skin and advanced cranially. A pop may be felt once the needle has passed into the epidural space.
4. After *negative* aspiration for CSF or blood, the local anesthetic can be delivered and the needle removed. It is important to assess the resistance to injection as an indicator for correct placement. There should be no resistance, nor should a skin wheal develop.

Delivery of 1 ml/kg of local anesthetic provides adequate dermatomal coverage with a duration of 4 to 6 hours. There is thought to be a greater separation of motor and sensory effects with ropivacaine. Many different additives can be used, such as epinephrine, clonidine, or opioids.

Femoral Nerve Block

Femoral nerve blocks are another commonly employed block in pediatric anesthesia practice for above-the-knee surgeries that require analgesia of the thigh, including for femur fracture:

1. With the child supine and the feet rotated outward, the needle is inserted at a slightly cephalad angle 0.5–1 cm below the inguinal ligament and 0.5–1 cm lateral to the femoral artery.
2. If a nerve stimulator is used, the desired response is contraction of the mid-quadriceps. If the thigh adductors contract, the needle is adjusted laterally and if the lateral muscles are stimulated, the needle is adjusted medially.
3. On ultrasound imaging, the femoral nerve often has a triangular, hyperechoic appearance and is located lateral to the femoral artery and superficial to the iliopsoas muscle.
4. Once the desired location of the needle is achieved, local anesthetic is injected incrementally with frequent aspiration for blood.

Local Anesthetics

The same considerations for local anesthetic use should be applied to children as to adults. The following are the maximum recommended doses of local anesthetics:

1. Lidocaine without epinephrine – 5 mg/kg
2. Lidocaine with epinephrine – 7 mg/kg
3. Bupivacaine – 3 mg/kg
4. Ropivacaine – 3 mg/kg

In any situation where local anesthetics are used, intralipid should be available due to its potential to reverse the cardiotoxic effects of local anesthetics.

Recovery

The anesthesiologist caring for children should keep in mind that they may be the only physician available to care for patients in both the recovery room and the operating room, and so steps should be taken to prevent common post-anesthetic complications. Most of the problems encountered in the pediatric patient in the recovery room are related to upper airway obstruction. As such, considering the resource-limited setting, it is probably advisable to avoid deep extubations, and to ensure adequate spontaneous ventilation and return of protective reflexes prior to extubation. Titrating analgesics effectively in the intra-operative period will make it less likely that the child will exhibit significant pain in the recovery room. Care should be taken when administering opioids post-operatively. A typical approach is to administer one-third of the typical dose of an opioid, and re-assess 5–10 minutes later and administer more if needed. Non-opioid analgesics such as acetaminophen or ibuprofen are also useful in the post-operative period. Adequate hydration should be ensured prior to ward transfer, and ideally the patient should be tolerating oral intake.

Pediatric Advanced Life Support

While the likelihood of a successful cardiopulmonary resuscitation (CPR) is extremely low in the trauma patient in cardiopulmonary arrest in an austere disaster setting, it is not low in the pediatric patient who arrests during the intra-operative period. The anesthesiologist caring for children in a disaster should be familiar with pediatric advanced life support (PALS) algorithms, as well as the appropriate techniques for basic life support (BLS) in children, such as the appropriate compressions to ventilation ratio and the appropriate depth and frequency of compressions.

A PALS algorithm card is an excellent resource for any anesthesiologist providing care to children. Of note, the card provides normal pediatric vital signs by age. The Stanford emergency manual is another useful cognitive aid that can be used to manage peri-operative critical events.[7]

Table 10.3 gives a list of suggested resources for pediatric anesthesia in the disaster setting. The reader is also referred to the World Health Organization's "Guide to Infrastructure and Supplies" for further information.[8]

Table 10.3 Suggested resources for pediatric anesthesia in a disaster setting

Anesthesia delivery systems and patient monitoring	<ul><li>Anesthesia ventilator</li><li>Vaporizer</li><li>Electric power source with manual override</li><li>Ventilator circuits</li><li>Pulse oximeter, spare probes</li><li>ECG monitor/dots</li><li>Automatic blood pressure</li><li>Capnograph, sampling lines, water traps, connectors, filters-fuel cells</li><li>Oxygen analyzer</li><li>Peripheral nerve stimulator</li><li>Temperature probe</li><li>Warming blanket</li><li>Electric overhead heater</li><li>Infant incubator</li></ul>
Airway management equipment	<ul><li>Adult and child resuscitators (e.g. Ambu® resuscitator)</li><li>Adult, child, and infant facemasks</li><li>Adult, child, and infant oral and nasopharyngeal airways</li><li>Adult, child, and infant LMAs</li><li>Oxygen source/concentrator</li><li>Laryngoscope Miller blades 1 and 2, or Macintosh blades 1–4</li><li>Sizes 2.0–8.0 endotracheal tubes, cuffed and uncuffed</li><li>Adult and child Magill's forceps</li><li>Adult and child intubating bougies</li><li>Suction tubing/Yankauer</li><li>Suction catheters</li><li>Portable/electric/foot sucker</li><li>Fiberoptic bronchoscope</li><li>Video laryngoscope</li><li>Cricothyrotomy kit</li></ul>
Vascular access	<ul><li>Examination gloves</li><li>Sterile gloves</li><li>16 G–24 G intravenous catheters</li><li>Central venous line kits</li><li>Portable ultrasound machine (laptop or handheld)</li><li>Handheld LED transilluminator</li><li>IV pressure infuser bag</li><li>IVF tubing</li><li>Infusion pumps</li><li>Intra-osseous access kit</li><li>Venous cut-down kits</li><li>Tape and occlusive dressings</li><li>Blood delivery/warming systems</li><li>Syringes of various sizes</li></ul>

Table 10.3 (cont.)

Emergency equipment	• Defibrillator • i-STAT is TM or (R) • Mechanical ventilator capable of ventilating pediatric patients • Flashlights and batteries • UPS (uninterrupted power supply) or similar power failure backup systems • Headlamp
Miscellaneous	• 10–16 Fr gastric tubes • 22 G and 25 G spinal needles
Standard anesthetic/ analgesic medications	• Midazolam PO/IV • Acetaminophen/hydrocodone PO • Tylenol with codeine • Eutectic mixture of lidocaine and prilocaine • Volatile anesthetics • Propofol, etomidate, ketamine • Fentanyl, morphine, hydromorphone IV • Succinylcholine, rocuronium, vecuronium • Neostigmine • Glycopyrrolate IV • Ondansetron IV • Dexamethasone IV • Bupivacaine, ropivacaine, lidocaine • Acetaminophen PO/PR • Ketorolac IV • Ibuprofen PO • Cefazolin, ceftriaxone, gentamicin, metronidazole, vancomycin, clindamycin IV • Ringer's lactate, normal saline, dextrose 5% containing fluids
Emergency drugs	• Epinephrine • Atropine • Sodium bicarbonate • Calcium gluconate • Magnesium sulfate • Amiodarone • Adenosine • Lidocaine • Dopamine • Phenylephrine • Ephedrine • Esmolol • Labetalol • Hydralazine

Table 10.3 (cont.)

	• Dextrose 50% • Digoxin • Naloxone • Furosemide • Dantrolene • Diphenhydramine • Albuterol • Insulin • Mannitol • Potassium chloride IV • HIV post-exposure prophylaxis kit and a point-of-care rapid test of HIV antibody
Communication Tools	• Two-way radios • Cell phones with local sim cards • At least one satellite phone per team in remote locations • Directory of local emergency and official phone numbers
Personnel	• Liaison officers or volunteers from local authority • Translators with some medical knowledge • Family reunification personnel
Record keeping	• Computerized (portable) or paper medical and anesthesia records • Standard advisory templates to give to patients/families (difficult airway/allergies) • Consent forms (with translation in local language)

References

1. Graves L, Chayen G, Peat J, OLeary F. A comparison of actual to estimated weights in Australian children attending a tertiary children's hospital, using the original and updated APLS, Luscombe and Owens, Best Guess formulae and the Broselow tape. *Resuscitation* 2014;**85**:392–396.

2. American Society of Anesthesiologists Committee on Standards and Practice Parameters. Standards for basic anesthetic monitoring. Updated October 28, 2015. www.asahq.org/stan dards-and-guidelines/standards-for-basic -anesthetic-monitoring (accessed September 2018).

3. Iovino F, Pittiruti M, Buononato M, et al. Central venous catheterization: complications of different placements. *Ann Chir* 2001;**126**(10):1001.

4. Verghese ST, McGill WA, Patel RI, et al. Ultrasound-guided internal jugular venous cannulation in infants: a prospective comparison with the traditional palpation method. *Anesthesiology* 1999;**91**(1):71.

5 American Society of Anesthesiologists. Practice guidelines for management of the difficult airway: An updated report. *Anesthesiology* 2003;**98**:1269–1277.

6. Marks RJ, Minty BD, White DC. Warming blood before transfusion: does immersion warming change blood composition? *Anaesthesia* 1985;**40**(6):541–544.

7. Stanford Anesthesia Cognitive Aid Group. Emergency manual. http://emergencyman ual.stanford.edu/downloads.html (accessed September 2019).

8. World Health Organization. Disaster management guidelines. www.who.int/sur gery/challenges/esc_disasters_emergen cies/en/ (accessed September 2019).

Laboratory Tests and Blood Banking

Dan Holmes and Felicity Stone

Pre-Operative Laboratory Testing

Although routine pre-operative laboratory testing is firmly established in anesthesia practice, common themes to emerge from the literature are that blood tests are inconsistently applied, consistently overused, and routine testing rarely changes anesthetic management.[1]

In the post-disaster environment, the availability of laboratory testing may range from nothing at all to a full laboratory service offering testing comparable to a modern hospital in a high-income country.[2] Minimum standards for disaster medical assistance teams (DMATs) mandate the availability of urinalysis, blood glucose, and rapid detection malaria tests, where applicable.[3] However, the increasing availability of portable, robust, and simple to use point-of-care (PoC) testing devices, including Hemocue (AB, Ängelholm, Sweden), iStat (Abbott, Libertyville, IL, USA), and ePoC (Alere, Waltham, MA, USA) mean that access to measurement of hemoglobin, renal function, electrolytes, and others is more readily available.

Rationale for Laboratory Tests

For a peri-operative laboratory investigation to be worthwhile, there should be a reasonable chance that the result will alter the management of the patient, whether through onward referral for further investigation, altering the anesthetic technique, or postponing/cancelling the procedure. Surgery taking place in the aftermath of a disaster is likely to be of an urgent nature, options for anesthesia more limited, and the risks of not operating more significant.

Anesthetists working in disaster medical teams are frequently involved in the management of acutely ill medical patients, and some blood tests – for example arterial blood gases (ABGs) in assessing hypoxia or hypercarbia in a patient with respiratory distress – can also have value in treating patients and assessing response.

In short, the anesthetist working in a disaster environment must remain flexible and be comfortable proceeding without information they may be used to having in their usual environment. However, in recognizing that the use of good clinical acumen is paramount, in certain circumstances targeted laboratory investigations might be useful. Some examples are outlined below.

General Considerations When Selecting Equipment

Many parts of the world most at risk from sudden-onset disasters are also prone to extremes of weather and challenging conditions. Heat, cold, humidity, precipitation, dust, sand, and other factors can all affect the performance of equipment leading to inaccurate results and risking patient harm. Limits of performance and robustness are important when selecting equipment. Other considerations include any requirement for a cold chain to store testing cartridges.

It is vital that equipment is properly maintained, particularly in view of the conditions in which it may be employed. Quality control and maintenance standards according to the manufacturers' recommendations are mandatory and should not be ignored because the equipment is used intermittently or infrequently, or because of a feeling that "something is better than nothing."

Specific Laboratory Tests

Hemoglobin

Hemoglobin can be estimated using a fingerprick test on cheap, simple color comparison cards.[4] Modern electronic devices such as those mentioned above use either single- or multi-test blood cartridges, or make non-invasive transcutaneous measurements (Pronto-7, Masimo Corp., Irvine, CA, USA).

With the increased trauma load after a natural disaster, the ability to measure hemoglobin concentration can help guide the appropriate use of intravenous fluids and blood products. Measuring hemoglobin may also help in managing obstetric hemorrhage and non-disaster-related trauma, both of which are common presentations to DMATs in the aftermath of a disaster. It is worth considering that in some low- and middle-income countries (LMICs) 25% of the population may be chronically anemic, including around 50% of young children and 40% of women.[5] The burden of anemia is particularly high in areas where diseases such as malaria and hookworm are endemic.

Urea, Creatinine, and Electrolytes

There are likely to be limited indications for peri-operative electrolyte testing in the setting of a disaster. However, in patients with crush injuries, such as after an earthquake, rhabdomyolysis may result in both acute kidney injury and profound hyperkalemia. Pre-operative optimization might include the use of intravenous fluids, insulin/dextrose, inhaled beta-2 agonists, and calcium, with ongoing treatment and monitoring intra- and post-operatively.

Other post-disaster situations where electrolyte measurements may provide useful information peri-operatively include in outbreaks of diarrhoeal illness, in malnourishment, in acute kidney injury due to severe sepsis, or in patients who present late with gastro-intestinal obstruction.

Blood Glucose

The burden of non-communicable diseases, including type 2 diabetes, is increasing worldwide, across low-, middle-, and high-income countries. Many patients remain untreated or under-treated. Poorly controlled diabetes leads to poor wound healing and secondary infection, necessitating repeated trips to the operating theatre. This in turn results in significant use of limited resources and a poor outcome for the patient.

Modern blood glucose monitors are small, easy to use, and inexpensive, and provide the ability to monitor (thus facilitating control of) blood sugar levels in the peri-operative period. This may lead to fewer procedures, improved wound healing, and reduced morbidity.

Arterial Blood Gas Analysis

Arterial blood gas (ABG) analysis is included in many PoC devices and provides information on the acid–base state of the patient, as well as the oxygen-carrying capacity of the blood. pO_2, pCO_2, and pH (or H^+ concentration) are standard tests and give the most useful information. They may be supplemented by serum lactate and other measurements.

The use of ABG analysis in selected surgical cases may help to inform decisions on medical and surgical management, fitness for surgery, prognosis, and futility and palliation. The presence of extreme metabolic acidosis in a patient being considered for laparotomy in a facility with no critical care facility may prompt transfer to another facility or palliation on the grounds of futility. Such decisions will rely on the combination of results with the clinical condition of the patient, the diagnosis, and the capability of the health care facility (for example the presence of an intensive care capacity in a type 3 facility).

ABGs may also be of use in the assessment and management of non-surgical patients with respiratory distress or metabolic derangement from systemic illness.

Coagulation Testing

Traditional coagulation tests such as prothrombin time (PT) and activated partial thromboplastin time (APTT) are some of the most over-ordered peri-operative investigations in high-income countries. These tests were developed to monitor specific anticoagulant therapies, and may not give an accurate picture of in vivo blood clotting.

The advent of viscoelastic PoC coagulation tests with easy to use cartridge systems has made "whole of coagulation" testing both user-friendly and somewhat more transportable, and has the potential to help peri-operative decision-making in the disaster setting. Clotting abnormalities, for example those due to low platelet numbers (or poor platelet function), can be corrected by transfusing either whole blood or, where available, fractionated blood products. Conversely, the ability to exclude medical bleeding through whole of coagulation testing may help in determining when bleeding is surgical in nature and requires a return to the operating theatre. Whilst still likely to be confined to the most sophisticated of DMAT laboratories at present, devices such as ROTEM (Tem International GmbH, Munich, Germany), TEG (Haemonetics Corp., Braintree, MA, USA), and Sonoclot (Sienco Inc., Arvada, CO, USA) may become more widely available to DMATs, particularly those dealing with trauma patients, in future.

Blood Transfusion

Introduction

Providing safe blood transfusion is challenging in the field hospital or disaster medicine setting. In 2013 the WHO released specific guidelines for the capabilities of DMATs, including blood transfusion services.[3] Inpatient surgical teams must provide "basic blood transfusion" (level 2 DMATs) or "enhanced blood transfusion" services (level 3 DMATs). This section outlines the major issues that must be considered regarding austere transfusion, reviews the basic physiology of transfusion medicine, and offers some of the possible approaches and techniques for providing transfusion in the field. Anesthesiologists are the clinicians most likely to be involved in transfusion and are well placed to take a lead role in the oversight of such a service.

Overview of Blood Transfusion and Major Disasters

Despite media coverage in the aftermath of large-scale disaster events, there is rarely a demand for blood products that cannot be readily met within a short time frame. Bloodstocks can be mobilized from stores nearby, from outside the immediate area, or collected from local repeat donors if blood banks remain functional.

The safest and most reliable source of blood almost always comes from a country's own supply, if it has been rigorously screened to international standards and stored appropriately. Ideally it is this supply that is mobilized and used in a disaster. However, damage to buildings and equipment, loss of cold chain through power outage, damage to transport infrastructure, or chronic lack of supply – particularly in remote locations – can all impact on the ability of the local health system to deliver safe blood products.[6]

Knowledge of epidemiology after disasters allows some forward planning of the likely needs for transfusion in different disaster settings, although other issues such as the burden of obstetrics and ongoing trauma (e.g. motor vehicle accidents), particularly in settings with a high prevalence of chronic anemia, are also relevant.

Triggers for transfusion in austere environments are different from those in a routine hospital setting. Hemorrhagic shock, severe anemia, or bleeding with severe coagulopathy remain clear indications for blood products. However, other indications – transfusion of blood on hemoglobin concentration alone or prophylactic pre-procedural correction of mild coagulation defects – must take into consideration the clinical condition of the patient. Blood products will likely be limited and insufficient to treat every patient, and risks heightened, meaning clear clinical guidelines for transfusion should be in place.[7]

Review of Basic Transfusion Physiology

The most important antigenic groups in human blood are ABO and rhesus (rh) groups. ABO describes the presence on red cells of A-antigen (the patient is blood type A), B-antigen (type B), both A and B antigen (type AB) or neither A nor B antigen (type O). By around three months of age humans develop plasma antibodies to those AB antigens not present on their own cells. People of group O therefore contain both anti-A and anti-B antibodies in their plasma, whereas those who are group A have only anti-B antibodies (Figure 11.1).

Although the rhesus group has many more antigens, only the most immunogenic – rh D – determines whether an individual is rhesus positive or negative. Unlike ABO antibodies, rhesus antibodies do not develop naturally, only once a rhesus negative patient comes into contact with rhesus positive blood; either through fetal blood in a parturient or via transfusion (alloimmunization – see below). Some populations are overwhelmingly (>99%) rhesus positive, including many parts of East and South-East Asia and the Pacific Islands, where rhesus incompatibility is less of an issue.

The patient who is A rhesus positive (A+) has both A antigen and D antigen present on the surface of their red blood cells, and has anti-B antibody in their plasma. A patient who is O rhesus negative (O−) has neither ABO nor rhesus antigen on their red cells, which is why O− red cells are "universal" – there is no antigen to be targeted by any recipient antibodies. Whole blood, however, contains both red calls and plasma, meaning there is no universal donor (nor universal recipient) for whole blood.

Transfusing incompatible ABO blood will bring plasma antibodies into contact with the corresponding red cell antigen, resulting in a hemolytic transfusion reaction that can cause cardiovascular collapse, multiple organ failure, and death. In vitro testing detects which of

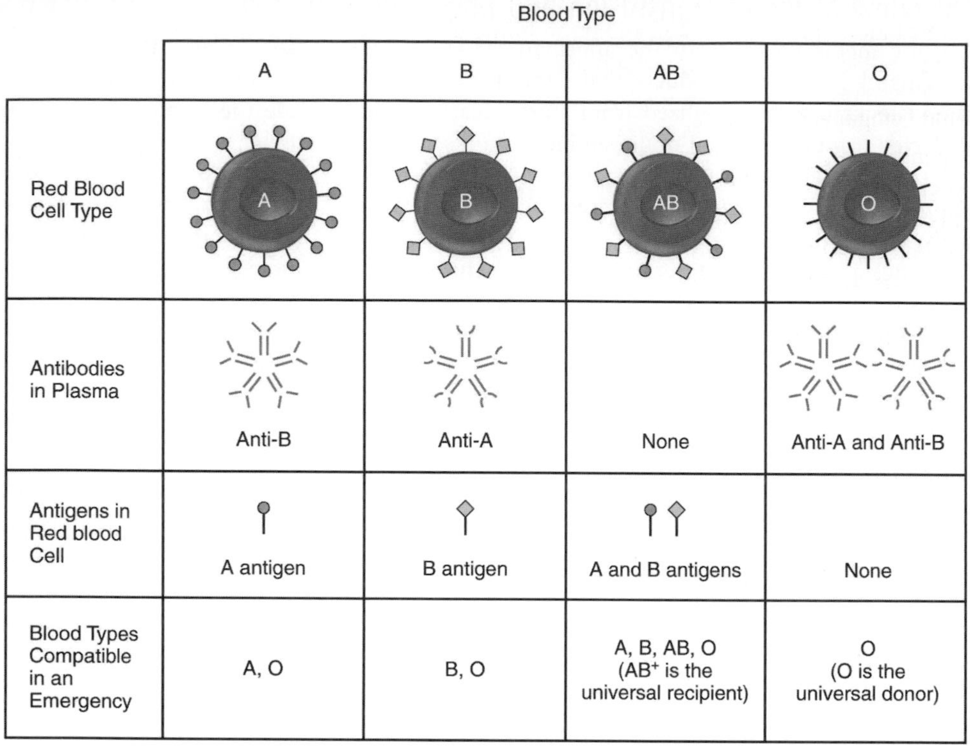

Blood Type

	A	B	AB	O
Red Blood Cell Type	A	B	AB	O
Antibodies in Plasma	Anti-B	Anti-A	None	Anti-A and Anti-B
Antigens in Red blood Cell	A antigen	B antigen	A and B antigens	None
Blood Types Compatible in an Emergency	A, O	B, O	A, B, AB, O (AB⁺ is the universal recipient)	O (O is the universal donor)

Figure 11.1 The ABO blood group system.

the ABO and rhesus-D antigens are present in both the patient's blood and the donor's blood ("grouping" or "typing"). However, there are many other less important antigen–antibody groups which may still cause clinically relevant or severe immune reactions, and thus ABO grouping should ideally be followed by mixing together serum from the potential recipient with the donor red cells to ensure no agglutination occurs (cross-matching) before transfusion takes place.

Using rhesus positive blood in rhesus negative patients can induce rhesus antibodies (alloimmunization) in the recipient. This does not cause an immediate reaction, but may cause problems with either future blood transfusions or in subsequent pregnancies in rhesus negative women. Rhesus positive blood should only be given to rhesus negative patients – particularly young women – as a last resort.

Transfusion Options for DMATs

Fresh or Stored Whole Blood

Whole blood collected and transfused locally using a "walking blood bank" is a strategy commonly used in military and other settings (e.g. cruise ships). Whereas the military often pre-screen staff for infectious disease and blood type, in a civilian field hospital this is less practical and blood will likely come from voluntary local donors. This means establishing robust processes and clear documentation, as outlined in the "Walking Blood Bank" section. Whole blood may be harvested and given immediately (fresh whole blood) or can be stored for up to five days in a specialized blood fridge.

Blood Component Therapy

Depending on resources available, whole blood can be separated into its components and stored as occurs in most hospital blood banks around the world. Sophisticated equipment and expertise is necessary, and is beyond most DMATs. Bringing blood components in from the donor country faces ethical, legal, and political challenges, and requires both a reliable cold chain and a large storage capacity.

Frozen Blood Products

Cryopreserved platelets, deep frozen red cells, and deep frozen plasma (at –80 °C) have a long half life (2, 7, and 10 years, respectively) and have been successfully used by some organizations.[8] Development in this area is promising, though large capital expense, heavy equipment, and logistical challenges currently limit the technology to sophisticated field hospital facilities.

Walking Blood Bank

It is likely that most civilian DMATs requiring a transfusion capability will establish a walking blood bank for harvesting whole blood. There are a number of considerations when establishing such a capability.

Personnel and Training

Although most members of a DMAT will have clinical training and awareness of blood transfusion, in a surgical team the anesthesiologist may have most regular exposure to administering blood products. Nursing or paramedical staff can be trained and assigned to the daily running of the service. The presence of a laboratory or transfusion technician as part of the team facilitates extended testing and improved expertise with blood grouping and infectious disease screening tests. This is essential where more sophisticated methods such as separation of whole blood to components or frozen blood products are used.

Collecting and preparing blood for transfusion may be an unfamiliar role to those tasked with it in a DMAT. The importance of initial education and regular retraining cannot be understated, along with clear manuals and guidelines being available on deployment.[9] Two-person checking of techniques, processes, results, and documentation may reduce errors and improve safety.

Establishing a Transfusion Committee and Donor Recruitment

Upon deployment, a committee should be formed of relevant personnel to establish and oversee the transfusion service, ensure ethics and safety requirements are met, and trouble-shoot problems that occur.

Donor recruitment will depend largely on local engagement, which may include addressing the acceptability of transfusion to the local community. Information exchange with local people through word of mouth, local media, or contact with voluntary groups, charities, NGOs, and other health care facilities may all be useful.

Pre-Donation Screening, Donor Suitability, and Donor Consent

There are many established pre-screening questionnaires available which can be adapted to suit local requirements. Questions must be clear and unambiguous, translated into local language (by interpreter), and meet agreed international standards. Bear in mind that donors may have discomfort in answering some questions accurately due to cultural and social factors. The aim of questionnaires is both to ensure the donor is healthy enough to donate blood, and to minimize the risk of transmissible disease to the recipient.

Physical examination should check for fever, lymphadenopathy, and other signs of chronic disease or immunosuppression. A hemoglobin measurement is required to ensure potential donors are not anemic. Contraindications to donation include anemia (hemoglobin concentration <11 g/dl), certain chronic illnesses, known or high risk of exposure to blood-borne viruses, and recent or ongoing acute illness or fever.

Informed donor consent must include the potential for uncovering blood-borne viral disease and considering the health and social consequences this may have.

Documentation

In maintaining high standards of governance, safety, and quality assurance, adequate record keeping is essential. Patient questionnaires, medical records, a donor registry, a blood bank registry, fridge temperature record (where applicable), blood labels, prescription forms, observation charts, and transfusion reaction report forms should all be completed. Digital photographs of infectious disease screening and blood typing tests may be kept. Although donations are anonymous, there must be an ability to trace recipients should there be any adverse events.

Infectious Disease Screening

Blood should be screened as per WHO guidelines for human immunodeficiency virus (HIV) using two separate tests, as well as hepatitis B, hepatitis C, syphilis, and any relevant blood-borne diseases such as malaria. A number of simple, rapid, and reliable PoC tests are available for these diseases. If tests are in any way equivocal, a risk-averse approach must be taken and the donor excluded. The potential for false negative results in those with recently acquired infection means excluding people with high-risk behavior or recent febrile illness. Preparations for a positive test must be made, including counseling and a referral plan. As with all equipment, manufacturers' instructions must be followed and factors such as performance limits in extremes of temperature and humidity considered when purchasing screening tests. Test cards often have a limited expiry in the range of 10–12 months.

Blood Typing

Various methods are available, from simple-to-use test cards impregnated with antiserum such as the Eldoncard (Eldon Biologicals, Gentofte, Denmark) to sophisticated laboratory machinery. The "tile" and "test tube" techniques are common in LMICs, and are both examples of methods involving adding specific reagents (antisera) to blood that will induce agglutination in the presence of specific red cell antigen. Thus anti-A reagent will cause agglutination in patients of type A or AB. This is repeated with anti-B and anti-D reagent and establishes the ABO and rhesus blood type (Figure 11.2). Equivocal reactions may be repeated, but should usually result in exclusion of the donor for safety reasons.

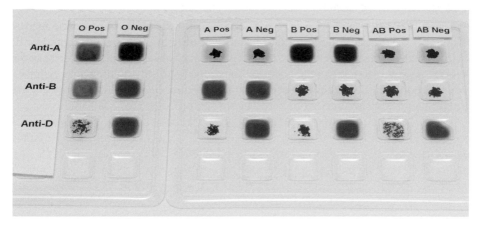

Figure 11.2 The tile method displaying agglutination in various blood types.

The method used must take into account team expertise, ease of use, the likelihood of user error, training and equipment required, reliability and safety, performance in extreme environments, need for cold chain (e.g. for antisera storage), and quality assurance.

Harvesting

Harvesting blood requires equipment that should ideally be set aside for sole use in the transfusion setting. Even in a resource-constrained environment, donors should be placed in a quiet, cooled, or shaded area, with a comfortable place to lie. Equipment for blood collection and treatment of complications such as transfusion reactions and vasovagal episodes must be immediately available. Donors should be looked after for a short period after donation and provided with sustenance.

Blood bags are placed on scales to allow assessment of the volume of blood collected. 450–500 ml is usually donated, although some donors, such as those who are physically small or have a mild anemia, may donate smaller volumes of around 200 ml. The bags are filled into the sampling "side tubes" and several sections clamped or tied off in order to allow small volumes of blood to be obtained for repeat screening, typing, or cross-match.

Recipient Consent

All patients regardless of context have the right to know about their treatment, the potential risks and benefits, and to refuse if they wish. The difficulties of a post-disaster setting do not excuse the denial of autonomy. True informed consent can be difficult with language and cultural barriers, but should be sought where possible. In emergency situations it is acceptable to proceed with lifesaving transfusion and discussion held with the patient as soon as practicable.

Transfusion

A medical practitioner should prescribe all transfusions with the indication recorded in the medical notes. Sterility should be maintained throughout, and regular observations (pulse, blood pressure, temperature) recorded on the anesthetic or transfusion chart.

Adverse Effects

All suspected transfusion reactions require cessation of the transfusion, followed by patient assessment. Most are mild allergic or febrile non-hemolytic transfusion reactions, and if the symptoms settle with simple measures the transfusion may be recommenced. Bear in mind, however, that any reaction has the potential to become a life-threatening emergency.

More serious reactions require emergency treatment as dictated by the clinical picture. The main points are summarised in Table 11.1.

Table 11.1 Immediate management of transfusion reactions
- *Stop the transfusion immediately*
- Keep the intravenous line open with 0.9% saline
- Repeat the patient and blood unit identity check
- Report to treating medical officer and transfusion committee

Signs and symptoms	Possible diagnosis	Management
≥38 °C and/or chills, rigors or 38 °C to <39 °C and no other symptoms	Febrile non-hemolytic transfusion reaction	• Exclude serious adverse events • Antipyretics • If no further symptoms recommence transfusion
<39 °C and other symptoms (e.g. hypotension, tachycardia) or ≥39 °C	Bacterial contamination or acute hemolytic transfusion reaction	• May become a medical emergency • IV antibiotics if sepsis • Maintain urine output
Hives, itching, rash <2/3 body (no other symptoms)	Mild allergic reaction	• Antihistamine/ corticosteroid • If subsides recommence transfusion
Hives, itching, rash >2/3 body (no other symptoms)	Severe allergic reaction	• Antihistamine/ corticosteroid
Hives, itching, rash plus airway obstruction, dyspnoea, hypotension	Anaphylaxis	• Medical emergency • Resuscitate • Epinephrine and corticosteroid
Dyspnea, shortness of breath, $\downarrow O_2$ saturation With/without hypertension, tachycardia	Transfusion-associated circulatory overload	• Sit patient upright • Oxygen • Diuretics
With/without hypotension	Transfusion-related acute lung injury	• May become a medical emergency • Chest X-ray for infiltrates • Oxygen • Possible intubation, ventilation

Table 11.1 (cont.)

Signs and symptoms	Possible diagnosis	Management
	Bacterial contamination or acute hemolytic transfusion reaction	• May become a medical emergency • IV antibiotics if sepsis • Maintain urine output

Safety and Governance

Blood transfusion in an austere environment is more risky than in a conventional hospital, meaning strict controls and procedures must exist regarding the processes described above. Both donor and recipient identification should be meticulous, as should blood product labelling. Legible comprehensive documentation allows safe practice to be maintained and follow-up of adverse events.

Storage of whole blood can be either fresh (best used immediately, but within 24 hours) or cold (refrigerated for up to five days) and safe expiry times adhered to. Blood fridges (which require a robust power supply) must be solely used for blood products, and temperature monitored and recorded.

The transfusion committee should meet regularly to record and address any complications, concerns, and safety issues.

References

1. Bryson GL, Wyand A, Bragg PR. Preoperative testing is inconsistent with published guidelines and rarely changes management. *Can J Anaesth*. 2006;**53**(3):236–241.

2. Finestone AS, Wolf Y, Bar-Dayan Y, et al. Medical auxiliary equipment in a field hospital: experience from the Israeli delegation to the site of the Turkish earthquake. *Br Med J* 1999;**319**:648.

3. Norton I, von Schreeb J, Aitken P, Herard P, Lajolo C. *Classification and Minimum Standards for Foreign Medical Teams in Sudden Onset Disasters*. Geneva: World Health Organization, 2013.

4. Critchley J, Bates M. Haemoglobin colour scale for anaemia diagnosis where there is no laboratory: a systematic review. *Int J Epidemiol* 2005;**34**(6):1424–1434.

5. De Benoist B, McLean E, Egli I, Cogswell M, (eds.) *Global Database on Anaemia 1993–2005*. Geneva: World Health Organization, 2008.

6. Abolghasemi H, Radfar MH, Tabatabaee M, Hosseini-Divkolayee NS, Burkle F. Revisiting blood transfusion preparedness: experience from the Bam earthquake response. *Prehosp Disaster Med* 2008;**23**(5):391–394.

7. World Health Organization. *The Clinical Use of Blood: Handbook*. Geneva: World Health Organization, 2002.

8. Neuhaus S, Wishaw K, Leikens C. Australian experience with frozen blood products on military operations. *Med J Aust* 2010;**192**:203–205.

9. Maari C, Gueguen M, Grouzard V, (eds.) *Blood Transfusion: A Manual for Doctors, Nurses and Laboratory Technicians*. Paris: Médecins Sans Frontières, 2010.

Chapter 12

High-Altitude Physiology and Anesthesia

Carlton Brown

Human physiology is well adapted to sea-level atmospheric pressure. Decreased atmospheric pressures at altitude have profound effects on human physiology and anesthetic delivery. Seemingly arcane, the need for high-altitude anesthesia and critical care in disaster response is unusually common. The seismology and meteorology of high-altitude mountainous environments leads to frequent natural disasters. Approximately 140 000 000 people worldwide live persistently at altitudes above 2500 meters (8000 feet). Additionally, millions of people transiently visit high altitudes for vacation hiking, skiing, sport climbing, or other recreational pleasures. These endemic and visiting populations are subject to the risks of natural disasters, in addition to their usual needs for surgical care at elevation. Anesthesiology providers are also asked to support military operations, aviation, mountain-climbing expeditions, and disaster-response humanitarian missions at extreme altitudes. These latter operations may be conducted in minimally developed areas with limited resources and involve high-risk behaviors, trauma, minimal time for acclimatization, and hostile environmental exposure. Expedition climbers and other adventurers have required surgical care at altitude in the past – not without anesthetic adventure and adverse outcome.[1] Safe and effective anesthesia care at high altitude requires an understanding of the normal and pathological effects of altitude and an appreciation for the anesthetic challenges in this environment.

Basic Science

Atmospheric pressure has a non-linear decrease as altitude increases. Half of the atmosphere is below 18 000 ft and the remaining half extends up to >100 000 ft. Increased altitudes are often categorized to denote their increasing effect of physiology:

- "High altitude" begins at 1500 m (~5000 ft) above sea level.
- "Very high altitude" begins at 3500 m (~11 500 ft)
- "Extreme altitude" begins at 5500 m (~18 000 ft)

Anesthetics delivered between 5000 and 11 500 ft require only modest changes from standard sea-level practices. Anesthetic care above 11 500 ft becomes increasingly problematic. The distinction and risks of "extreme altitude" are self-explanatory.

Fractional atmospheric oxygen concentration remains approximately 21% at all altitudes. As atmospheric pressure decreases with elevation, the absolute partial pressure of oxygen in air declines according to Dalton's Law – "The sum of all the partial equals the total pressure." (*Pbar* × 0.21) calculates the atmospheric oxygen pressure at any altitude. The alveolar gas equation defines a partial pressure for alveolar oxygen based on barometric pressure. A simplified form of the equation is:

$$P_{Alveolar}O_2 = FiO_2(P_{Bar} - 47mmHg) - \left(\frac{PaCO_2}{RQ}\right)$$

where $P_{Alveolar}$ is the partial pressure of oxygen in the alveolus (mmHg) – "PAO$_2$," FiO_2 is the fractional concentration of oxygen in inhaled gas (21% unless enhanced), P_{Bar} is the barometric (atmospheric) pressure (mmHg), 47 mmHg is the vapor pressure of water at body temperature (altitude does *not* change), $PaCO_2$ is the partial pressure of CO_2 in the alveolus (mmHg), and RQ is the respiratory quotient (moles CO_2 produced per moles O_2 consumed – typically about 0.82 for normal diet).

Using the alveolar gas equation, the effects of altitude and carbon dioxide on alveolar and arterial oxygen become very evident (calculations assume PaCO$_2$ = 40 – no compensation with hyperventilation):[2]

At sea level – P_{Bar} is 760 mmHg, PAO$_2$ is 101 mmHg, and hemoglobin saturation (SaO$_2$) is 98%.

At 5000 ft – P_{Bar} is 632 mmHg, PAO$_2$ is 73 mmHg, and SaO$_2$ is 95%

At 10 000 ft – P_{Bar} is 522 mmHg, PAO$_2$ is 51 mmHg, and SaO$_2$ is 86%.

At 15 000 ft – P_{Bar} is 438 mmHg, PAO$_2$ is 32 mmHg, and SaO$_2$ is 62%.

At 20 000 ft – P_{Bar} is 364 mmHg, PAO$_2$ is 17 mmHg, and SaO$_2$ is 24%.

(This last altitude is only sustainable with hyperventilation/hypocarbia or supplemental oxygen.)

With PaCO$_2$ = 20 mmHg – note the effect of hyperventilation on saturation

At 20 000 ft – P_{Bar} is 364 mmHg, PAO$_2$ is 42 mmHg, and SaO$_2$ is 78%.

Demographics

All people are subject to the normal physiological effects of altitude. Rapid ascent to high altitude without adequate acclimatization additionally risks altitude-related illnesses. Physiologic adjustment to altitude requires both time and patience.

Adaptation

Acute adaptation to high altitude involves hyperventilation and increased cardiac output. Lower P_{Bar} leads to lower PAO$_2$, decreased SaO$_2$, and PaO$_2$. Increased hypoxic ventilatory drive from low PaO$_2$ leads to hyperventilation. Hyperventilation leads to decreased PaCO$_2$ and PACO$_2$, enhancing alveolar oxygen tension (per above illustration). As hyperventilation is the primary means of acute adaptation to ascent, the ability to rapidly tolerate hypobaric environments depends largely on sufficient pulmonary reserve. The degree of hypocapnia can be striking. End-tidal CO_2 on Mt Everest has been measured at 7.5 mmHg, clearly low enough to modify cerebral and other organ blood flow. Decreased gas density offsets some of the adverse work of breathing from hyperventilation. Cardiac output is increased by sympathetic signaling due to hypoxemia, particularly through increased heart rate. This acute response may be detrimental to individuals with ischemic or valvular cardiac disease or with pre-existing pulmonary hypertension.

Longer-term adaptation occurs over days to weeks. Mechanisms include:

- Increased 2,3-DPG levels due to hypoxic stress, shifting O_2–Hgb dissociation curve toward the right and facilitating O_2 unloading in tissues
- Increased erythropoiesis – polycythemia toward >50% Hct
- Increased cardiac output secondary to hypoxemia

- Renal compensation for the alkalosis of hypocarbia – largely bicarbonate wasting to improve left-shifted O_2–Hgb dissociation curve
- Genetic differences modify adaptive responses
- The complete mechanism of adaptation is not fully elucidated.

Pathophysiology at Altitude

Both anesthesia providers and their patients arriving acutely at high altitudes are susceptible to hypobaric illnesses. Over-exertion, poor hydration, and young age may contribute to risk. Physical fitness and gender do not seem to affect incidence. Sudden exposure to very high or extreme altitudes (>11 500 ft) can be fatal. Unconsciousness can occur within minutes and death may follow without supplemental oxygen. Although discussion of these illnesses may seem tangential to "high-altitude anesthesia," these conditions may affect either the provider or the patient. Prolonged emergence, refractory hypoxemia, and other adverse anesthetic patient outcomes may be explained by these mechanisms. Providers impaired by these conditions constitute a substantial hazard to their patients. *Cerebral hypoxia impairs judgment – perhaps your judgment!*

Acute high-altitude exposure can cause several forms of illness, overlapping in both pathophysiology and clinical presentation:

- acute mountain sickness (AMS)
- high-altitude pulmonary edema (HAPE)
- high-altitude cerebral edema (HACE).

Acute Mountain Sickness

AMS is the mildest mild form of hypobaric illness.

Symptoms

- Early symptoms (12–24 hours): headache refractory to standard analgesics, nausea, anorexia, lassitude, sleep disturbances, peripheral edema. Judgment may be impaired.
- Late symptoms: can progress to shortness of breath, intense snoring, vomiting, hallucinations, and severely impaired cognitive function.
- Advanced symptoms: severe dyspnea, cyanosis, decreased SaO_2, ataxia.

Treatment

- If severe, definitive treatment is descent! Often descent of only 500–1000 m leads to complete resolution of symptoms. Most symptoms resolve in several days, even at altitude.
- Rest, hydration, analgesics, oxygen all can help.
- Acetazolamide 250 mg q 8–12 hours improves symptoms and SaO_2 (especially during sleep).
- Dexamethasone 4 mg q 6 hours.

Prevention

- Ascend slowly (not always possible in military or disaster operations)
- Oxygen, particularly at night while sleeping
- Daily altitude gain of no more than 300 m above 3000 m
- After ascending 1000 m spend two consecutive nights

- Rest on arrival at altitude, avoiding over-exertion, adequate hydration
- Acetazolamide 250 mg q8 hours beginning at least 24 hours before ascent and continued for two to three days after reaching highest altitude.

Two additional forms of altitude-induced illness are, though less common, more severe and life threatening.

High-Altitude Pulmonary Edema (HAPE)

HAPE is a malignant form of AMS with similar early symptoms and is life threatening. It may occur in healthy individuals after rapid ascent above 2500 m (8200 ft). It is thought to be a form of right-heart failure caused by exaggerated hypoxemic pulmonary vasoconstriction and high cardiac output. Right atrial and pulmonary artery pressures are elevated. If a patent foramen ovale (PFO) is present, atrial flow reversal may occur. Alterations of pulmonary capillary permeability may also be involved. An individual with a previous episode of HAPE may be particularly susceptible to this condition. They should approach returning to altitude with caution, as altitude re-exposure has induced recurrence.

Symptoms

- Dyspnea, tachypnea, chest pain, rales, tachycardia, dry cough, followed by the production of pink frothy sputum
- Respiratory failure and death can quickly ensue
- CXR shows patchy infiltrates, which spare lung bases and costophrenic angles
- Elevated pulmonary artery pressure secondary to hypoxia
- ECG shows right heart strain
- LV function is normal.

Treatment

- Rapid descent to lower altitude!!
- Supplemental O_2
- Morphine? (controversial due to depression of ventilation)
- Nifedipine SR 20 mg q 12 hours
- Nitric oxide, hydralazine, phentolamine sublingual nifedipine, sildenafil may reduce pulmonary pressures
- PEEP or BiPAP, if available
- If descent is not possible, consider Gamow bag.

High-Altitude Cerebral Edema (HACE)

HACE is another severe form of AMS and is very life threatening. It is thought to be due to increased cerebral blood flow and alterations in blood–brain barrier permeability due to severe hypoxemia. Early symptoms are similar to AMS but progress to gross CNS dysfunction. Judgment is severely impaired.

Early Symptoms

- Headache
- Anorexia

- Nausea
- Emesis
- Papilledema, retinal hemorrhage, photophobia
- Fatigue
- Irritability
- Decreased socialization

Late Symptoms

- Ataxia
- Irrationality
- Hallucinations
- Visual disturbances
- Focal neurological deficits
- Abnormal reflexes.

Diagnosis

- Patients may have concurrent HAPE symptoms.
- Death may be imminent when symptoms of HACE become severe.
- Lumbar puncture may show markedly elevated CSF pressure.
- CT suggestive of brain edema – particularly in the corpus callosum.

Treatment

- Immediate, rapid descent!!!
- Dexamethasone 10 mg IV or IM, then 6 mg q 6 h
- Supplemental O_2, may be helpful if pulmonary symptoms are present
- Diuretics may reduce brain edema, but may worsen an already dehydrated state.

If immediate descent is not possible to treat HACE or HAPE, relative hyperbaric conditions may be temporarily induced in a Gamow bag. Reasons delaying descent include high winds, weather, limited manpower, hostile fire, absent communications, or limited extraction assets (including the service ceilings of helicopters). *Actual descent is always the preferred treatment for life-threatening hypobaric illness.*

Gamow Bag (Figure 12.1)

- Portable, lightweight, fabric hyperbaric chamber.
- Can generate 103 mmHg of pressure above ambient pressure.
- Simulates a descent of 4000 to 9000 ft at moderate altitudes.

Cold Injuries and Complications

Particularly for patients coming from combat, natural disasters, or other outdoor exposure into the OR, hypothermia is a major anesthetic consideration. Ambient temperature decreases with altitude. The "standard lapse rate" is 3.5 °F per 1000 feet of altitude. By example, if an area is 72 °F at sea level, it will be simultaneously 40 °F colder (i.e. 32 °F) at 11 500 ft. Hypothermia alters pharmacokinetics, pharmacodynamics, control of ventilation, level of consciousness, and other important aspects of anesthetic care. Warming of

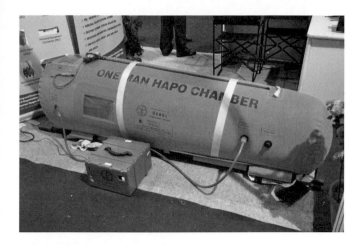

Figure 12.1 Gamow bag, portable, lightweight, fabric hyperbaric chamber.

severely hypothermic patients should be completed, if possible, before attempting surgical or anesthetic intervention. Anesthesiologists are often asked to participate in rewarming, given experience and equipment used in intraoperative thermoregulation. Surgical urgency may force active treatment of hypothermia while undergoing surgical stabilization.

Two common cold-induced injuries include:

- Frostbite – this is a frequent cause for urgent surgical intervention at extreme altitude
- Hypothermia – defined as core temperature below 35 °C.

Treatment

- Handle gently
- Oxygen (warmed, humidified)
- IV fluids (warmed)
- Monitor: core temperature, oxygen saturation, cardiac rhythm
- Dysrhythmias may be refractory to treatment until patient is rewarmed
- May complicate surgical and anesthetic care.

Rewarming

- Passive: allow patients to rewarm passively and slowly
- Active: rewarm with external (water immersion, radiant heat, forced warm air heating blankets) and core techniques (heated IV fluids, body cavity lavage, cardiopulmonary bypass pump)
- Resuscitation with lactated Ringer's solution might be avoided as the cold liver inefficiently metabolizes lactate
- Neither passive nor active rewarming has been shown to yield superior outcomes.

Indications for Rapid Rewarming

- Cardiovascular instability
- Moderate or severe hypothermia (<32.2 °C)

- Inadequate rate or failure to passively rewarm
- Endocrine insufficiency
- Traumatic or toxicological peripheral vasodilation
- Secondary hypothermia impairing thermoregulation.

Dehydration

Altered breathing at high altitudes results in systemic dehydration. Hyperventilation to compensate for hypoxemia results in increased minute ventilation. This hyperventilation may be affected through mouth breathing, bypassing normal nasal mucosal hydration and moisture recovery. Further, the vapor pressure of water at body temperature (47 mmHg) remains constant at altitude. At reduced ambient pressures, the fraction of exhaled water vapor is increased relative to that at sea level. Many areas of high altitude have low relative humidity due to meteorological conditions. For all these reasons, personnel at altitude lose substantially more free water through breathing than at sea level. Dehydration limits increased cardiac output as a compensation mechanism for altitude, modifies response to anesthetic drugs, and may increase the risk of hypobaric illness. Dehydration may also increase the risk of DVT, stroke, thrombophlebitis, pulmonary embolism, and generalized hypercoagulability. Major surgery may worsen this condition. Aggressive volitional hydration is required to offset this normal physiologic loss of free water at altitude. Alcoholic beverages are inappropriate for this purpose due to the augmented cerebral effects of alcohol from hypoxia and the diuretic effects of alcohol.

Anesthetic Management at Altitude

The difficulty and risk of anesthetic care is proportional to altitude. Descent to the lowest practical altitude to render care will enhance patient safety and decrease anesthetic misadventure. It may not always be practical to descend and some anesthetics must be administered at high or extreme altitudes. Administration of anesthetics above 18 000 ft is known to be very hazardous (case reports) and should be considered only in the absence of any practical alternatives.

Anesthetic Management Considerations

Oxygen

Increasing FiO_2 can compensate for the effect of reduced barometric pressure, both during and after anesthetic administration[3]. It is suggested that 30% inspired oxygen be a minimum at 5000 ft and that 40% oxygen be a minimum at 10 000 ft for both intra-operative and post-operative care. Remembering that the alveolar gas equation gives the *highest* level of alveolar oxygen available, V/Q mismatch induced by low FRC, low cardiac output, residual neuromuscular block, hypercarbia, and other physiological effects of surgery and anesthesia may substantially reduce actual arterial blood oxygen concentrations (PaO_2). High cardiac output may cause incomplete equilibration of alveolar and capillary oxygen due to short transit times in the lung. A major risk of anesthesia at high altitude is that anesthetized patients can become hypoxic in spite of normally adequate inspired oxygen concentrations. Oxygen availability increases in importance with increasing altitude – both as a matter of logistics and physiology. The availability of compressed (tank) oxygen may be limited and resupply may be unreliable. Portable oxygen generators (concentrators) do work at increased altitude if adequate energy sources (battery or generator) are available.

Nitrous oxide is largely irrelevant at altitude. In austere surgical settings, it may simply be unavailable. Further, the potential benefit of N_2O as part of an inhaled anesthetic is decreased by 50% at 5000 feet and is essentially insignificant by 10 000 ft. Diffusion hypoxemia after nitrous administration further compromises tenuous oxygenation in the immediate post-operative period.

Regional Anesthesia

Given the relative scarcity of gaseous or liquid oxygen in austere environments it is reasonable to conduct surgery using regional techniques. Inhaled agents and opioids blunt hypoxic ventilatory drive, even into the post-operative period. At altitude, maximizing the use of regional anesthesia not only decreases use of scarce resources, but may improve patient safety post-operatively. Minimizing opioid use decreases the risk of post-operative respiratory depression. Some reports have suggested that spinal anesthesia may have an increased risk of post-dural puncture headache, perhaps due to ICP changes with hypoxemia or dehydration. Other studies have not duplicated this finding. If regional anesthesia cannot be used, utilizing compressed air to power ventilators, using piston ventilators, or using TIVA and spontaneous ventilation will spare scarce compressed oxygen.

Pharmacology

Opioids depress ventilation and may compromise oxygenation through hypercarbia and a lack of hypoxic ventilatory drive. Modest hypercarbia (or even normocarbia) that would be tolerable at sea level is life-threatening at extreme altitude. Ketamine may be a better analgesic agent than opioids. Local and regional techniques may minimize the need for systemic analgesia. Patients may be taking acetazolamide, sildenafil, calcium channel blockers, or other medications to mitigate hypobaric illness. These may have some bearing on anesthetic choices and patient response.

Vaporizers

Actual vaporizer performance at extreme altitude (>18 000 ft) is speculative. Certain engineering principles are known to apply, but little research has been reported at extreme hypobaric pressures. Experimental data are available on vaporizer performance up to 10 000 ft. Studies of vaporizer output from 3 atm hyperbaric to 10 000 ft all suggest that the fractional flows of gas through proportional flow vaporizers remain constant. This reflects a design principle of maintaining laminar flow in the proportioner mechanism so that the division of gas flow depends largely on the viscosity of the gas mixture rather than density. Viscosity, the stress–strain and sheering relationship between gas molecules, is largely independent of pressure. Intermolecular distances in gases are large and do not change substantially with altitude. Density reflects the number of molecules and their molecular weight. Gas density falls rapidly with altitude, and measurements or functions that depend upon density are substantially modified. Extremely high fresh gas flow through a vaporizer might induce turbulent flow, in which case density (versus viscosity) would modify vaporizer output. Moderation of fresh gas flows should yield more predictable vaporizer behavior.

Effect of Altitude on Vaporizer Output

As stated above, modern vaporizers largely maintain the fractional relationship between their bypass and saturation chamber gas flows. Assuming this constant ratio, one can predict vaporizer output partial pressures. The vapor pressure of any liquid anesthetic agent depends only on temperature and substance and is independent of total atmospheric pressure. Even with all vaporizer input fresh gas being "thin air," the same volume of fresh gas is directed into the saturation chamber by the dial setting. The amount of anesthetic vapor picked up in the saturation chamber is the same as at sea level for the same volume of gas flowing through that chamber. The saturated gas carries the same amount of anesthetic when rejoining the bypass gas – whether at sea level or altitude. The anesthetic output vapor pressure does become a higher fractional part of reduced atmospheric pressure. By example, sevoflurane has a saturated vapor pressure (at 20 °C) of 157 mmHg. This would normally be 157/760 mmHg or 21% of atmospheric pressure. At 10 000 feet with P_{Bar} = 522 mmHg, however, that calculation would be 157/522 mmHg or 30%. Even with this apparently higher fraction, *the absolute partial pressure of sevoflurane is actually the same!* MAC values for anesthetics are typically reported as the "volume/volume %" at sea level. Sevoflurane has a MAC of "2.1%" of a sea-level atmosphere. This could equally be reported as "2.1% of 760 mmHg" or 16 mmHg of sevoflurane. With decreased atmospheric pressure, the same partial pressure of an anesthetic represents a higher "vol/vol%" of total atmospheric pressure. MAC in "vol/vol%" for sevoflurane at 10 000 ft. would be 16/522 mmHg or 3.1%. Modern proportional flow vaporizers yield an anesthetic partial pressure consistent with their dial settings. At sea level, a dial setting of 1% yields 7.6 mmHg of an agent. At altitude, the same dial setting also yields 7.6 mmHg of agent, but at a higher fractional part of a "thin" atmosphere. Bottom line – at altitude, vaporizer output is very close to the same absolute partial pressure of agent as at sea level![4] As partial anesthetic agent pressure in the CNS is the actual meaning of MAC, no change in dial settings of the vaporizer is necessary to obtain the same anesthetic effect[5]. If the vol/vol% is measured at altitude, it will be higher, but the absolute partial pressure similar to sea level. Many modern anesthetic gas analyzers have barometric corrections and will display a measured agent as it would appear at sea level. (Check the operating manual for any particular gas analyzer.)

One major exception to constant partial pressure output is a desflurane vaporizer. Desflurane vaporizers are not proportional flow vaporizers. They use measured bypass gas flow and a calibrated injection of desflurane vapor to create an output concentration. Desflurane requires that the vaporizer setting be adjusted to the vol/vol % MAC for actual atmospheric pressure at altitude. For example, if the MAC is 6% desflurane at sea level, the vaporizer would have to be set to 12% at 18 000 feet (an atmospheric pressure of ½ sea-level atmospheric pressure or 380 mmHg.) (Measured desflurane levels may be corrected to sea-level display – again, check your gas analyzer manual.)

Flow Meters

Traditional gas flow meters (Thorpe tubes) are affected by altitude. At low flows, where the interaction between the glass tube and the bobbin is very narrow, work done on the bobbin is largely dependent on laminar flow (tubular resistance). At low flows Thorpe tubes are reasonably accurate, as gas viscosity is minimally affected by altitude. At higher flows, however, the work done on the bobbin induces turbulent flow and force applied to the bobbin depends on gas density (orifice resistance). At higher flows Thorpe tubes tend to underestimate gas flow because of the reduced density. The effects of reduced density at these higher flows are not necessarily equal between oxygen and nitrous oxide. Caution should be exercised in calculating FiO_2 from flow-meter settings. The effects of altitude on other types of flow meters (such as hotwire flow meters) used internally in modern anesthesia machines is complex and beyond the scope of this discussion.

Caveats

Under no circumstances must an anesthetic agent reach its boiling point in a proportional flow vaporizer, as vaporizer output will become impossible to control. The definition of boiling point is atmospheric pressure equal to vapor pressure. (Desflurane is a known hazard, as it boils at less than 5000 ft even at 20 °C and its vaporizers are designed accordingly). With reduced atmospheric pressure and elevated ambient temperatures other anesthetics may boil at altitude (namely halothane and isoflurane). This may preclude the use of proportional flow vaporizers at extreme altitudes in warm conditions.

References

1. Firth PG, Pattinson KT. Anaesthesia and high altitude: a history. *Anaesthesia* 2008;**63**:662–670.

2. Cornell University. Calculator for pulmonary gas effects of altitude. www-users.med.cornell.edu/~spon/picu/calc/o2satcal.htm (accessed September 2019).

3. Sutton JR, Reeves JT, Wagner PD, et al. Operation Everest II: oxygen transport during exercise at extreme simulated altitude. *J Appl Physiol* 1998;**64**:1309,

4. International Anesthesia Research Society. Vaporizer output at altitude. www.openanesthesia.org/vaporizer_output_at_altitude/ (accessed September 2019).

5. Moon RF, Camporesi EM. Clinical care in extreme environments: at high and low pressure and in space. In: Miller RD, Eriksson LL, Fleisher LA, Wiener-Kronish JP, Young WL (eds.) *Miller's Anesthesia* 7th edn. London, UK: Churchill Livingstone; 2009: 2674–2704.

Chapter 13

Disaster: Mental Health Effects, Responses, and What Clinicians Can Do

Shaukat A. Khan and Kirsten M. Wilkins

Descriptions of disasters and their psychological impact as severe trauma on humans appear in ancient literature, such as Homer's *Iliad* and *Odyssey*, and various religious texts. The historian Herodotus, in the sixth century BC, described a soldier who suffered from permanent blindness after he witnessed the death of a fellow soldier. More recently, soldiers who fought in the civil war suffered from a set of physical and emotional symptoms known as "Soldier's Heart" or Da Costa's syndrome, a possible predecessor of what we now refer to as post-traumatic stress disorder. While most disaster victims do not develop psychopathology, depending on the intensity and severity of the trauma, many survivors suffer from varying degrees of emotional problems. The common post-disaster psychiatric disorders are post-traumatic stress disorder (PTSD), major depression, and alcohol use disorder.[1] Although disaster-related emotional traumas have been known for years, the clinical evaluation and treatment of these traumas within the disaster situation are relatively recent developments. Modern disaster psychiatry dates back to the 1942 "Cocoanut Grove" night-club fire in Boston which killed 492 people and left a community in grief. Erich Lindeman,[2] Stanley Cobb,[3] and Alexander Adler[4] published papers describing the psychiatric complications, symptomatology, and the management of acute grief related to this event.

There are several definitions of disaster. The definition offered by WHO is as follows: a "severe disruption, ecological and psychosocial, which greatly exceeds the coping capacity of the affected community."[5] There are different types of disasters based on etiology. Disaster may be caused by natural events, also known as "Acts of God" (e.g. flood, typhoon, tsunami, earthquake), by accidents or technological malfunctions (e.g. aircraft crash or power plant explosion), or by deliberate acts of human with ill-motives (e.g. gun-violence or terrorism). The frequency of disasters is increasing, which can be attributed to changes in climate, geopolitical situations, increasing use of technology, etc. According to EM-DAT, an emergency disaster database maintained by the Office of US Foreign Disaster Assistance (OFDA), natural disasters are steadily increasing in recent decades. This increase is both due to natural (e.g. climate change) and man-made factors (e.g. population movements, unplanned urbanization, deforestation, etc.). While better disaster preparedness and prevention programs have reduced the number of deaths from natural disasters, more people are left injured or displaced by the disasters.[6] These facts underscore the need for increased involvement of health care professionals in the disaster relief.

Mental health professionals are becoming increasingly active within disaster response. More than 700 psychiatrists responded to the 9/11 attacks (Disaster Psychiatry Outreach, personal communication, 2010). Following the earthquake and tsunami in the Indian

Ocean, hurricane Katrina in 2005, and the earthquake in Haiti in 2010, psychiatrists continued to volunteer in disaster relief. In the aftermath of the Newtown shooting disaster, under the leadership of Connecticut Psychiatric Society, more than 50 psychiatrists served, all together providing over 400 hours service. Mental health professionals can play important roles in various areas, as such, their participation in disaster relief should be encouraged. However, they should be aware that disaster psychiatry is not the same as trauma psychiatry, particularly in the immediate aftermath of disaster. The emphasis of disaster psychiatry is normality of responses not psychopathology. The primary focus is helping the population of high-risk groups, rather than individual treatment modalities. Disaster psychiatry aims to promote the overall medical health status of an affected community. It facilitates application and management of post-disaster aid (human services needs, financial, etc.) Disaster psychiatry is not an office-based practice, and disaster survivors with whom the provider interacts are not generally defined as "patients." Though disasters can lead to decompensation in stable psychiatric patients, many individuals who might benefit from mental health support are in fact experiencing normal reactions to extraordinary circumstances. Often the psychiatric presentations ("symptoms") in disaster survivors do not reach the threshold of psychiatric diagnostic criteria ("syndrome"). The skills required early on in disaster response, therefore, differ from those used in traditional trauma treatment. In addition, a mental health professional volunteering in a disaster situation may be asked to play other unusual roles, such as performing administrative, consultative, educational, and general medical duties.

Before committing to relief efforts, health professionals should be affiliated with a recognized organization, aware of major issues impacting those affected by disasters and knowledgeable about the appropriate intervention. There should be a clear understanding of the concerted purpose, and of one's own motivation for responding. Responders themselves should be in good health to operate in a variety of circumstances, and should be careful not to become a burden to the relief effort.

Phases of Disaster

It is generally accepted that there are three phases of response and recovery after a disaster hits a community:

1. Impact: first 24–48 hours of acute phase (hours to days)
2. Acute: Extends up to 2 months after the event
3. Post-acute: 2 months after the event and beyond (weeks to months and years).

Appropriate preparation for disaster should begin before the disaster hits a community (pre-disaster). The mental health intervention should begin as soon as possible in the acute phase and should continue in the post-acute phase and beyond.

Pre-Disaster Preparation

In the pre-disaster phase, prospective disaster-relief mental health workers should devote themselves to understanding the logistical issues related to disaster response and relief activities. They should familiarize themselves with the roles of different disaster response organizations, as well as the roles of the persons within an organization's hierarchy of response. If possible they should be involved in hospital/clinic disaster planning at their own institutions by being a part of the institution's emergency management committee. They should educate members in the emergency management committee regarding possible mental health consequences of disaster victims, and consider the welfare of individuals with serious mental illnesses in a disaster. Before being deployed for disaster relief, it is important for the health professional to be familiar with the characteristics of the affected community, including its strengths, weaknesses, and cultural characteristics.

Appropriate measures should be in place to meet the responder's own medical needs. Disaster responders are not immune to disaster-related stress. Leaving behind family members to go on an assignment can be very stressful. In addition, staying in a shelter with others, working in an unfamiliar and challenging setting with an unfamiliar culture or population, language barriers, and exposure to traumatic situations and/or stories can all add to the stress.

Effects of Trauma

One has to keep in mind that most disaster victims do not develop psychopathology. According to National Comorbidity Survey the rate of lifetime history of exposure to at least one traumatic event is 60.7% in men and 51.2% in women; exposure to a second trauma is between 25% and 50%. The prevalence of PTSD in the general population is 1.3% (DSM III), 8–9% (DSM III R, DSM IV); women are affected two times more than men. Since there is significant change in the diagnostic criteria of PTSD in DSM 5, the prevalence rate may be different now.

"Stress theory" generally assumes that external *demands*, (e.g. the traumatic events) as primary stressors evoke responses that draw on inner or external *resources*. Loss of resources, in either *concrete* (social, financial) or *symbolic* (beliefs, expectations) ways, may significantly impact the recovery trajectory.[7] In addition to a psychological reaction to the exposure to trauma, genetics and neurobiology all play a part in long-term psychopathology caused by trauma. Dysregulation of stress hormone, neuropeptide Y, pre-cortical executive function, amygdala, hippocampal, and HPA axis function,[8] and over-consolidation of fear-related (emotional) memory may all be associated with psychopathology caused by trauma.

Acute Phase Assessment

Individuals react to disaster in various ways in response to the combination of different factors. Stress is a common reaction among the survivors and workers. The contributing factors to stress include the characteristics of the disaster itself as well as the characteristics of the victims. The acute phase intervention begins with assessment of the disaster victims. The basic assessment includes assessment of exposure and assessment of needs.

Assessment of exposure should include:

1. Proximity and duration of event
2. Personal injury and/or loss of possessions
3. Ongoing insecurity or threat
4. Demographic: age, gender, family composition, cultural, ethnic, racial background
5. Medical injury or exposure
6. Past psychiatric and substance abuse history
7. Pre-disaster problems with living, health, finances, social support etc.

Other factors, such as pre-disaster preparedness, post-disaster living situation, and availability and/or quality of disaster relief services or medical care, may all determine the level of stress in the disaster victims.

The most important aspect in the assessment of needs is identifying survivors who need immediate medical or psychiatric treatment. The following (psychiatric) situations need urgent triage:

1. Suicidality
2. Homicidality/harm to others
3. Inability to care for self
4. Acute exacerbation/recurrence of psychiatric symptoms
5. Substance relapse/acute intoxication.

Assessment of needs should also include:

1. Continuation of ongoing medical/psychiatric care
2. Food, water, shelter
3. Safety, reuniting with family/community
4. Psychological, psychiatric, spiritual care.

Determining psychological impact requires careful assessment with knowledge about common physical, emotional, cognitive, behavioral, and spiritual reactions to disaster. Mental health professionals also need to distinguish between symptoms and syndromes, distress, and diagnosis.

Common initial psychiatric symptoms include anxiety, insomnia, and mood dysregulation (irritability); less common but equally important symptoms are agitation, psychosis, dissociation, medically unexplained somatic complaints, and relapse with substance abuse.

The acute phase psychiatric diagnoses include:

1. PTSD
2. Acute stress disorder (ASD)
3. Major depression
4. Substance use disorder
5. Acute bereavement
6. Adjustment disorder
7. Panic disorder
8. Exacerbation of personality disorder
9. Brief psychotic disorder
10. Delirium.

Acute Phase Interventions

Acute phase mental health intervention could be psychological or pharmacological. Key goals of acute phase intervention are to assure safety, reduce symptom burden, reduce anxiety and distress, and improve functioning.

Acute phase psychological interventions should be empathic, supportive, and practical. Targeted mental health interventions should be provided for enhancing resilience and addressing impairment, symptoms, and acute issues. Referrals should be made as needed.

Psychological First Aid (PFA)

"Psychological first aid" is a very helpful tool, and every disaster psychiatrist should be aware of it. According to the Red Cross Instructor Manual, "The idea with Psychological First Aid is simply to provide basic care, comfort, and support to those individuals who are experiencing disaster-related stress." PFA was developed by the National Child Traumatic Stress Network (NCTSN) and the National Center for PTSD (NCPTSD). The first and second editions of the PFA operation guide were released in 2005 and 2006, respectively, and the guide is now available online.[9] The PFA has received widespread acceptance, including adoption by the American Red Cross, public health agencies, and the military, state, and local governments. It has been translated into several different languages. PFA is an evidence-informed modular approach to help children, adolescents, adults, and families in the immediate aftermath of disaster and terrorism,[10] designed to reduce the initial distress caused by traumatic events and to foster short- and long-term adaptive functioning and coping. It is a set of early and practical responses, which can be started immediately at the scene of an incident and continued for several days or weeks. Many of these responses are not psychological in nature but are a common-sense approach related to meeting basic needs for physical safety, connectedness, security, and survival, thus improving function and mental health response. The principles and techniques of PFA meet four basic standards. They are: (1) consistent with research evidence on risk and resilience following trauma, (2) applicable and practical in field settings, (3) appropriate for developmental levels across the lifespan, and (4) culturally informed and delivered in a flexible manner.[9]

The elements of PFA are as follows:

1. Engagement
2. Information gathering
3. Identifying needs
4. Relaying accurate and timely information
5. Offering practical assistance
6. Promoting connectedness
7. Providing safety and comfort
8. Making collaborative services available
9. Encouraging good coping skills
10. Giving realistic assurance
11. Making appropriate referrals.

The short-term purpose of PFA is to promote a sense of safety, calmness, self and collective efficacy, connectedness, and hope, with the long-term goal of minimizing the long-term effects of exposure to traumatic experiences and acute stress.[10]

The "evidence-informed"[10] PFA is a very effective intervention tool for mental health workers; however, its social, religious, and cultural limitations must be kept in mind when using it in disaster situations. Health care providers can also practice some elements of PFA to help themselves during a disaster assignment.

Other Psychological Interventions

In addition to psychological first aid, other individual and/or group psychotherapies utilized among disaster victims include supportive psychotherapy, grief counseling, anxiety management, cognitive behavioral therapy (CBT), and dialectical behavioral therapy (DBT). Among the short-term therapies, the most evidence-based is cognitive behavioral therapy. CBT focuses on alleviating suffering by modifying maladaptive thoughts (e.g. over-generalization) and behaviors, thought processes, and symptoms associated with re-exposure memories. Although it is still practiced in the aftermath of disaster or non-disaster-related trauma, critical incident stress debriefing (CISD) as an intervention in the aftermath of disaster is not recommended anymore. Repeated controlled trials have failed to show its effectiveness to reduce acute subjective distress or long-term risk of PTSD.[11] In addition to other therapies mentioned above, eye movement desensitization and reprocessing (EMDR) as a long-term psychotherapy has also been an effective intervention.[11]

The majority of survivors, however, eventually recover from initial shock, even though there is no formal intervention.

Pharmacological Treatment Options

In the acute disaster setting, treatment is directed at specific symptoms rather than specific syndromes or disorders, as mentioned earlier.

There is no US Food and Drug Administration (FDA) approved medication for ASD. The standard clinical practice, however, is to prescribe anxiolytic, sedative, or antipsychotic medications for "off-label" use to treat anxiety, insomnia, and/or agitation, similar to such practice in emergency psychiatry or primary care settings.[9] Much of the current psychopharmacological intervention in the acute phase of disaster is guided by targeting the postulated disease mechanism of ASD and PTSD that includes dysregulation of the hypothalamic-pituitary-adrenal axis and of the norepinephrine, glutamate, and serotonin systems. But one has to remember that not all ASD leads to PTSD and PTSD may occur acutely.

Medications, if prescribed, are usually done so on a short-term basis to reduce target symptoms, usually guided by prior clinical experience in disasters and research evidence from its use on other acutely stressed populations. The following is a list of medications which may prove to be helpful additions in a disaster psychiatrist's tool box: lorazepam, clonazepam, diphenhydramine, hydroxyzine, zolpidem, eszopiclone, trazodone, citalopram, mirtazapine, fluoxetine, risperidone, olanzapine, and quetiapine.[11] Very careful evaluation is required before administering benzodiazepines. It is important to remember that there are many contraindications in administering benzodiazepines including (but not limited to) substance use disorder and traumatic brain injury.

Education

Education is a very important component of many individual, group, and community interventions offered in the aftermath of disaster. Education should be relatively brief, non-stigmatizing, and low cost; it should cover the following points:[10]

1. Understand a range of post-trauma responses
2. View post-trauma response as expected and understandable
3. Recognize circumstances under which one should consider further counseling
4. Know how and where to get additional help
5. Increase use of social support

6. Decrease use of problematic form of coping (e.g. alcohol)
7. Increase ability to help family members.

Conclusion

Mental health workers have played important roles in the relief efforts in recent disasters, and it is expected that their involvement in disaster relief will continue to increase. Armed with adequate pre-disaster preparations, knowledge about disaster, and the skills of managing acute and post-acute disaster situations, mental health providers will be able to play more effective roles as clinicians and relief workers. The American Medical Association (AMA) acknowledges that "National, regional and local responses to epidemics, terrorist attacks, and disasters require extensive involvement of physicians. Because of their commitment to care for the sick and injured individuals, individual physicians have an obligation to provide urgent medical care during disasters. This ethical obligation holds even in the face of greater than usual risks to their own safety, health or life."[12] The organization also makes a cautionary statement, "The physician workforce, however, is not an unlimited resource; therefore, when participating in disaster responses, physicians should balance immediate benefits to an individual patient with the ability to care for patients in the future."[12] The American Psychiatric Association (APA) is playing an important role, not only by responding to disaster situations, but also by training psychiatrists with required skills. Many district branches are already supporting the APA's effort in disaster response and training.

Certain issues have come up while responding to disaster situations, such as clinician's time, insurance coverage, leadership issues, preparedness training, confidentiality, charting, clinician's license status, etc. These issues may also need to be addressed before responding to a disaster situation.

Are We Prepared?

In one study, 21% of disaster responders reported willingness to care for victims in the event of an outbreak of an unknown but potentially deadly illness, 80% of responders believed they were well-prepared to play a role in a bioterrorism event; 40.5% of responders in the aftermath of 9/11 attack developed at least one psychiatric diagnosis in 13 months.[13,14] These facts emphasize the need for educating physicians in disaster medicine/psychiatry. Without coordination and a planning affiliation with an established agency, the providers may be a part of the "secondary disaster", not a part of the solution.

References

1. Disaster Psychiatry Outreach. *The Essentials of Disaster Psychiatry: A Training Course for Mental Health Professionals.* New York: Disaster Psychiatry Outreach, 2008.

2. Lindemann E. Symptomatology and management of acute grief. *Am J Psychiatry* 1944;**151**:155–160.

3. Cobb S, Lindemann E. Neuropsychiatric observations. *Ann Surg* 1943;**117**:814–824.

4. Adler A. Disintegration and restoration of optic recognition in visual agnosia: analysis of a case. *Arch Neurol Psychiatry* 1944;**51**:243–259.

5. World Health Organization Risk reduction and emergency preparedness. www.who.int/hac/techguidance/preparedness/emergency_preparedness_eng.pdf (accessed September 2019).

6. Than K. Scientists: natural disasters becoming more common. 2005www.livescience.com/414-scientists-natural-

disasters-common.html (accessed September 2019).

7. Raphael B, Wilson JP. *Psychological Debriefing: Theory, Practice and Evidence.* New York: Cambridge University Press, 2000.

8. Averill LA, Smith RP, Katz CL, Charney DS, Southwick SM. Neurobiology of disaster exposure: fear, anxiety, trauma, and resilience. In: Ursano RJ, Fullerton CS, Weisaeth L, Raphael B (eds.), *Textbook of Disaster Psychiatry*, 2nd edn. Cambridge, UK: Cambridge University Press; 2017: 60–75.

9. US Department of Veteran Affairs. *Psychological First Aid Manual.* www .ptsd.va.gov/professional/treat/type/psy ch_firstaid_manual.asp (accessed September 2019).

10. Ursano RJ, Fullerton CS, Weisaeth L, Raphael B (eds.). *Text Book of Disaster Psychiatry*. Cambridge, UK: Cambridge University Press, 2017.

11. Stoddard FJ, Pandya A, Katz CL. *Disaster Psychiatry: Readiness, Evaluation, and Treatment.* Arlington, VA: American Psychiatric Publishing, 2011.

12. American Medical Association. Code of Medical Ethics Opinion 9.067 Physician Obligation in Disaster Preparedness and Response. https://journalofethics.ama-assn.org/article/ama-code-medical-ethics-opinions-quarantine-and-physician-duty-treat/2010-09 (accessed September 2019).

13. Centers for Disease Control and Prevention. Mental health status of World Trade Center rescue and recovery workers and volunteers: New York City, July 2002– August 2004. *MMWR Mob Mortl Wkly Rep* 2004;53(35):812–815.

14. SAMHSA. First responders: behavioral health concerns, emergency response, and trauma. Disaster Technical Assistance Center Supplemental Research Bulletin, 2018. www .samhsa.gov/sites/default/files/dtac/sup plementalresearchbulletin-firstresponders-may2018.pdf (accessed September 2019).

Considerations When Working with Children and Families

Steve J. Brasington

A child's response to disaster is influenced by developmental stage, parental coping, and family stability. Parents are expected to monitor the eating, sleeping, and socializing of very young children, while students in elementary school require less monitoring. Yet school children still depend on adults for support. When adults experience injury, loss of income, or displacement, family routines are inevitably disrupted. Teens may be overwhelmed if expected to fill parenting roles during times parents are emotionally unavailable or stressed. Parents with developmental problems manifested by educational or vocational failure tend to impose their difficulties on their children. Importantly, heads of households need to keep children engaged in schoolwork, involved with healthy peers, and committed to steady routines around eating, sleeping, playing, and studying.

Clinicians should assess and monitor risks to normal child development across all phases of a disaster.[1,2] Studies indicate symptoms of anxiety and depression are the most common vulnerabilities in a disaster. Notably, the greater the proximity to the event, the greater the likelihood that emotional reactions will persist. Researchers found that over two years following the 9–11 terrorist attacks in New York, "Younger children (6–11 years) were more likely to present with anxiety, problems concentrating, social isolation, and withdrawal, whereas older children (12–17 years) were more likely to exhibit numbing, avoidance reactions, and substance abuse."[3] Children at risk may show signs of sleep disturbance, conflicts with caregivers, and poor school adjustment. Children at low risk usually experience little distress or change in functioning.

First aid to persons in psychological distress involves mobilizing support and assistance. Government, private, and volunteer organizations comprise the system of disaster care. Command and control of the response includes coordination of responders like the American Red Cross, who partner with other agencies providing disaster relief. Local agencies unique to the community serve in familiar settings like places of worship or halls operated by service organizations. Media and public service announcements can provide information on the availability of these support services – especially services available to children and families. Importantly, repeated viewing of media coverage in shelters may induce excessive or visible anxiety in both children and their parents.

Researchers analyzing the response to Hurricane Andrew concluded that adults who diverted children from watching excessive television while out of school reduced emotionally troubling images in their children. School is a major life activity for children. A school psychologist is often the key person to whom faculty, staff, and parents turn to when confronted with events that overwhelm the coping ability of students. School psychologists in some locations have been trained as mental health partners in disaster response.

Importantly, they may be familiar with the most vulnerable students and families and the services they already receive in the local system of care. School psychologists serve as a vital resource for helping children and families feel supported and more in control of their lives.

Children and adolescents do best when routines are preserved. The routine of sleep is crucial for healthy functioning. Investigators from the Department of Epidemiology and Public Health London, England found that young children with regular bedtimes have fewer behavioral problems than youngsters who did not. Clinicians should support family routines that encourage adequate sleep and rest. When children present with sleep problems, melatonin is recommended over prescription sleep aids for the restoration of earlier bedtimes and earlier wake up times. For children and adolescents taking prescription medications, adult should limit access to psychotropic or controlled medications to prevent non-medical use. Parents need to be reminded of the importance of proper storage and safeguarding of medications with abuse potential, such as stimulants or anti-anxiety pills. Investigators at the University of Michigan noted over 70% of adolescents recently prescribed controlled medications had unsupervised access to prescriptions pills at home.[4]

The Ministry of Social Development in New Zealand reviewed the literature on family resilience and noted certain qualities allow families to cope with adversity and challenges to their well-being.[5] Families with strong emotional bonds, who are able to find meaning in difficult circumstances do better than families unable to make sense of events altering the family's sense of place or future in the community. Although families with teenagers may demonstrate less cohesion, families with adolescents actively seeking autonomy do not necessarily show impaired functioning during a crisis. On the contrary, adolescents often have networks of support and communication that provide robust connections to resources. Importantly, social media used by teens may provide a methodology for rapid location of persons separated from families. Teens may provide a ready source of energy and optimism, when resolution of a disaster is prolonged.

Economic calamity for parents may aggravate abuse or neglect of children. The presence of clinicians at a disaster may provide opportunity for recognition of child maltreatment. Recognition may be difficult under ordinary circumstances. Marital problems, intimate partner violence, and financial stress contribute to child maltreatment. Inquire about safety and welfare. Ask, "How are things at home?" Clues to potential problems include responses like, "Mom and Dad yell all the time." Ask, "What do you wish was different that would make you feel better?" You might get an answer like "I wish dad would not drink so much." If the mother is being assaulted, the chances increase that the children are witnessing abuse. Use systems in place for reporting domestic violence. When confronted with evidence of child maltreatment, engage social services or child protective services. When circumstances prevent a definitive determination of abuse, engage trained volunteers to provide crucial support to families, whose crisis may not rise to the level of investigation by protective services.

Some families are raising special needs children. These children may have mobility issues or have limited flexibility involving daily routines. The importance of maintaining consistent routines is vital for these youngsters. In a policy statement regarding youth preparedness for disaster the American Red Cross advised parents, "How you react to an emergency gives them clues on how to act. If you react with alarm, your child may become more scared. They see your fear as proof that the danger is real. If you seem overcome with a sense of loss, your child may feel their losses more strongly." A resource for parents is a mobile application developed by the American Red Cross called "Monster Guard" (www.redcross.org/monsterguard). Sponsored by the Disney Corporation, this application includes games in addition to tips on how to manage real-life emergencies. Games can be particularly helpful for anxious kids or older kids with developmental challenges overwhelmed by new environments. For mobile devices to function, these devices must be charged and re-charged. Portable chargers or special radios are available with hand-cranks to energize batteries when off the grid.

Informed consent is different for youth, especially if they are under the age of 16. By age 16 some jurisdictions recognize that an individual may demonstrate sufficient maturity and intellectual capacity to grasp the nature of the procedure, the implications of the proposed procedure (reversible or non-reversible), the alternatives, and possible risks by expressing a choice in his or her own best interest. When a person is unable to make a reasoned decision due to intellectual delay or cognitive impairment, he or she would be considered unable to give expressed informed consent, even if that individual has reached the age of consent. Under these circumstances, a court order would be necessary unless delay would compromise the life of the patient. Magistrates may need to be involved if an older teen is refusing a procedure his or her parents advocate, but the individual has not reached his or her eighteenth birthday. For example, standard trauma practice may require amputation, but the young person objects. Ideally, the child, the parents, and the clinician agree on the best intervention. When a parent's refusal to provide consent for a non-elective procedure places an underage child at risk, the physician may seek an injunction or order. Legal counsel is advised when in doubt about the doctor's authority to provide care.

Disasters may produce conditions conducive to human trafficking. A toll free hotline for human trafficking, 1–888-373-7888, is provided by the National Human Trafficking Resource Center. This hotline is designed as a coordination mechanism between law enforcement and government. According to the Polaris Project half of the 27 million people trafficked globally are children. The website http://globalmodernslavery.org/ provides a directory of antitrafficking agencies based on location. These locations tend to be at international entry points, such as port cities. Notably, coastal regions are often subjected to hurricanes and flooding. Important indicators and red flags for human trafficking include poor mental and physical health among persons under the age of 18, who seem reluctant to speak freely, who are not free to come and go and who lack sufficient funds, typical photo identification or permanent address. Disaster responders should look for signs of trafficking amongst young people who appear without family or legitimate employment.

References

1. Pfefferbaum B, Pfefferbaum RL, Van Horn RL. Involving children in disaster risk reduction: the importance of participation. *Eur J Psychotraumatol* 2018;**9** (sup2):1425577.

2. Dudley N, Ackerman A, Brown KM, Snow SK. Patient- and family-centered care of children in the emergency department. *Pediatrics* 2015;**135**(1):e225–e272.

3. Covell NH, Allen G, Essock SM, et al. Service utilization and event reaction patterns among children who received Project Liberty counseling services. *Psychiatr Serv* 2006;**57**:1277–1282.

4. Ross-Durow PL, McCabe SE, Boyd CJ. Adolescents' access to their own prescription medications in the home. *J Adolesc Health* 2013;**53**:260–264.

5. Mackay R. Family resilience and good child outcomes: an overview of the research literature. *Social Policy J NZ* 2003;**20**:98–118.

15 Chemical and Radiologic Exposures in Trauma and Disasters

Joseph McIsaac and Corry Kucik

Abbreviations

TIC = Toxic industrial chemicals
CW = Chemical weapons
PPE = Personal protective equipment
CHEMM = Chemical Hazards Emergency Medical Management
REMM = Radiation Emergency Medical Management
WISER = Wireless Information System for Emergency Responders
RDSL = Reactive decontamination skin lotion
NIOSH = National Institute for Occupational Safety and Health
PAPR = Powered air-purifying respirators
APF = Assigned protection factors
PEEP = Positive end-expiratory pressure
ATLS = Advanced trauma life support
TOXALS = Advanced life support for acute toxic injury
MSDS = Material safety data sheets
HCN = Hydrogen cyanide
H_2S = Hydrogen sulfide
CO = Carbon monoxide
Pb = Lead
EDTA = Ethylenediaminetetraacetic acid
DMSA = Dimercaptosuccinic acid
NA = Nerve agents
DNA = Deoxyribonucleic acid
rad = Radiation absorbed dose
Gy = Grays
rem = Roentgen-equivalent man
Sv = Sievert
W_R = Weighting factor
ALC = Absolute lymphocyte counts
Ca-DTPA = Calcium diethylenetriaminepentaacetic acid
uHCG = Urine human chorionic gonadotropin
ANC = Absolute neutrophil count
HSV = Herpes simplex virus
CDC = Centers for Disease Control
IDSA = Infectious Disease Society of America
G-CSF = = Granulocyte colony-stimulating factor

GM-CSF = Granulocyte-macrophage colony-stimulating factor
SCF = Stem cell factor
RSO = Radiation safety officer
OR = Operating room

Introduction

Ethanol and recreational drugs are by far the most common chemical exposures associated with trauma. This chapter, however, covers other possibly associated exposures: toxic industrial chemicals (TIC), chemical weapons (CW), and radiation.

Limited exposures occur commonly in the industrial setting. The Bhopal disaster of 1984; mustard use during the Iran–Iraq War; the recent use of chlorine and sarin in Syria; the recent use of VX and Novichok in targeted assasinations; and the 2011 Fukushima earthquake, tsunami, and nuclear disaster are examples of combined trauma/toxic exposure. Indeed, chemical weapons of World War I are common industrial chemicals such as phosgene, chlorine, and cyanide, which are still used in vast quantities.

Combined trauma-exposure management begins with advanced trauma life support (ATLS) guidelines, balanced by the need for caregiver personal protective equipment (PPE) and rapid decontamination. After resuscitation, toxidrome treatment and advanced management commence. No specific antidotes exist for most chemical exposures; supportive care through emergency, operative, and critical care phases is key.

Common toxic injury patterns include inhalational injury, chemical burns, and metabolic poisoning. Frequently, two or more types are present. When combined with conventional trauma, they synergistically increase morbidity and mortality. In a mass casualty disaster setting, exposure to toxic chemicals or radiation add a further layer of complication that endangers responders as well.

Resources for Agent Identification and Management

The US Department of Health and Human Services' Chemical Hazards Emergency Medical Management (CHEMM) website (http://chemm.nlm.nih.gov/index.html) allows "first responders, first receivers, other healthcare providers, and planners to plan for, respond to, recover from, and mitigate the effects of mass-casualty incidents involving chemicals." The site has tools for rapid toxidrome (i.e. clinical syndromes) identification, patient management, and planning. Similarly, the Radiation Emergency Medical Management (REMM) website (www.remm.nlm.gov/index.html) focuses on radiation events. Additional resources include Wireless Information System for Emergency Responders (WISER, http://wiser.nlm.nih.gov) and CHEMTREC® (www.chemtrec.com/), a commercial service focused on industrial and transportation accidents involving chemicals. WISER is available for download to mobile devices. Finally, a chemical-induced illness pocket card ("Chem card") can be downloaded at www.healthquality.va.gov/biochem/bio_poc_chem.pdf (Figure 15.1).

Decontamination and Personal Protective Equipment (PPE)

Decontamination begins as soon as possible, preferably pre-hospital. Simply removing clothing can dramatically reduce both patient and caregiver exposure. Large volumes of water (with or without detergent) remove more persistent agents. Water should be avoided

CHEMICAL TERRORISM GENERAL GUIDANCE* Pocket Guide

Diagnosis: Be Alert to the Following
- Groups of individuals becoming ill around the same time
- Any sudden increase in illness in previously healthy individuals
- Any sudden increase in the following non-specific syndromes:
  - Sudden unexplained weakness, collapse, apnea, or convulsions in previously healthy individuals
  - Dimmed or blurred vision
  - Hypersecretion syndromes (such as drooling, tearing, and diarrhea)
  - Inhalation syndromes (eye, nose, throat, chest irritation; shortness of breath)
  - Burn-like skin syndromes (redness, blistering, itching, sloughing)
- Unusual temporal or geographic clustering of illness (for example, patients who attended the same public event, live in the same part of town, etc.)

Understanding Exposure
- Exposure may occur from any state of matter. Route of exposure may delay onset of symptoms
- Chemical effects are dependent on:
  - volatility and amount of a chemical
  - water solubility (higher solubility leads to more mucosal and less deep lung deposition and toxicity)
  - increased fat solubility and smaller molecular size increase skin absorption

August 2003

VA access card: http://www.oqp.med.va.gov/cpg/cpg.htm
DoD access card: http://www.qmo.amedd.army.mil

Produced by the Employee Education System for the Office of Public Health and Environmental Hazards, Department of Veterans Affairs

Confirmation and Sources of Assistance and Support
- Contact your local poison control center
- Contact your local industrial hygienist or safety officer
- Department of Justice (DOJ) Domestic Preparedness National Response Hotline (800-424-8802)
- If you need further help in clinical diagnosis or management, call DOJ Chembio Help Line (800-368-6498)
- Review US Army Chemical Casualty Care handbook (go to http://ccc.apgea.army.mil or internally at vaww.oqp.med.va.gov/cpg/BCR/BCR_base.htm)
- CDC/ATSDR Hotline (770-488-7100)

Decontamination Considerations
- Chemical warfare agents always require removal of clothing and decontamination of the patient, usually with soap and water. Avoid bleach
- Treating contaminated patients in the emergency department before decontamination may contaminate the facility
- Assume patients are contaminated unless otherwise documented
- Time is of the essence

Institutional Reporting
- If reasonable suspicion of chemical attack, contact your hospital leadership (Chief of Staff, Hospital Director, etc)
- Immediately discuss hospital emergency planning implications

Public Health Reporting
- Contact your local public health office (city, county, or state)
- If needed, contact the FBI (for location of nearest office, see http://www.fbi.gov/contact/fo/fo.htm)

*The information in this card is not meant to be complete but to be a quick guide; please consult other references and expert opinion, and check drug dosages, particularly for pregnancy and children.

CHEMICAL TERRORISM AGENTS AND BIOLIGICAL TOXINS

Agents	Symptom Onset	Symptoms	Signs	Clinical Diagnostic Tests	Decontamination	Exposure route and treatment	Differential diagnostic considerations
Nerve agents	Vapor: seconds Liquid: minutes to hours	**Moderate exposure**: Muscle cramping, runny nose, difficulty breathing, eye pain, dimming of vision, sweating, diarrhea **High exposure**: Loss of consciousness, flaccid paralysis, seizures **Delayed Onset**: The onset of symptoms may be delayed up to 18 hours, especially with local exposures.	Pinpoint pupils (miosis); often absent without conjunctival exposure to vapor. Excessive lacrimation Pulmonary secretions Wheezing Muscle twitching & rippling under the skin (fasciculations) Sweating Hypersalivation Diarrhea Seizures, apnea	Red blood cell or serum cholinesterase (whole blood) **Treatment based on signs and symptoms; Use lab tests only for later confirmation** Collect urine for later confirmation and dose estimation	Rapid disrobing, Water wash with soap and shampoo	**Inhalation & dermal absorption** Atropine 2 – 6 mg IV or IM 2-PAMCl 600–1800 mg injection or 1.0 g infusion over 20-30 minutes Additional atropine 2 mg q 3-5 min to decreased secretions. One additional 2-PAMCl 600mg injection or 1.0 g infusion over 20-30 minutes at 1 hr if necessary Diazepam or lorazepam to prevent seizures in patients with severe enough exposure to require 6mg of atropine at one time Ventilation support	Pesticide poisoning from organophosphorous agents and carbamates cause virtually identical syndromes
Cyanide	Seconds to minutes	**Moderate exposure**: Dizziness, nausea, headache, eye irritation **High exposure**: Loss of consciousness	**Moderate exposure**: non-specific findings, gasping, flushing, (typically not cyanosis **High exposure** convulsions, cessation of respiration	Cyanide (blood) or thiocyanate (blood or urine) levels in lab; increased arteriovenous oxygen difference **Treatment based on signs and symptoms; Use lab tests only for later confirmation**	Clothing removal	**Inhalation & dermal absorption** Oxygen (face mask) Amyl nitrite Sodium nitrite (300mg IV) and sodium thiosulfate (12.5g IV)	Similar CNS illness results from: Carbon monoxide (from gas or diesel engine exhaust fumes in closed spaces) H_2S (sewer, waste, industrial sources) Sulfur mustard symptoms of pain usually delayed; Lewisite symptoms usually immediate
Blister Agents (Sulfur mustard)	2 – 48 hours	Burning, itching, or red skin Mucosal irritation (prominent tearing, and burning and redness of eyes) Shortness of breath Nausea and vomiting	Skin erythema Blistering Conjunctivitis and lid swelling Upper airways sloughing Pulmonary edema Marrow suppression with lymphocytopenia	Often smell of garlic, horseradish, and mustard on body Oily droplets on skin from ambient sources No specific diagnostic tests	Clothing removal Large amounts of water	**Inhalation, dermal absorption, & oral ingestion** Thermal burn type treatment Supportive care For Lewisite and Lewisite/ Mustard mixtures: British Anti-Lewisite (BAL or dimercaprol)	Diffuse skin exposure with irritants, such as caustics, sodium hydroxides, ammonia, etc., may cause similar syndromes. Sodium hydroxide (NaOH) from trucking accidents
Pulmonary agents (phosgene etc.)	1 – 24 (rarely up to 72) hours	Shortness of breath Chest tightness Wheezing Mucosal and dermal irritation and redness	Pulmonary (non-cardiogenic) edema with some mucosal irritation (signs after symptoms)	No tests available but source assessment may help identify exposure characteristics (majority of trucking incidents exposing contaminants to humans have labels on vehicle)	None usually needed	**Inhalation** Supportive care Specific treatment depends on agents Consider steroids	Inhalation exposures are the single most common form of industrial agent exposure (eg: phosgene, chlorine) Mucosal irritation, airways reactions, and deep lung effects depend on the specific agent
Ricin (castor bean toxin)	18 – 24 hours	**Ingestion**: Nausea, diarrhea, vomiting, fever, abdominal pain **Inhalation**: chest tightness, coughing, weakness, nausea, fever	Clusters of acute lung or GI injury; circulatory collapse and shock	ELISA (from commercial laboratories) using respiratory secretions, serum, and direct tissue	Clothing removal Water rinse	**Inhalation & Ingestion** Supportive care For ingestion: charcoal lavage	Tularemia, plague, and Q fever may cause similar syndromes, as may CW agents such as stapylococcal enterotoxin B and phosgene
T-2 mycotoxin	2 – 4 hours	Dermal & mucosal irritation; blistering, necrosis Blurred vision, eye irritation Nausea, vomiting, and diarrhea Ataxia Coughing and dyspnea	Mucosal erythema and hemorrhage Red skin, blistering Tearing, salivation Pulmonary edema Seizures and coma	ELISA from commercial laboratories Gas chromatography/Mass spectroscopy in specialized laboratories	Clothing removal Water rinse	**Inhalation & dermal contact** Supportive care For ingestion: charcoal lavage Possibly high dose steroids	Pulmonary toxins (O_3, NO_x, phosgene, NH_3) may cause similar syndromes though with less mucosal irritation.

Figure 15.1 Chemical-induced illness pocket card.

when flammable metals (e.g. lithium, sodium, potassium) are suspected; in such cases, mineral oil is used until debridement is possible. Adsorbents (e.g. sand, cat litter) are also effective. Topical decontamination of military agents can be accomplished using reactive decontamination skin lotion (RDSL, www.rsdecon.com/). First responders should wear PPE Level C or higher when treating contaminated patients (www.remm.nlm.gov/osha_e pa_ppe.htm). Level A or B is indicated for unknown agents or high concentrations. Additional decontamination at the hospital is indicated for persistent agents or when field decontamination was incomplete.

Lifesaving medical treatment takes precedence over decontamination. The "ABCs" should be managed throughout the decontamination process. Level C PPE respiratory protection includes hooded NIOSH-certified powered air-purifying respirators (PAPR) with assigned protection factors (APF) of ≥1000 and appropriate chemical/radiological filters. These respirators should be used by hospital personnel receiving contaminated victims. OR procedures can be performed wearing PAPR when needed. Double gloving with at least one nitrile glove is recommended when dealing with chemical exposure victims.

Several studies demonstrate the difficulty of performing manual medical procedures (intubation, venipuncture) while wearing PPE. Maneuvers requiring less fine motor skill (e.g. laryngeal mask airway or intraosseous needle placement) should be considered, especially in mass casualties.

Inhalational Injuries

Acute inhalation injuries are frequently a consequence of industrial or household accidents. Agents released into confined spaces result in relatively high concentrations. Larger releases may result from bulk stored agents at industrial sites or during transportation accidents.

Several mechanisms of toxicity exist. Acute asphyxiants (e.g. carbon dioxide, argon, methane, nitrogen) simply displace oxygen and prevent its uptake, resulting in hypoxemia, anerobic metabolism, and metabolic acidosis. Water-soluble agents (e.g. chlorine, ammonia) at low concentrations cause upper airway mucosal injury, while higher concentrations penetrate deeper into the airway and may induce bronchospasm and mucosal sloughing. Less-soluble agents cause injury to lung parenchyma, resulting in necrosis or pulmonary edema. Pulmonary edema is also common with nitrogen oxides, isocyanate, and phosgene. Different inhalational injury mechanisms are commonly superimposed. Survivors often develop chronic obstructive pulmonary disease.

Mainstays of acute asphyxiant therapy are supportive oxygenation, ventilation, and bronchodilators. Positive end-expiratory pressure (PEEP) helps reduce pulmonary edema, while diuretics are of limited value, and steroids have been shown to be ineffective. Serial chest X-rays, arterial blood gases, and pulmonary function tests allow clinicians to follow the disease course closely. Once the acute phase subsides, therapy follows conventional critical care management guidelines.

Chemical Burns

Chemical injuries cause 3% of burn admissions but 30% of burn deaths. Degree of injury frequently parallels exposure time. Decontamination should occur as soon as possible at the scene and emergency department to limit the extent of injury; the incidence of full thickness burns increases fivefold when irrigation is not initiated within 10 minutes. General decontamination procedures includes clothing removal and flushing with water or adsorbents;

however, water is contraindicated in case of reactive metals or phenol injury. Tissue destruction occurs due to saponification of fats by alkali, coagulative necrosis by acids, and protein denaturation by organic materials and reactive metals. Chemical warfare agents produce both local and systemic toxicity. The extent of chemical injury is frequently under-estimated.

Management includes ATLS followed by burn center admission, if available. The "ABCs" should generally not be delayed due to the presence of chemicals. However, caregivers should wear PPE. The advanced life support for acute toxic injury (TOXALS) protocol, introduced by Baker in 1996, is one method for managing acute chemical injury.

Identification of the chemical agent allows for more specific treatment and prognostica-tion. Material safety data sheets (MSDS) and chemical placards on transport vehicles should be noted. Firefighters are often excellent sources of chemical information in the pre-hospital setting. Poison control centers, CHEMM, WISER, and CHEMTREC are also useful. Consultation with or transfer to a burn center should be considered if possible.

Hydrogen fluoride binds calcium, penetrating deeply into tissues and bone. Patients with skin involvement should receive topical calcium gluconate and monitoring for hypo-calcemia. Hand injuries are treated with fasciotomy and intra-arterial calcium gluconate infusions. Injury is often more extensive than initially thought. Burn center and surgical consultation is always indicated.

Mustard (bis-(2-chloroethyl) sulfide) binds to DNA, interrupting rapidly dividing cells such as epithelium and resulting in inflammation, pain, and blistering. Moist areas (e.g. eyes, genitals) are easily affected, while pulmonary and systemic effects are also possible. After decontamination, treatment is largely supportive. Irrigation, topical antibiotics, and systemic analgesics reduce symptoms and scarring. Small skin blisters can be left intact, while large bullae should be unroofed, irrigated, and treated with a topical antibiotic in the same manner as a thermal burn. Fluid loss into blisters may be significant, necessitating volume resuscitation. Pulmonary mucosal injury is managed supportively. Large mustard exposures depress bone marrow within 3–5 days; resuscitative surgery should occur before immune compromise occurs or after the white count rebounds. Gut sterilization can be considered if leukopenia develops.

Lewisite (2-chlorovinyl dichloroarsine) is similar to mustard, but immediate pain is the prominent symptom. There are no immunologic effects. Treatment includes early dimer-caprol application and supportive care.

Metabolic Poisons

Hydrogen cyanide (HCN), hydrogen sulfide (H_2S), and carbon monoxide (CO) are classic inhaled metabolic poisons. They act at the cellular level, inhibiting oxygen binding or utilization. Supplemental or hyperbaric oxygen are therapeutic mainstays for CO. Sodium nitrite and sodium thiosulfate are indicated for HCN toxicity, while only sodium nitrite treats H_2S.

Heavy metals like lead (Pb) respond to chelation therapy. Calcium disodium ethylene-diaminetetraacetic acid (EDTA) and dimercaptosuccinic acid (DMSA) are effective.

Nerve agents (NA), such as tabun (GA), sarin (GB), soman (GD), and VX, are another metabolic toxin class. Organophosphate toxidromes may also occur from pesticide expo-sures. Both types of agents bind and inhibit cholinesterase, resulting in excess acetylcholine and over-stimulation of nicotinic and muscarinic receptors resulting in miosis, lacrimation, salivation, bronchospasm, dyspnea, vomiting, incontinence, seizures, central apnea, and respiratory paralysis. Patients require respiratory support and treatment with atropine and an oxime (pralidoxime, obidoxime, HI-6). Seizures are treated with benzodiazepines or propofol. Benactyzine, aprophen, azaprophen, trihexyphenidyl, procyclidine, biperiden, and scopolamine have been demonstrated to terminate soman-induced seizures at lower concentrations than diazepam. There is recent literature supporting the use of magnesium sulfate and ketamine, as well. Heavy exposures require substantial critical care resources. Caregivers should wear Level C PPE until patients are fully decontaminated to avoid exposure.

Delayed onset of succinylcholine and vecuronium action has been reported in NA-exposed swine. Prolongation of muscle-relaxant effect may also occur. All NA-exposed patients should be considered to have a "full stomach." Etomidate and ketamine are appropriate induction hypnotics in these patients. While propofol and thiopental are also acceptable, they may result in profound cardiac depression, bradycardia, and vasodilation. Opioids may be used, however morphine may exacerbate bronchospasm. Fentanyl and morphine may also induce bradycardia, while remifentanyl action may be prolonged by NA inhibition of non-specific tissue esterases.

The use of Novichok agents in the UK in 2018 has introduced a new class of neurotoxins to the world. They are thought to be more potent than the classic nerve agents and harder to treat. To date, all treatment protocols remain highly classified, but three patients ultimately survived a severe exposure. It is presumed that the treatment followed roughly that of standard nerve agent protocols, with additions.

Severe opioid intoxication is another recent development, especially with potent synthetic fentanyl derivatives. These may require very high doses of naloxone.

Multiple other toxins exist. Some biologic agents (e.g. botulinum, anthrax toxin) are treated with early administration of antitoxin. Others, such as ricin, are treated supportively (an antiricin monoclonal antibody has been licensed but is not yet in production). The CHEMM website can guide casualty care.

Radiation Injuries

A person exposed to ionizing radiation is said to be irradiated. External irradiation does not make a person radioactive; thus, this patient poses no threat to healthcare providers. Contamination occurs when radioactive material comes to rest on a person or item; it poses a threat until it is removed. However, unlike chemical or biological agents, there is no documentation of a health care provider ever receiving radiation injury while caring for a contaminated patient. Internal contamination occurs when radioactive material is ingested, inhaled, or inspissated in wounds. Internal contamination may be confined to the lungs or gastrointestinal tract or distributed throughout the body. Therefore, decontamination may require irrigation of oral and nasal passages, expectorants, emetics, gastric or pulmonary lavage, or medications that block absorption or incorporation of radioactive contaminants.

Radiological effects decrease with decreased time of exposure, increased distance from the source, and increased shielding. First responders should wear protective gear (especially respiratory protection) and rotate team members in order to minimize potential exposure and heat stress. Personal dosimeters should be considered.

Radiation may be particles (alpha, beta, neutrons) or electromagnetic waves (X-rays, gamma rays). Alpha particles are positively charged equivalents of helium nuclei (two

Table 15.1 Weighting factors associated with various types of ionizing radiation

Type of ionizing radiation	W_R
Alpha particle	20
Beta particle, X- and gamma rays	1
Neutron	5–20 (depends on inherent energy level)

Adapted from the National Council on Radiation Protection and Measurements Report No. 116, 1993.

neutrons, two protons) that quickly interact with nearby electrons and have a very short range. They tend to be dangerous only if inhaled, ingested, or absorbed from wounds. Beta particles are in essence free electrons. They have a larger range than alpha particles, can be stopped by thin solids (e.g. an aluminum sheet), and can cause eye damage or pruritus, paresthesias, and erythema if allowed to stay on the skin for long periods. Just like alpha particles, internal contamination with beta particles can be harmful. Neutrons are emitted from atomic fission, and are only encountered after a nuclear detonation. Their penetrance is significant, and they easily cause considerable damage to deoxyribonucleic acid (DNA). Gamma and X-rays are neutral energy packages that travel at the speed of light. They penetrate deep tissues; dense materials (e.g. lead, concrete) can block them.

Humans receive cosmic or terrestrial radiation every day. Increased doses are received during an airplane flight or a radiologic study. Absorbed radiation is typically measured in radiation absorbed dose (rad) or in grays (Gy), where 100 rad = 1 Gy = 1 J/kg. Expression in terms of *equivalent doses* accounts for different biological effects of various radiation types. The Roentgen-equivalent man (rem) and the sievert (Sv) reflect absorbed dose (rad or Gy) multiplied by a weighting factor (W_R), where 100 rem = 1 Sv.

For example, gamma and X-rays have a W_R of 1, while alpha particles have a W_R of 20. (Table 15.1). Therefore, for an absorbed dose of 100 rad of undifferentiated radiation,

100 rad (gamma) $\times$ 1 (W_R for gamma) = 100 rem or 1 Sv
100 rad (alpha) $\times$ 20 (W_R for alpha) = 2000 rem or 20 Sv

Thus, *type* of exposure markedly affects biological results.

Acute radiation syndrome (or radiation sickness) occurs hours to weeks after a rapid whole-body exposure. When sufficient radiation doses reach internal organs, DNA can be irreversibly damaged, with rapidly dividing cell lines (marrow, gastrointestinal mucosa) suffering most acutely. Different dose ranges produce different manifestations, including hematopoietic, gastrointestinal, and cardiovascular/central nervous system subtypes. Each syndrome tends to progress through prodromal, latent, and manifest illness stages, culminating in either death or recovery. Higher doses predictably cause higher morbidity, as well as a faster transit through stages of illness (Table 15.2). "$LD_{50/60}$" describes the dose that will kill 50% of an exposed population within 60 days. $LD_{50/60}$ is decreased (i.e. increased death with decreased dose) in extremes of age, chronic malnutrition or comorbidity, trauma, or infection. When combined with burns, trauma, infection, or chemical exposure, a radiation injury that would have otherwise been survivable will have significantly greater morbidity. A

Table 15.2 Approximation of relative hazard given exposure

Dose	Relative Hazard
About 10 mGy or 10 mSv (1 rad or rem) or less	No acute effects and only a very small chance of subsequent cancer
About 0.1 Gy or 0.1 Sv (10 rad or rem)	No acute effects, subsequent additional risk of cancer about 0.5%
About 1 Gy or 1 Sv (100 rad or rem)	Nausea, vomiting possible, mild bone marrow depression, subsequent risk of cancer 5%
Greater than 2 Gy or Sv (200 rad or rem)	Definite nausea, vomiting, medical evaluation and treatment required

From the American College of Radiology, Disaster Preparedness for Radiology Professionals Response to Radiological Terrorism, 2006.

Table 15.3 Using presence, onset, and duration of vomiting to estimate absorbed dose

Estimated dose (Gy)	Time of onset (hours)	Duration (hours)
0.5–2	2–24 or longer	<24
2–3	2–6	12–24
3–5	1–2	24
>5	<1	48

Adapted from Dickerson, W. "Acute Radiation Syndrome," Medical Effects of Ionizing Radiation Course, Armed Forces Radiobiology Research Institute, 14DEC06.

generally accepted $LD_{50/60}$ for untreated radiation injury is 3–4 Gy; optimal medical treatment can increase survival in most patients receiving $LD_{50/60}$ of 6 Gy, or less.

Radiological injuries present difficulties even in a single patient; incomplete information on the radiological incident, variations in the time course of non-specific findings, and patient anxiety or psychosomatic illness will confound diagnosis and prognosis. Large patient loads will present after an industrial or terrorist incident, making clinical judgment, rigorous triage, rapid laboratory analysis, and conservation of resources crucial in deciding which patients will receive treatment and which will not recover despite the best care possible. Tables 15.3 and 15.4 can be used to predict dose, and therefore, prognosis, on the basis of clinical findings.

The hematopoietic syndrome occurs at radiation doses above 0.7 Gy, affecting erythropoiesis, myelopoiesis, and thrombopoiesis. Lymphocyte counts fall precipitously with higher doses, and serial absolute lymphocyte counts (ALC) help predict outcome. Red cell levels may return to normal quickly, while lymphocyte and platelet levels may remain low, imparting an increased risk of infection, bleeding, and poor wound healing. Prodromal nausea, vomiting, anorexia, and malaise may last days. During a

Table 15.4 Likely outcomes with optimum care after sustaining a radiation injury

Dose range (Gy)	Prognosis
0.5–1.0	Excellent
1.0–2.0	Probable survival (>90%)
2.0–3.5	Likely survival (>75%)
3.5–5.5	Death likely in 3–6 weeks
5.5–7.5	Death likely in 2–3 weeks
7.5–10.0	Death in 1–3 weeks
10.0–20.0	Death in 5–12 days
>20.0	Death in 2–5 days

Adapted from the Textbook of Military Medicine, Part I, Volume 2, Medical Consequences of Nuclear Warfare, 1989, 22

latent stage of 1–6 weeks, the victim appears to improve despite continuing hematopoietic stem cell depletion. Ensuing frank illness may last months, yielding immunosuppression, neutropenic fevers, malaise, hemorrhage, and infection. Recovery may occur if sufficient stem cells regenerate.

The gastrointestinal syndrome can occur when radiation damages the rapidly growing endothelial cells of the small intestine, causing mucosal sloughing, loss of neural control, submucosal edema, malabsorption, fluid loss, and electrolyte abnormalities. Within a few hours of a radiation dose of 6–10 Gy, the victim develops profound nausea, vomiting, cramping, diarrhea, fatigue, tachycardia, and hypotension lasting a few days. A latent stage of roughly one week is then followed by the return of symptoms, along with immunosuppression and anemia from a superimposed hematopoietic syndrome. Transmigration of intestinal flora can lead to sepsis, shock, and death, generally within two or three weeks. Survival data for the gastrointestinal syndrome is scant; death from hemorrhage or infection is likely despite optimal care. Clinicians thus face therapeutic and ethical dilemmas, and must judge whether limited resources might be better used on those with better chance of recovery. In any event, palliative measures such as antiemetics and narcotics are indicated.

The cardiovascular/central nervous system syndrome develops after doses exceeding 20 Gy. Profound, intractable symptoms occur within minutes, including dysesthesias, mental status changes, seizures, nausea, vomiting, bloody diarrhea, hypotension, autonomic dysregulation, coma, and cardiovascular collapse. Death occurs regardless of treatment, generally within three days. When history, physical, and radiation readings confirm such an overwhelming dose, the patient should be categorized as expectant and given comfort measures, particularly in the setting of multiple casualties.

Patient Care Approaches

Patients with potentially survivable radiation injuries may not develop symptoms for three to four weeks – more than enough time for any traumatic cause of mortality to take its toll.

As in any emergency response, providers must address life-threatening injuries first, while not becoming casualties themselves. Standard algorithms should be used to secure the airway, ventilate, and control hemorrhage, with decontamination following as soon as practicable. Once triage, stabilization, and decontamination take place, patients are admitted for longitudinal care and monitoring. Radiation dose can be estimated based on the size and type of exposure (nuclear, radiological dispersal device, orphan source), whether there was an explosion yielding embedded sources, the radionuclide involved (e.g. cesium, iodine, cobalt), time course of radiation-related symptoms, distance from the source, exposure duration, and whether any shielding was present. Continuous radiological surveys and laboratory analysis can help estimate exposure. Patients that have received a critically high dose and are unlikely to survive should receive comfort and spiritual support. Expert consultation is available from the Centers for Disease Control (800-CDC-INFO), the Radiation Emergency Assistance Center/Training Site (865–576–3131), or the Armed Forces Radiobiology Research Institute (301–295–0530).

Severe internal contamination can cause acute radiation syndrome, while prolonged low-grade internal exposure can lead to distribution throughout the body, profound damage to organs, and cancer induction. Absorption is markedly faster through mucous membranes and lungs than through intact skin. If the eyes are affected, they should be rinsed gently but copiously. If significant lung exposure has occurred, bronchoscopic lavage may be of benefit. Radioactive contamination of the gastrointestinal tract is treated similarly to oral poisoning. Recently swallowed contamination can be lavaged by means of an oro- or nasogastric tube. Laxatives can speed transit of gastrointestinal contamination, decreasing exposure time. Osmotic laxatives such as polyethylene glycol or magnesium citrate are more effective than bulk laxatives such as psyllium, but may cause increased abdominal discomfort, obscuring clinical findings. Activated charcoal selectively binds chromium, while alginates, barium sulfate, and aluminum-based antacids (e.g. Maalox®, Gaviscon®) can bind strontium-90. The ion exchange resin Prussian blue (ferric ferrocyanide, Radiogardase®) binds cesium-137 and thallium. Adult dosing for Prussian blue is 3 g three times a day, while a pediatric dose is 1 g three times a day.

Blocking and diluting agents (e.g. potassium iodide, potassium perchlorate) saturate target organs, crowding out harmful radionuclides. Mobilizing agents (e.g. oral ammonium chloride plus intravenous calcium gluconate) increase metabolism of ingested contaminants, hastening their elimination. Chelating agents (e.g. deferoxamine, calcium diethylenetriaminepentaacetic acid [Ca-DTPA]) form complexes with metallic ions, removing them from circulation. Each should begin as soon as possible, guided by daily dose assessments and urinary levels.

Laboratory monitoring can reveal marked lymphocyte depletion soon after injury. Complete blood counts with white cell differential, taken every 6 hours for 48 hours, aid in determining dose and prognosis. Urinalyses help determine baseline renal function and track the degree of radionuclide-induced kidney damage. Urine human chorionic gonadotropin (uHCG) measurement is appropriate in all women of childbearing age. Pregnant victims should be counseled by an obstetrician regarding potential teratogenesis. Fetal sensitivity to radiation is highest 3–7 weeks post-conception.

Opportunistic infections pose extreme risk in irradiated, neutropenic patients. A fine line must be maintained between intervention and infection control; invasive procedures, including line placement and surgery, should be avoided if possible, particularly during the neutrophil nadir two days post-exposure. If wounds must be left open, topical antibiotics should be considered. Hygiene and nosocomial risk minimization must be enforced. Stable patients can be discharged before the neutrophil nadir, with outpatient follow-up performed away from the hospital's nosocomial risk. Positive pressure isolation rooms will benefit inpatients. If fever develops during the neutropenic phase, empiric antibiotics should be started, tailored to the hospital's bacterial susceptibility profile and culture results. Prophylaxis should start when the absolute neutrophil count (ANC) falls to 0.5×10^9 cells/l, continuing until ANC rebounds above 1.0×10^9 cells/l. Empiric 21-day intravenous regimens include quinolones (ciprofloxacin, levofloxacin) for Gram-negative infection, possibly supplemented by penicillin, amoxicillin, piperacillin, or vancomycin for Gram-positive coverage. A third- or fourth-generation cephalosporin (ceftriaxone, cefepime), imipenem, or an aminoglycoside (gentamicin, amikacin) may be substituted for the quinolone if needed. If afebrile, antibiotics should end after seven days. Oropharyngeal mucositis or known/suspected herpes simplex virus (HSV) infection should prompt addition of acyclovir. If clostridial enterocolitis develops, a 500 mg dose of metronidazole three times a day for one to two weeks should begin. Fluconazole should be used for fungal infections.

If immune compromise and gastrointestinal symptoms develop, gut decontamination should be considered. Normal gut flora may be affected by radiation, causing overgrowth of Enterobacteriaceae, possible transmigration, and sepsis. Effective options include oral ciprofloxacin, polymyxin B, or trimethoprim-sulfamethoxizole. Though rarely used due to gastrointestinal side effects, oral neomycin is also effective. Immunization status should be addressed after acute-phase treatments. Revaccination against *Streptococcus pneumoniae*, *Neisseria meningitidis*, and *Haemophilus influenzae B* should be given for positive serologies or functional hyposplenism, guided by Centers for Disease Control (CDC) and Infectious Disease Society of America (IDSA) protocols. Live vaccines should be deferred for two years (Table 15.5).

Nutritional demands must be tempered by possible bowel mucosa injury. Similarly to burns, trauma, or infection, radiation induces hypermetabolic stress. Increased needs are satisfied enterally or parenterally. Regular diets are avoided initially, replaced by soft elemental diets that minimize mechanical, acidic, and enzymatic damage to remaining mucosa, decrease bacterial growth, and encourage normal function. Enteral glutamine may aid in mucosal rehabilitation. If bowel function is impaired (e.g. malabsorption, obstruction) or mucosal breakdown is likely, parenteral nutrition should be used, necessitating central access and infective risk. Dietary consultation en masse for similar patients may help in a mass casualty (Table 15.6).

Cytokines (Table 15.7) are potent inducers of inflammation and hematopoiesis. Subcutaneous or intravenous granulocyte colony-stimulating factor (G-CSF, Filgrastim) or granulocyte-macrophage colony-stimulating factor (GM-CSF, Sargramostim) given after a 3 Gy dose can augment cell production and minimize neutropenia. Lower thresholds (2 Gy) are used in extremes of age (<12, >60). Cytokines such as stem cell factor (SCF), thrombopoietin, and interleukins (IL-1 through IL-16) are investigational.

Surgical Treatment and Anesthetic Management
Co-existing trauma is likely in patients that are close to an explosion or that survive secondary (flying object striking patient) or tertiary (shock wave throws patient

Table 15.5 Infection control and treatment

Modality	Treatment	Comments
Infection control measures		Strict contact and droplet precautions Proper hand washing Positive pressure room Minimize invasive procedures Early discharge if appropriate

Antibiotics	• Quinolone (ciprofloxacin, levofloxacin)
	   OR
	• 3rd/4th generation cephalosporin
	   OR
	• Imipenem
	   OR
	• Aminoglycoside (gentamicin, amikacin)
	   AND
	• Gram-positive coverage (penicillin, amoxicillin, vancomycin)
		Broad-spectrum, prophylactic antibiotics during the neutropenic period, continue until ANC recovers

	• Acyclovir	If HSV positive or suspected
	• Fluconazole	If fungal infection present
	• Topical antibiotics	For open wounds in neutropenic phase
	• Flagyl 500 mg PO q8 x7-14 days	To treat *C. difficile* if occurs
	• Consider gut prophylaxis	For risk of translocation of intestinal bacteria
Vaccines	• *Streptococcus pneumoniae* • *Neisseria meningitidis* • *Haemophilus influenzae B*	As hyposplenism or serology dictates (see CDC and IDSA guidelines) No live vaccines for two years

Table 15.6 Nutritional support

Route	Characteristics
Enteral	Provides adequate calories Promotes mucosal growth and patency Hastens return of normal bowel function Decreases acidic and enzymatic damage Prevents overgrowth of abnormal flora Risk of mechanical wall stress
Parenteral	Can provide adequate calories (if total parenteral nutrition) Viable option if gut not functioning Minute design of intake possible Infective risk of central line Risks villous atrophy and bacterial transmigration

Table 15.7 Cytokine therapy

Drug	Dosage
G-CSF (Filgrastim)	• 5–10 µg/kg SQ/IV qD 　OR • 200–400 µg/m²/day
GM-CSF (Sargramostim)	• 2.5–5.0 µg/kg SQ/IV qD 　OR • 100–250 µg/m²/day
PEG G-CSF (Pegfilgrastim)	• 6 mg SQ q week

against fixed object) blast trauma, requiring general, orthopedic, plastic, vascular, or neurosurgical intervention. Anesthetic plans assume a full stomach necessitating rapid sequence induction, definitive airway control, close hemodynamic management including invasive monitors, and fluid and blood component therapy. When decontamination is suboptimal, anesthesiologists should wear PPE as indicated by a radiation safety officer (RSO). Whenever possible, intravascular lines should be started in uncontaminated parts of the body. Resources may be limited, including surgical instruments, anesthesia machines, ventilators, monitors, drugs, endotracheal tubes, fluids, blood, medical gases, and even electricity. Likewise, personnel, including anesthesiologists and nurse anesthetists, surgeons and surgical technicians, operating room (OR) and recovery nurses, will also represent precious commodities. Maximum use of ancillary personnel, including technicians, medical students, volunteers, and the walking wounded, is critical.

Interventions performed outside the OR with minimal anesthetic requirement will do the most good for the most patients. Properly employed light sedation, hypnotics, and regional anesthesia that maintain spontaneous ventilation will help alleviate shortages. The decision to go to the OR must be tempered by the relative likelihood of surgical success, the needs of other patients, and equipment availability. Supplies may need to be washed and reused. In extreme cases, two or more surgeries may be performed in the same suite with a single anesthesia provider caring for them simultaneously.

Wounds are assumed to be contaminated. Higher priority is given to wounds than to intact skin, because of the possibility of blood-borne spread of radionuclides. The aggressiveness of debridement should be tempered by bleeding, co-morbidities, number of wounds, amount of inspissated material, relative radiotoxicity of the species involved, and competing OR demands.

Radiation-induced lymphopenia can cause immunosuppression, delayed wound healing, increased rates of infection, and failure of primary closure. If possible, definitive treatment should be undertaken within 36 hours of injury, before the white cell count decreases significantly. Surgical protocols that require multiple OR trips may be catastrophic for these patients, who may benefit more from wide excision, amputation, and early primary closure with sufficient margins of healthy, non-irradiated tissue. Hyperbaric oxygen therapy may be beneficial. Primary closure of wounds still containing radioactive material will yield infection and dehiscence.

Wounds should be draped with impermeable material to limit contamination spread. If sufficient PPE is not available, runoff and dressings should go into a shielded container. Radiation safety personnel should periodically inspect ORs. Radiation readings should guide focused debridement. Grossly contaminated wounds may require serial returns to the OR before primary or graft-assisted closure. Once normal radiation levels are reached, the wound can be treated normally.

Long-range health concerns after radiation exposure come in two varieties: deterministic effects, wherein a definitive (often linear) causal relationship exists between exposure and sequelae, and stochastic effects, in which a causal relationship cannot be proven but where exposure increases the likelihood of development. With deterministic effects, disease severity increases with dose. Examples include cutaneous injury, cataract formation, sterility, leukopenia, and decreased immunity. By contrast, probability of stochastic effects such as cancer increases with dose suffered, while severity may be attenuated by host and environmental factors. Survivors of radiation injuries remain at risk for multiple health problems for years to come, and should have close health surveillance. Women of childbearing age and men at risk for radiation-induced sterility should be offered genetic counseling, while exposed pregnant women should receive obstetrical advice. Support groups exist for patients who suffer radiation-associated diseases. Social services should help patients find support long before discharge.

Biological Disasters

Biological disasters typically come in the form of epidemics or pandemics. The rate of spread, the degree of infectivity, and the disability/lethality of the disease determine how it is handled. Highly infective diseases with high mortality, like SARS and Ebola, require elaborate isolation and personal protection procedures. Less morbid and less lethal infections can be dealt with through routine precautions. Anesthesia personnel encounter these situations during pandemics when they are called to intubate patients in respiratory distress or to manage patients in the ICU. In addition, they may also be exposed to patients who require emergency surgery for trauma or other acute conditions. The ASA Committee on Trauma and Emergency Preparedness recommends use of the Precautionary Principle: using higher levels of personal protective equipment (PPE) until a newly emerging disease is fully characterized. This is especially true when aerosol-generating procedures are performed (intubation, suctioning, bronchoscopy, and flushing a toilet with patient waste.) The Ebola Guidelines can be found at www.asahq.org/resources/clinical-information/ebola-information.

When highly infectious patients require surgery (and it has been determined to be unavoidable), it is better to move equipment and supplies to the isolation room (or ward). The equipment should remain there until full decontamination can be guaranteed. Staff will need to don PPE before entering, decontaminate, and doff their PPE when leaving. This is still preferable over moving infectious patients through the halls. Thought should be given to maintaining "hot" passageways for the exclusive use of isolation patients. Alternatively, all affected patients could be concentrated at "epidemic hospitals". Many authorities advocate single patient drills followed by a mass casualty drill to test the feasibility of plans (Boxes 15.1 to 15.3).

Box 15.1 Principles of Personal Protective Equipment (PPE)

- Respiratory protection
  - N95
  - PAPR (powered air-purifying respirator)
- Barrier protection
  - Multiple layers of gloves and impermeable coverings
  - Donning and doffing technique
- Post-doffing sanitization
  - Self, equipment, room
  - Tompkins, Anesthesia and Analgesia: October 2010 – Volume 111 – Issue 4 – pp. 933–945

Box 15.2 Environmental Issues

- Air flow (negative vs positive)
- Air filtering (HEPA)
- Infectious waste disposal
- What happens to suctioned air?
  - How do you sterilize the suction system?
- Waste water disposal/decontamination
  - DON'T FLUSH THE TOILET!
  - Disinfect first

Box 15.3 Isolation for Surgery

- Patient and equipment do not move
- Only staff PPE logistics to worry about
- Works best for small numbers of patients
- Consider designation of an "Epidemic Hospital" if large numbers of infected patients
- Ethical implications
  - Who do we expend limited resources on?
  - Ethics committees, State laws

Key Points

- Mass casualties lead to unavoidable shortages. Efficient use of personnel (including technicians, students, volunteers, and walking wounded) and supplies (including alternate anesthetic techniques, wash and reuse of equipment) is critical. Anesthesiologists may need to care for multiple patients simultaneously.
- Decontamination limits exposure, but should not delay resuscitation. Caregivers should wear PPE until decontamination is performed.

- Most chemical exposures require supportive care only. Some chemical injuries have specific treatments. The CHEMM website is an excellent resource for first responders/ first receivers.
- Irradiation is exposure to radiation, and does not make the patient a threat to health care providers. Contamination occurs when radioactive material comes to rest on or inside a patient; it poses a threat until removed.
- Radiological damage decreases with shorter exposure time, increased distance from the source, and increased shielding.
- Acute radiation syndrome occurs after exposure of more than 1 Gy. The hematopoietic syndrome affects bone marrow, leading to immunosuppression, neutropenic fevers, hemorrhage, and infection. The gastrointestinal syndrome causes mucosal sloughing, malabsorption, and possible transmigration of gut flora. Death from hemorrhage or infection is likely despite care. The cardiovascular/central nervous system syndrome results in mental status changes, seizures, hypotension, autonomic dysregulation, and cardiovascular collapse within minutes. It is uniformly fatal.

Bibliography

Armed Forces Radiobiology Research Institute. *Medical Management of Radiological Casualties Handbook*, 2nd edn. Bethesda, MD: Armed Forces Radiobiology Research Institute, 2003.

Baker DJ. The pre-hospital management of injury following mass toxic release: a comparison of military and civilian approaches. *Resuscitation* 1999;42:155–159.

Centers for Disease Control and Prevention. Acute radiation syndrome: a fact sheet for physicians. www.cdc.gov/nceh/radiation/eme rgencies/arsphysicianfactsheet.htm (accessed September 2019).

Hamilton M, Conley J, Grychowski K, Lundy P. Management problems in combined chemical/ trauma casualties. www.researchgate.net/publi cation/267402352_Anaesthetic_Management_ Problems_in_Combined_ChemicalTrauma_C asualties?opdsd=1 (accessed September 2019).

McIsaac III JH, Kucik I. Chemical and radiologic exposures in trauma. In: Varon AJ, Smith CE, eds., *Essentials of Trauma Anesthesia*. Cambridge: Cambridge University Press; 2012: 156–170.

National Council on Radiation Protection and Measurements. Report No. 65, *Management of Persons Accidentally Contaminated with Radionuclides*, 7th edn. Bethesda, MD: NCRP, 1997.

Pellmar TC, Ledney GD. Combined injury: radiation in combination with trauma, infectious disease, or chemical exposures. Published in the proceedings of the NATO Human Factors and Medicine (HFM) Panel Research Task Group (RTG) 099 Meeting, "Radiation Bioeffects and Countermeasures," Bethesda, MD, USA, June 21–23, 2005. https://apps.dtic.mil/dtic/tr/fulltext/u2/a4387 64.pdf (accessed October 2019).

Seth, R, Chester D, Moiemen N. A review of chemical burns. *Trauma* 2007;9:81–94.

Tucci MA, Camporesi EM. Risks and effects of radiation terrorism. *Semin Anesth Periop Med Pain* 2003;22(4):268–277.

Vijayan VK. Toxic trauma affecting the lungs with special reference to the Bhopal disaster. *Pulmon* 2006;8(2):44–50.

Weinbroum AA, Rudick V, Paret G, Kluger Y, Ben Abraham R. Anaesthesia and critical care considerations in nerve agent warfare trauma casualties. *Resuscitation* 2000;47:113–123.

Chapter 16

Pain in Disasters

Tracey Jackson and Matthew Pena

Optimal management of severe pain in a traditional hospital setting can be a challenging process. [1-3] Yet, attempting to manage pain in an out-of-hospital, combat, or austere environment is even more demanding.[4-8] Because early intervention in both acute pain[9] and chronic pain[10] is associated with improved outcomes, timely and aggressive treatment may reduce the prevalence or severity of chronic pain and lead to enduring improvements in patients' quality of life.[11]

Multiple physical challenges in disaster and austere environments exist. Extremes in weather and terrain, difficulties obtaining adequate facilities and equipment, logistical challenges, and personnel safety add to the difficulties of treating pain in disaster situations.[12] Natural disasters and terrorist acts have proven the need for health care providers to be properly trained in pain management principles in these environments.[13] However, data indicate that in both normal conditions and during major emergencies, the majority of health care providers are culturally and professionally unprepared to adequately treat acute pain conditions.[14,15] Unfortunately, there is an inadequate level of training among health care professionals and the source of aid is frequently limited, especially in the immediate aftermath of a disaster.[16]

No guidelines or validated protocols provide adequate indications for the treatment for pain in case of massive emergencies.[16] Unfortunately, most trauma care algorithms, even at major trauma centers, do not include a systematic approach to pain assessment. Furthermore, empirical studies of pain assessment in trauma patients are virtually nonexistent.[17]

The understanding that pain is not just a symptom of disease but at times is a disease process in itself is indicative of a fundamental change occurring in the field of medicine.[19] In recent decades, the concept of pain had been outlined as a multifactorial disease that takes into account environmental, personal, physiological, and psychological elements influencing the individual responses.[20] The patients' self-report of pain is a critical component of a comprehensive pain assessment, which includes clinical assessment and pain history and treatment. Pain scores, although imperfect as a stand-alone assessment tool, provide a clinician with an idea of triage priority, of what type of analgesic to use, how well any intervention has worked and what may be required subsequently, the patient's perception of general quality of care, and alters the patient's experience of the pain because the pain is recognized as being "real" by another person.[18,21-23]

Multiple pain assessment tools exist as self-reported forms and scales[24,25]. However, the use of these pain assessment tools has not been studied in the disaster setting, and future research should focus on accurate pain assessment during disaster settings to help aid in the diagnosis and adequate treatment of pain. In emergency departments, the intensity of pain

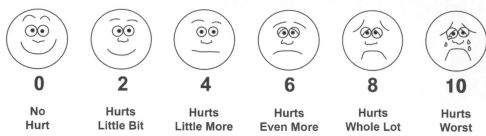

Figure 16.1 Wong-Baker FACES Pain Rating Scale. (Wong-Baker FACES Foundation (2019). Wong-Baker FACES® Pain Rating Scale. Retrieved 06 June 2019 with permission from www.WongBakerFACES.org.)

is gauged using an 11-point verbal numerical rating scale (VNRS), although few studies support the validity of the VNRS.[26-30] The visual analog scale (VAS) is often considered the gold standard in pain research and is more sensitive to changes in pain intensity.[31-34] The VAS may be useful in the disaster setting to bypass cultural and language barriers that may exist in these austere settings (Figure 16.1).

Pain inadequately treated may modify the characteristics of the pain itself. Pain is no longer considered just a symptom, but itself becomes an autonomous pathology heavily influencing the social life and psychosocial aspects of a person (Figure 16.2).[16] Improved understanding of the pathophysiology of pain and its associated morbidity has only recently begun to alter physician attitudes. There is an evolving appreciation that poorly managed pain can develop into a disease of the nervous system with the potential for lifelong disability and morbidity consequences for the patient.[35]

Essential Medications

The World Health Organization (WHO) defines essential medicines as those that satisfy the priority health care needs of the population. A list of essential medicines has been devised, and medicines are selected with regard to disease prevalence, evidence on efficacy and safety, and comparative cost-effectiveness. In 1977, WHO devised a Model List of Essential Drugs to use as a guide for the development of national and international essential medicine lists. Since then, the list has been updated and expanded on a regular basis. Essential medicines are one of the most cost-effective elements in modern health care and their potential health impact is remarkable.[36]

The Model List of Essential Drugs compiled by the World Health Organization may be useful to prepare and treat pain in disaster situations. The Model List medications useful in the treatment of pain include:[36]

Anesthetics: halothane, isoflurane, nitrous oxide, oxygen, ketamine, propofol, bupivacaine, lidocaine

Analgesics: aspirin, ibuprofen, acetaminophen (paracetamol), codeine, morphine, meperidine, methadone

Psychotropics: midazolam, diazepam, carbamazepine, valproate, phenytoin, amitriptyline.

Anti-infectives: including antibiotic, antifungal, and antiviral medications

Other: dexamethasone, hydrocortisone, fluoxetine, cyclizine, phenobarbital, valproic acid

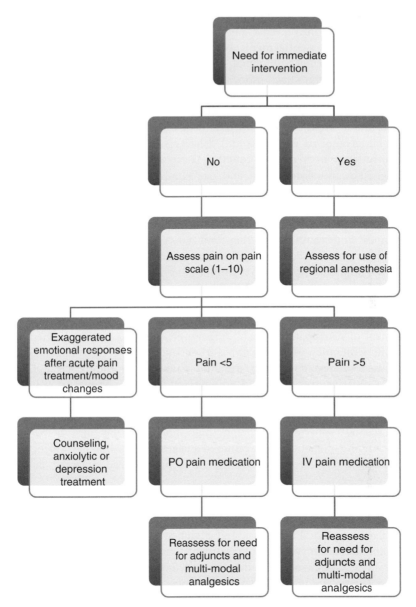

Figure 16.2 Treatment algorithm for acute pain acquired in disaster situations.

During a disaster situation, opioids, the mainstay of acute pain management, become less available but are essential for the treatment of patients with acute pain.[37,38] Insufficient administration of opioids may be due to difficulties in finding, storing, prescribing, and dispensing these drugs, as many low–middle-income countries lack the funds needed to provide even the most basic health services. Shortage of analgesic drugs after a disaster can be related to difficulties in internal transport and transfer of drugs to and from disaster staging areas. Inconsistent availability of these medications may result in pain that is under-treated and difficult to control, especially in the long term.[39] Therefore, opioids should be considered primary and essential medications in a disaster setting.[40,41] New formulations of opioids, such as transdermal, sublingual, or transmucosal compositions may facilitate the administration of therapies, act more quickly, and may prove to be more effective overall.[42-46] The lack of availability of opioid drugs can seriously compromise the possibility to adequately treat pain, and may lead to subsequent ongoing and costly disability.

The multi-modal approach to pain treatment utilizes multiple analgesic medications with different mechanisms of action and delivery method. For example, opioids, non-steroidal anti-inflammatory drugs, N-methyl-D-aspartate (NMDA) receptor antagonists, alpha-2 antagonists, antineuropathics, and local anesthetics may be used in various combinations to achieve a synergistic effect improving overall pain control while minimizing adverse effects. In cases of primary nerve injury or neuropathic pain, drugs like gabapentin and tricyclic antidepressants may be more fiscally and clinically appropriate than procedural or surgical interventions. In the combat situation, oral opioids, cyclooxygenase (COX)-2 selective non-steroidal anti-inflammatory drugs, and acetaminophen can be self-administered by soldiers who sustain a painful injury.[47,48] Ketamine has also been used in the combat setting, partially due to its large margin of safety, and in subanesthetic doses has been shown to provide profound pain relief, potentiate the effects of opioids, and prevent opioid hyperalgesia.[49-53] There is substantial evidence for the use of tricyclic antidepressants in the treatment of neuropathic pain.[54-59] However, their use may be limited due to side effects. The antiepileptics sodium valproate, phenytoin, and carbamazepine have been successfully used to treat chronic neuropathic pain.[60-64] Clonidine, an alpha-2 agonist, acts both as a sedative and an opioid adjunct and has been shown to reduce one-year surgical mortality.[65] In addition to the opioid adjuncts, benzodiazepines can significantly calm trauma patients and decrease pain scores, distinct from the sedation and anxiolysis that benzodiazepines provide.[68] Utlizing multi-modal therapy may help decrease the incidence of complications of opioid-centered analgesia, including dependence, addiction, ileus, post-operative respiratory depression, and opioid-induced hyperalgesia.[66,67]

Other Interventions

The use of a multi-modal approach is appropriate for pain management in a disaster setting. Regional analgesia, epidural analgesia, and peripheral nerve blocks, as well as local field blocks, acupuncture, and psychosocial treatments, are available to help treat acute pain as well as decrease the likelihood of the development of chronic pain.

Regional analgesia, epidural analgesia, or peripheral nerve blocks have been used in the polytrauma patient to provide improved analgesia, improved outcomes, and lead to higher patient satisfaction.[69-71] Nerve blocks, with and without ultrasound guidance, can also be invaluable as part of a multi-modal approach to pain reduction in disasters. Emergency ultrasound-guided nerve blocks have proven utility in combat and disaster settings[72-74] to induce a reversible loss of sensation with minimal central nervous system and cardiovascular adverse effects. The primary goal of emergency ultrasound-guided nerve blocks is pain reduction with a simple, single-injection nerve block that is safe, rapid, and easily learned to provide acute pain reduction. Successful use of ultrasound-guided blocks of the femoral nerve, popliteal block, median, ulnar, and radial nerves (forearm block), and the interscalene brachial plexus has been described in the emergency medicine literature.[75-83]

Ultrasound guidance for nerve blocks has been shown to be either equivalent to or better than other nerve localization techniques and may decrease complication rates and improve performance time and time to onset of blocks.[84,85] In addition, ultrasound guidance prevents the need for potentially painful motor stimulation of injured extremities and can be used across a language barrier. With improved portability, ultrasound is increasingly recognized as a valuable tool in resource-limited and disaster settings for tasks as diverse as triage, surgical decision-making, obstetric care, and procedural efficiency.[86-89]

The inherent difficulties of disaster settings raise challenges to documentation, sterile technique, and monitoring for adverse effects such as local anesthetic systemic toxicity (LAST) that will require further investigation. This becomes challenging in a setting in which multiple physicians working across language barriers may evaluate the patient in a given period, the basic tools of charting are difficult to procure, and patient condition may necessitate urgent transfer. Detailed training protocols need to be developed for emergency physician providers to ensure proficiency and understanding of the potential complications.[90] Patients who have received a block will need to be identified with an unambiguous and universal system that allows clear communication between the multidisciplinary team caring for them and centers to which they may be transferred.

The indication, nerve block(s) performed, technique, approach, sedating medication used, and sedation level achieved (if applicable), local anesthetic and quantity, use of epinephrine, and complications should be carefully documented and reliably stored for later reference.[91] The choice of local anesthetic used should be based on the safety profile and accessibility of long- and short-acting agents. The addition of vasoconstrictors, such as epinephrine, to local anesthetics can serve as an early marker of intravascular injection and can significantly slow the systemic absorption, thereby improving the safety profile and prolonging the analgesia. The potential infectious risks of practicing ultrasound-guided nerve blocks in a non-sterile setting, as well as the possible risk of delaying the diagnosis of compartment syndrome, should be further explored, although preliminary data from military operations in Iraq and Afghanistan suggest that the benefits outweigh the risks, despite these challenges.[92] Health care providers should be aware of the risks associated with different types of blocks and treatment. Nerve injury is also of concern and known to be exacerbated by high-pressure injection; however, because ultrasound guidance allows good visualization, intraneural injection is usually avoidable, making a rare occurrence even more unlikely. Teams providing blocks should be prepared to recognize and treat LAST, a potential complication that usually occurs within minutes of injection and is most commonly associated with an inadvertent intravascular injection leading to nervous system and cardiovascular system effects, such as agitation, auditory changes, seizures, coma, respiratory arrest, tachycardia, dysrhythmias, cardiovascular collapse, and asystole.[93]

Ideally, nerve blocks should be performed in a controlled setting with cardiorespiratory monitoring. In a disaster setting, however, this may not be possible. Close clinical monitoring of the patient's mental status, with vigilance for potential symptoms of toxicity, will allow the early diagnosis of LAST in many patients.[94] Monitoring the patient's pulse rate and oxygen saturation with a pulse oximeter, particularly if epinephrine is used, during and in the immediate 30 minutes after a single injection block may also aid in the early identification of inadvertent intravascular injection, improving the safety of blocks in an austere setting.[94-96] Local wound infiltration or basic nerve blocks such as fascia iliacus,[97] intercostal,[98] or suprascapular[99] blocks can also provide profound analgesia.[13]

Acupuncture has also been shown to successfully reduce pain in a variety of settings.[100,101] Common indications include pain in musculoskeletal disorders,[102-104] fatigue,[107,108] and depression.[109-111] Auricular acupuncture techniques are well-described for acute and chronic pain and anxiolysis after physical and psychological trauma, including amputation and post-traumatic stress disorder (PTSD) in military settings.[105,106] There is also evidence in civilians that acupuncture may be effective in the treatment of other complex pain diseases such as irritable bowel syndrome (IBS),[112,113] fibromyalgia,[114] and post-traumatic stress disorder.[115] Studies have shown acupuncture is well tolerated by patients, safe, effective, and cost-effective compared to routine care.[116,117]

Relationships between disaster events and subsequent psychopathology have been widely established.[118] Psychopathology is commonly associated with chronic pain, particularly affective disorders, anxiety disorders, and substance-abuse disorders.[119] Psychiatric syndromes such as depression and anxiety disorders, and also somatically mediated complaints, may be exacerbated by the impact of catastrophic events. After disasters, a dramatic rise in pain intensity has been observed. The significant rise in pain was postulated to be due to an acute stress reaction, which could have stimulated a sympathetic-mediated physiological response that resulted in a magnified perception of pain. In addition, these patients may have suffered from post-traumatic stress disorder (PTSD), which caused an exacerbation of symptoms when confronted with media exposure of the event. In addition, women have been noted to experience higher increases in pain scores than men after stressful events.[120-122] In a distressed population, there is an increased risk of other musculoskeletal complaints, as manifested by escalating work-related injuries, work absence, and lost productivity.[123] Pain and its effects (e.g. disruptions of activities of daily living, such as work and recreation) result in emotional changes.[119] These emotional changes can produce significant increases in anxiety, depression, and anger. This emotional distress can then lead to increased psychophysiological stress and tension, which substantially affect pain threshold and exacerbations, ultimately affecting physical functioning and change. This cycle can alter pain threshold and exacerbations, leading to further increases in psychosocial morbidity that can, in turn, produce disruptions in activities of daily living (e.g. anxiety and depression may decrease interest and motivation in getting involved in work and social activities). Disaster or terrorism situations, either as an event or a threat, can interact in or activate this cycle at any point.[124] Psychosocial treatment through counseling, antidepressants, anxiolytics, and pain treatment (Table 16.1) should be implemented early to help treat and prevent perpetuation of pain related to psychosocial changes. Because many of the psychological pathologies that manifest after exposure to disaster situations are not diagnosed for months to years after the event, information regarding early intervention with the use of counseling, anxiolytics, and antidepressants is based on retrospective studies in which these interventions are rarely, if ever, instituted and are severely lacking.

Conclusion

Given the evidence that early intervention in both acute pain[9] and chronic pain[10] is associated with improved outcomes, timely treatment of these problems may lead to enduring improvements in patients' quality of life and corresponding reductions in the psychosocial sequelae that are closely associated with chronic pain conditions.[9,125] Accurate assessment of pain is necessary to adequately treat pain.[126] As we improve in our success in the early identification of pain-related problems we also must expect increased demands on

Table 16.1 Essential medications used to treat pain

Drug class	Medications	Indications

Anesthetics	Inhalational
	• halothane
	• isoflurane
	• nitrous oxide
	• oxygen
	Intravenous
	• ketamine
	• propofol
	• local anesthetics
	  • bupivacaine
	  • lidocaine
		• Surgical or procedural intervention
		• Acute pain treatment
		• Local anesthetics: peripheral or neuraxial blocks

Analgesics	Oral • aspirin • ibuprofen • acetaminophen (paracetamol) • codeine Intravenous • morphine • meperidine	• Acute and chronic pain treatment
Benzodiazepines	Intravenous • midazolam • diazepam	• Anxiety
Antiepileptics	Oral • carbamazepine • valproate • phenytoin • amytriptyline	• Neuropathic pain
Antibiotics	Intravenous or PO • amoxicillin • penicillin • cloxacillin • chloramphenicol • ciprofloxacin • doxycycline • erythromycin • gentamycin • metronidazole • spectinomycin • sulfadiazine • cotrimoxazole • trimethoprim	• Bacterial infections

Table 16.1 (cont.)

Drug class	Medications	Indications
Antidepressants	Oral • fluoxetine (SSRI)	• Neuropathic pain • Prevention and/or treatment of central sensitization
Steroid	Intravenous • dexamethasone	• Inflammation
Antihistamine	Oral, intravenous, or intramuscular • cyclizine	• Nausea, vomiting, dizziness

pain care resources for acute treatment and prevention of chronic disabling pain. By anticipating the needs of patients with pain in disasters and implementing corresponding changes in health care systems responsible for their care we may be able to minimize suffering while maximizing potential for improvement.[127]

References

1. American Pain Society. Pain assessment and treatment in the managed care environment: a position statement from the American Pain Society. *Case Manager* 2000;**11**(5):50–53.

2. Ducharme J. Acute pain and pain control: state of the art. *Ann Emerg Med* 2000;**35**:592–603.

3. Wilson J, Pendelton J. Oligoanalgesia in the emergency department. *Am J Emerg Med* 1989;**7**:620–623.

4. National Association of EMS Physicians. Prehospital pain management: a position paper from the National Association of EMS Physicians. *Prehospital Emerg Care* 2003;**7**:482–488.

5. Butler F, Hagmann J, Butler E. Tactical combat casualty care in special operations. *Mil Med* 1996;**161**:3–16.

6. Butler F, Hagmann J, Richards D. Tactical management of urban warfare casualties in special operations. *Mil Med* 2000;**165**:1–48.

7. Weiss E. Medical considerations for wilderness and adventure travelers. *Med Clin North Am* 1999;**83**:885–902.

8. Bowen T. *Emergency War Surgery: Second United States Revision of the Emergency War Surgery NATO Handbook*. Washington, DC: United States Government Publication Office.

9. Smith D, McMurray N, Disler P. Early intervention for acute back injury: can we finally develop an evidence-based approach? *Clin Rehabil* 2002;**16**(1):1–11.

10. Jordan K, Mayer T, Gatchel R. Should extended disability be an exclusion criterion for tertiary rehabilitation? Socioeconomic outcomes of early versus late functional restoration in compensation spinal disorders. *Spine* 1998;**23**(19):2110–2116.

11. Clark M, Scholten J, Walker R, Gironda R. Assessment and treatment of pain associated with combat related polytrauma. *Pain Med* 2009;**10**(3):456–469.

12. Macintyre P, Rowbotham D, Walker S. Acute pain management in field and disaster situations. In: Macintyre P, Rowbotham D, Walker S. *Clinical Pain Management: Acute Pain*. London: Hodder Arnold; 2008: 376–385.

13. Black I, McManus J. Pain management in current combat operations. *Prehosp Emerg Care* 2009;**13**(2):223–237.

14. Rupp T, Delaney K. Inadequate analgesia in emergency medicine. *Ann Emerg Med* 2004;**43**:494–503.

15. Jones J. Assessment of pain management skills in emergency medicine residents: the role of a pain education program. *J Emerg Med* 1999;**17**:349–354.

16. Guetti C, Angeletti C, Paladini A, Varrassi G, Marinangeli F. Pain and natural disaster. *Pain Pract* 2013;**13**(7):589–593.

17. Edwards WT. Posttrauma pain. In: Loeser J, Bonica J (eds.), *Bonica's Management of Pain*, 3rd edn. Philadelphia, PA: Lippincott Williams & Wilkins; 2001:788–793.

18. Wolf N. *The Beauty Myth: How Images of Beauty are Used Against Women.* New York: Vintage, 1998.

19. Buckenmaier C. The role of pain management in recovery following trauma and orthopaedic surgery. *J Am Acad Orthop Surg* 2012;**20**(Suppl 1): S35–S38.

20. Vervest A, Schimmel G. Taxonomy of pain of the IASP. *Pain Med* 1988;**34**:318–321.

21. Murray M, Bullard M, Grafstein E. Revisions to the Canadian emergency triage priority. *Can J Emerg Med* 2004;**6**:421.

22. Kovach C, Weissman D, Griffie J, Matson S, Muchka S. Assessment and treatment of discomfort for people with late-stage dementia. *J Pain Symptom Manage* 1999;**18**:412–419.

23. Thomas S, Andruszkiewicz L. Ongoing visual analog score display improves emergency department pain care. *J Emerg Med* 2004;**26**:389–394.

24. Cleeland C, Ryan K. Pain assessment: global use of the Brief Pain Inventory. *Ann Acad Med Singapore* 1994;**23**(2):129–138.

25. Atkinson T, Rosenfeld B, Sit L, et al. Using confirmatory factor analysis to evaluate construct validity of the Brief Pain Inventory (BPI). *J Pain Symptom Manage* 2011;**41**(3):558–565.

26. Berthier F, Potel G, Leconte P, Touze M, Baron D. Comparative study of methods of measuring acute pain intensity in an ED. *Am J Emerg Med* 1998;**16**:132–136.

27. Bijur P, Latimer C, Gallagher E. Validation of a verbally administered numerical rating scale of acute pain for the use in emergency department. *Acad Emerg Med* 2003;**10**:390–392.

28. Carpenter J, Brockopp D. Comparison of patients' ratings and examination of nurses' responses to pain intensity rating scales. *Cancer Nurs* 1995;**18**:292–298.

29. Choiniere M, Amsel R. A visual analogue thermometer for measuring pain intensity. *J Pain Symptom Manage* 1996;**11**:299–311.

30. Deloach L, Higgins M, Caplan A, Stiff J. The visual analogue scale in the immediate postoperative period: intrasubject variability and correlation with a numeric scale. *Anesth Analg* 1998;**86**:102–106.

31. Myles P, Troedel S, Boquest M, Reeves M. The pain visual analog scale: is it linear or nonlinear? *Anesth Analg* 1999;**89**:1517–1520.

32. Myles P, Urquhart N. The linearity of the visual analogue sclae in patients with severe acute pain. *Anesth Intensive Care* 2005;**33**:54–58.

33. Paul-Dauphin A, Guillemin F, Virion J, Briancon S. Bias and precision in visual analogue sclaes: a randomized controlled trial. *Am J Epidemiol* 1999;**150**:1117–1127.

34. Price D, McGrath P, Rafii A, Buckingham B. The validation of visual analogue scales as ratio scale measures for chronic and experimental pain. *Pain* 1983;**17**:45–56.

35. Joshi G, Ogunnaike B. Consequences of inadequate postoperative pain relief and chronic persistent postoperative pain. *Anesthesiol Clin North America* 2005;**23**:21–36.

36. World Health Organization. WHO model lists of essential medicines. www.who.int /medicines/publications/essentialmedi cines/en/ (accessed September 2019).

37. Sepehri G, Meimandi M. Pattern of drug prescription and utilization among Bam residents during the first six months after the 2003 Bam earthquake. *Prehosp Disaster Med* 2006;**21**:396–402.

38. Mulvey J, Oadri A, Magsood M. Earthquake injuries and the use of ketamine for surgical procedures: the Kashmir experience. *Anaesth Intensive Care* 2006;**34**(4):489–494.

39. Tamayo-Sarver J, Dawson N, Cydulka R, Wigton R, Baker D. Variability in emergency physician decision making about prescribing opioid analgesics. *Ann Emerg Med* 2004;**43**:483–493.

40. Chou R, Fanciullo J, Fine P, et al. Clinical guidelines for the use of chronic opioid therapy in chronic non-cancer pain. *J Pain* 2009;**10**:113–130.

41. Marinangeli F, Narducci C, Ursini M, et al. Acute pain and availability of analgesia in the prehospital emergency setting in Italy: a problem to be solved. *Pain Pract* 2009;**9**:282–288.

42. Dale O, Hjortkjaer R, Kharasch ED. Nasal administration of opioids for pain management in adults. *Acta Anaesthesiol Scand* 2002;**46**:759–770.

43. Kendall J, Reeves B, Latter V. Multicentre randomised controlled trial of nasal diamorphine for analgesia in children and teenagers with clinical fractures. *Br Med J* 2001;**322**:261–265.

44. Galinski M, Dolveck F, Borron S, et al. A randomized, double-blind study comparing morphine with fentanyl in prehospital analgesia. *Am J Emerg Med* 2005;**23**(2):114–119.

45. Rickard C, O'Meara P, McGrail M, et al. A randomized controlled trial of intranasal fentanyl vs intravenous morphine for analgesia in the prehospital setting. *Am J Emerg Med* 2007;**25**(8):911–917.

46. Angeletti C, Guetti C, Papola R, et al. Pain after earthquake. *Scand J Trauma Resusc Emerg Med* 2012;**20**:43.

47. Buttar N, Wang K. The "aspirin" of the new millennium: cyclooxygenase-2 inhibitors. *Mayo Clin Proc* 2000;**75**:1027–1038.

48. Doody S, Smith C, Webb J. Nonpharmacologic interventions for pain management. *Crit Care Nurs Clin North Am* 1991;**3**:69–75.

49. Wedmore I, Johnson T, Czarnik J, Hendrix S. Pain management in the wilderness and operational setting. *Emerg Med Clin North Am* 2005;**23**:585–601.

50. Himmelseher S, Durieux M. Ketamine for perioperative pain management. *Anesthesiology* 2005;**102**:211–220.

51. Subramaniam K, Subramaniam B, Steinbrook R. Ketamine as adjuvant analgesic to opioids: a quantitative and qualitative systemic review. *Anesth Analg* 2004;**99**:482–495.

52. Nadeson R, Tucker A, Bajunaki E, Goodchild C. Potentiation by ketamine of fentanyl antinociception. I. An experimental study in rats showing that ketamine administered by non-spinal routes targets spinal cord antinociceptive systems. *Br J Anaesth* 2002;**88**:685–691.

53. Koppert W, Sittl R, Scheuber K, et al. Differential modulation of remifentanil-induced analgesia and post infusion hyperalgesia by S-ketamine and clonidine in humans. *Anesthesiology* 2003;**99**:152–159.

54. Gram LF. Antidepressants: Receptors, pharmacokinetics and clinical effects. In: Burrows G, Norman T, Davies B, eds., *Antidepressants*. Amsterdam: Elsevier Science Publishers; 1983: 81–95.

55. Max M, Lynch S, Muir J, et al. Effects of desipramine, amitriptyline, and fluoxetine on pain in diabetic neuropathy. *N Engl J Med* 1992;**326**(19):1250–1256.

56. Max M, Culnane M, Schafer S, et al. Amitriptyline relieves diabetic neuropathy pain in patients with normal

or depressed mood. *Neurology* 1987;**37**(4):589–596.

57. Max M, Schafer S, Culnane M, et al. Amitriptyline, but not lorazepam, relieves postherpetic neuralgia. *Neurology* 1988;**38**(9):1427–1432.

58. Sindrup S, Gram L, Skjoid T, Froland A, Beck-Nielsen H. Concentration-response relationship in imipramine treatment of diabetic neuropathy symptoms. *Clin Pharmacol Ther* 1990;**47**:509–515.

59. Kishore-Kumar R, Max M, Schafer S, et al. Desipramine relieves postherpetic neuralgia. *Clin Pharmacol Ther* 1990;**47**(3):305–312.

60. Ross E. The evolving role of antiepileptic drugs in treating neurogenic pain. *Neurology* 2000;**55**:S41–S46.

61. McQuay H, Carroll D, Jadad A, Wiffen P, Moore A. Anticonvulsant drugs for management of pain: a systematic review. *BMJ* 1995;**311**:1047–1052.

62. Burchiel K. Carbamazepine inhibits spontaneous activity in experimental neuromas. *Exp Neurol* 1988;**102**:249–253.

63. Campbell F, Graham J, Zikha K. Clinical trial of carbazepine in trigeminal neuralgia. *J Neurol Neurosurg Psychiatry* 1966;**29**:265–267.

64. McCleane G. Intravenous infusion of phenytoin relieves neuropathic pain: a randomized, double-blinded, placebo-controlled, crossover study. *Anesth Analg* 1999;**89**:985–988.

65. Wallace A, Galindez D, Salahieh A, et al. Effect of clonidine on cardiovascular morbidity and mortality after noncardiac surgery. *Anesthesiology* 2004;**101**(2):284–293.

66. Angst M, Clark J. Opioid-induced hyperalgesia: a qualitative systematic review. *Anesthesiology* 2006;**104**:570–587.

67. Celerier E, Rivat C, Jun Y, et al. Long-lasting hyperalgesia induced by fentanyl in rats: preventative effect of ketamine. *Anesthesiology* 2000;**92**(2):465–472.

68. Colloca L, Benedetti F. Nocebo hyperalgesia: how anxiety is turned into pain. *Curr Opin Anaesthesiol* 2007;**20**:435–439.

69. Ong B, Arneja A, Ong E. Effects of anesthesia on pain after lower-limb amputation. *J Clin Anesth* 2006;**18**:600–604.

70. Richman J, Liu S, Courpas G, et al. Does continuous peripheral nerve block provide superior pain control to opioids? A meta-analysis. *Anesth Analg* 2006;**102**(1):248–257.

71. Malchow R, Black I. The evolution of pain management in the critically ill trauma patient: emerging concepts from the global war on terrorism. *Crit Care Med* 2008;**36**(Suppl 7):S346–S357.

72. Malchow R. Ultrasonography for advanced regional anesthesia and acute pain management in a combat environment. *US Army Med Dep J* 2009; Oct–Dec:64–66.

73. Buckenmaier C, Rupprecht C, McKnight G, et al. Pain following battlefield injury and evacuation: a survey of 110 casualties from the wars in Iraq and Afghanistan. *Pain Med* 2009;**10**:1487–1496.

74. Buckenmaier C, McKnight G, Winkley J, et al. Continuous peripheral nerve block for battlefield anesthesia and evacuation. *Reg Anesth Pain Med* 2005;**30**:202–205.

75. Blaivas M, Adhikari S, Lander L. A prospective comparison of procedural sedation and ultrasound-guided interscalene nerve block for shoulder reduction in the emergency department. *Acad Emerg Med* 2011;**18**:922–927.

76. Stone M, Wang R, Price D. Ultrasound-guided supraclavicular brachial plexus nerve block vs procedural sedation for the treatment of upper extremity emergencies. *Am J Emerg Med* 2008;**26**:706–710.

77. Stone M, Muresanu M. Ultrasound-guided ulnar nerve block in the management of digital abscess and hand cellulitis. *Acad Emerg Med* 2010;**17**:e3–e4.

78. Stone M, Carnell J, Fischer J, Herring A, Nagdev A. Ultrasound-guided intercostal

nerve block for traumatic pneumothorax requiring tube thoracostomy. *Am J Emerg Med* 2011;**29**(6):e1–e2.

79. Herring A, Stone M, Fischer J, et al. Ultrasound-guided distal popliteal sciatic nerve block for ED anesthesia. *Am J Emerg Med* 2011;**29**:697.

80. Herring A, Stone M, Nagdev A. Ultrasound-guided suprascapular nerve block for shoulder reduction and adhesive capsulitis in the ED. *Am J Emerg Med* 2011;**29**:963.

81. Herring A, Stone M, Nagdev A. Ultrasound-guided abdominal wall nerve blocks in the ED. *Am J Emerg Med* 2012;**30**(5):759–764.

82. Frenkel O, Herring A, Fischer J, Carnell J, Nagdev A. Supracondylar radial nerve block for treatment of distal radius fractures in the emergency department. *J Emerg Med* 2011;**41**(4):386–388.

83. Beaudoin F, Nagdev A, Merchant R, Becker B. Ultrasound-guided femoral nerve blocks in elderly patients with hip fractures. *Am J Emerg Med* 2010;**28**(1):76–81.

84. Choi S, Brull R. Is ultrasound guidance advantageous for interventional pain management? A review of acute pain outcomes. *Anesth Analg* 2011;**113**:596–604.

85. Walker K, McGrattan K, Aas-Eng K, Smith A. Ultrasound guidance for peripheral nerve blockade. *Cochrane Database Syst Rev* 2009;**7**(4):CD006459.

86. Shah S, Dala A, Joseph G, Rogers S, Dyer G. Impact of portable ultrasound in trauma care after the Haitian earthquake of 2010. *Am J Emerg Med* 2010;**28**(8):970–971.

87. Ma O, Norvell J, Subramanian S. Ultrasound applications in mass casualties and extreme environments. *Crit Care Med* 2007;**35**:S275–S927.

88. Mazur S, Rippey J. Transport and use of point-of-care ultrasound by disaster medical assistance team. *Prehosp Disaster Med* 2009;**24**:140–144.

89. Sippel S, Muruganandan K, Levine A, Shah S. Use of ultrasound in the developing world. *Int J Emerg Med* 2011;**4**:72.

90. Cheung J, Chen E, Darani R, et al. The creation of an objective assessment tool for ultrasound-guided regional anesthesia using the Delphi method. *Reg Anesth Pain Med* 2012;**37**(3):329–333.

91. Gandhi K, Patel V, Maliakal T, Xu D, Flisinski K. Universal documentation sheet for peripheral nerve blocks. *J New York School Reg Anesth* 2009;**12**:23–24.

92. Stojadinovic A, Auton A, Peoples G, et al. Responding to challenges in modern combat casualty care: innovative use of advanced regional anesthesia. *Pain Med* 2006;**7**(4):330–338.

93. Cox D, Durieux M, Marcus M. Toxicity of local anesthetics. *Best Pract Res Clin Anesthesiol* 2003;**17**:111–136.

94. DiGregorio G, Neal J, Rosenquist R, Weinberg G. Clinical presentation of local anesthetic systemic toxicity: a review of published cases, 1979 to 2009. *Reg Anesth Pain Med* 2010;**35**(2):181–187.

95. Ciechanowicz S, Patil V. Lipid emulsion for local anesthetic systemic toxicity. *Anesthesiol Res Pract* 2012;**2012**:131784.

96. Lippert S, Nagdev A, Stone M, Herring A, Norris R. Pain control in disaster settings: a role for ultrasound guided nerve blocks. *Ann Emerg Med* 2013;**61**(6):690–696.

97. Candal-Couto J, McVie J, Haslam N, Innes A, Rushmer J. Pre-operative analgesia for patients with femoral neck fractures using a modified fascia iliaca block technique. *Injury* 2005;**36**:505–510.

98. Karmakar M, Ho A. Acute pain management of patients with multiple fractured ribs. *J Trauma* 2003;**54**:615–625.

99. Ritchie E, Tong D, Chung F, et al. Suprascapular nerve block for postoperative pain relief in arthroscopic shoulder surgery: a new modality? *Anesth Analg* 1997;**84**:1306–1312.

100. Bullock M, Pheley A, Kiresuk T, Lenz S, Culliton P. Characteristics and complaints of patients seeking therapy at a hospital-based alternative medicine clinic. *J Altern Complement Med* 1997;**3**(1):31–37.

101. Cassidy C. Chinese medicine users in the United States. *J Alt Comp Med* 1998;**4**(1):17–27.

102. Haake M, Muller H, Schade-Brittinger C, et al. German acupuncture trials (GERAC) for chronic low back pain: randomized, multicenter, blinded, parallel-group trial with 3 groups. *Arch Intern Med* 2007;**167**(17):1892–1898.

103. Berman B, Ezzo J, Hadhazy V, Swyers J. Is acupuncture effective in the treatment of fibromyalgia. *J Fam Pract* 1999;**48**(3):213–218.

104. Tukmachi E, Jubb R, Dempsey E, Jones P. The effect of acupuncture on the symptoms of knee osteoarthritis–an open randomized controlled study. *Acupunct Med* 2004;**22**(1):14–22.

105. Niemtzow R, Gambel J, Helms J, et al. Integrating ear and scalp acupuncture techniques into the care of blast-injured United States military service members with limb loss. *J Alt Comp Med* 2006;**12**(7):596–599.

106. Goertz C, Niemtzow R, Burns S, et al. Auricular acupuncture in the treatment of acute pain syndromes: a pilot study. *Mil Med* 2006;**171**(10):1010–1014.

107. Vickers A, Rees R, Zollman C, et al. Acupuncture of chronic headache disorders in primary care: randomised controlled trial and economic analysis. *Health Technol Assess* 2004;**8**(48):1–35.

108. Pilkington K, Kirkwood G, Rampes H, Cummings M, Richardson J. Acupuncture for anxiety and anxiety disorders–a systematic review. *Acupunct Med* 2007;**12**(1-2):1–10.

109. Allen J, Schnyer R, Hitt S. The efficacy of acupuncture in the treatment of major depression in women. *Psychol Sci* 1998;**5**:397–401.

110. Allen J, Schnyer R, Chambers A, et al. Acupuncture for depression: a randomized controlled trial. *J Clin Psychiatry* 2006;**67**(11):1665–1673.

111. Manber R, Schnyder R, Allen J, Rush A, Blasey C. Acupuncture: a promising treatment of depression during pregnancy. *J Affect Disord* 2004;**83**(1):89–95.

112. Fireman Z, Segal A, Kopelman Y, Sternberg A, Carasso R. Acupuncture treatment for irritable bowel syndrome: a double-blind controlled study. *Digestion* 2001;**64**(2):100–103.

113. Jena S, Witt C, Brinkhaus B, Wegscheider K, Wilich S. Acupuncture in patients with headache. *Cephalgia* 2008;**28**(9):969–979.

114. Duncan B, White A, Rahman A. Acupuncture in the treatment of fibromyalgia in tertiary care. *Acupunct Med* 2007;**25**(4):137–147.

115. Hollifield M, Sinclair-Lian N, Warner T, Hammerschlag R. Acupuncture for posttraumatic stress disorder. *J Nerv Ment Dis* 2007;**195**(6):504–513.

116. Lao L. Safety issues in acupuncture. *J Altern Complement Med* 1996;**2**:27–31.

117. Burke A, Upchurch D, Dye C, Chyu L. Acupuncture use in the United States: findings from the National Health Interview Survey. *J Alt Comp Med* 2006;**12**(7):639–648.

118. Rubonis A, Bickman L. Psychological impairment in the wake of disaster: the disaster-psychopathology relationship. *Psychol Bull.* 1991;**109**:384–399.

119. Dersh J, Polatin P, Gatchel R. Chronic pain and psychopathology: Research findings and theoretical considerations. *Psychosom Med* 2002;**64**:773–786.

120. Young M, O'Young BJ, Stiens S, Hoffberg H. Terrorism's effect on chronic pain perception: an analysis of a multi-center cohort. *Pract Pain Manag* 2002;**2**:9–12.

121. Sokal J, Young M, O'Young B, Gatchel R. The impact of stress and anxiety on pain. *Adv Dir Rehab* 2003;**12**:25–27.

122. Bleich A, Gelkopf M, Solomon Z. Exposure to terrorism, stress-related mental health symptoms, and coping behaviors among a nationally representative sample in Israel. *JAMA* 2003;**290**(5):612–620.

123. Wesley A, Polatin P, Gatchel R. Psychosocial, psychiatric and socioeconomic factors in chronic occupational musculoskeletal disorders. In: Mayer T, Gatchel R, Polatin P (eds.), *Occupational Musculoskeletal Disorders: Function, Outcomes and Evidence.* Philadelphia, PA: Lippincott, Williams & Wilkins; 2000: 577–608.

124. Polatina P, Young M, Mayerd M, Gatchele R. Bioterrorism, stress, and pain: the importance of an anticipatory community preparedness intervention. *J Psychosom Res* 2005;**58**:311–316.

125. Donta S, Clauw D, Engel C, et al. Cognitive behavior therapy and aerobic exercise for Gulf War veterans' illnesses: a randomized controlled trial. *JAMA* 2003;**289**(11):1396–1404.

126. Resnik D, Rehm M. The undertreatment of pain: scientific, clinical, cultural, and philosophical factors. *Med Health Care Philos* 2001;**4**(3):277–288.

127. Clark M. Post-deployment pain: a need for rapid detection and intervention. *Pain Med* 2004;**5**(4):333–334.

Radiology in the Austere or Disaster Environment

David Besachio and Daniel Sutton

Radiology in the austere environment is an evolving entity. The extent to which the anesthesiologist will have to be aware of issues related to radiology is highly dependent upon the environment in which he or she will work. Capabilities may be limited to a portable ultrasound (US) carried by the provider in a backpack with an imaging screen the size of a modern smartphone to full magnetic resonance imaging (MRI) capabilities that may be seen in higher echelons of care, typically in a military setting. Each modality has its uses and limitations for the anesthesiologist and awareness of the capabilities, safety issues, and limitations of each modality allows maximal extraction of imaging in providing quality care in the "disaster" or austere environment. This chapter will focus on issues related to radiation safety in plain radiography (X-ray) and fluoroscopy, radiation protection, US familiarization, and image quality, and some issues surrounding computed tomography (CT) and MRI.

Radiation Safety

In recent years, greater attention has been placed on the importance of radiation safety within the radiology community.[1] Ionizing radiation refers to radiation that is produced from displacement of an electron from the outer shell of an atom. In biological systems, this can result in the formation of free radicals, subsequent damage to deoxyribonucleic acid (DNA), and resultant disease. In the recent past, the greatest amount of ionizing radiation any typical individual received was due to natural background sources (e.g. radon, solar). In the United States, the population dose of ionizing radiation is approximately the same as that from background sources.[2] While radiation-related injuries are rare, they have been reported with both fluoroscopy and CT in recent years.[3] Techniques that utilize ionizing radiation include X-ray, fluoroscopy, and CT. Radiation dose is often dependent on the use of proper technique with each of these modalities. The essence of radiation protection of which the anesthesiologist should be aware can be simplified to understanding three basic principles: time, distance, and shielding.

With any modality that utilizes ionizing radiation, the amount of time that the patient or anesthesiologist is exposed will be proportional to the total radiation dose received. While fluoroscopy time is rarely under control of the anesthesiologist, he or she can influence the total exposure time received by the entire team and the patient, especially in the trauma setting, through cooperation with the radiologic technician in ensuring appropriate patient positioning, which will ultimately minimize the need for repeat exposures due to poor positioning.

Radiation exposure decreases with the square of the distance from the ionizing radiation source (i.e. the inverse square law). Understanding this principle is one of the greatest single methods by which the anesthesiologist can minimize radiation dose to themselves or their team. While the anesthesiologist may not be able to completely leave their patient during radiation exposure, even a small amount of distance separating them from the radiation source will markedly decrease dose.

Shielding is a more obvious principle of which most anesthesiologists are aware. Wearing protective lead aprons is also a method by which radiation exposure may be minimized. Keep in mind that much of the dose received by health care providers around a patient being radiated is not from the main beam generated by the X-ray machine but rather by scatter radiation emanating from the patient. The greatest dose therefore occurs at the patient level indicating the best protection practice for the anesthesiologist is to shield the most radiosensitive organs: the thyroid and gonads. A thyroid shield and lead apron covering the anesthesiologist to the knee level is necessary.

Modalities

A full discussion on imaging interpretation for all modalities is beyond the scope of this text; however, some basic imaging safety, interpretation pearls, and techniques are discussed below.

Radiography

Radiography is one of the more readily available modalities seen in austere environments and disaster scenarios. Generator-powered portable radiographic units, while rudimentary, are nevertheless effective and widely available (Figure 17.1). These units are typically operated by a technician with working knowledge of appropriate positioning of the unit and patient for various exams to ensure the best radiographic image. Most modern

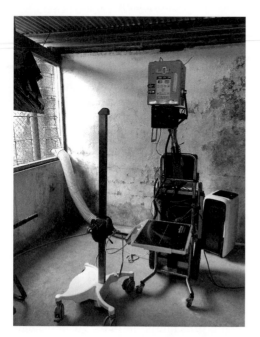

Figure 17.1 Portable radiographic unit (image courtesy of Commander David Besachio, Medical Corps, US Navy).

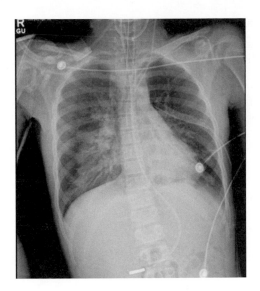

Figure 17.2 Standard portable chest radiograph demonstrating tube and line positioning in a supine patient (image courtesy of Daniel Sutton, MD).

radiographic units require little modification of technique due to systems-wide availability of automatic exposure settings. In general, if visualization is limited, increasing the kilovoltage potential and/or milliampere-seconds may improve image penetration and/or quality, albeit at the expense of increased patient dose and potential provider exposure.

The most common imaging modality used by the anesthesiologist will be the chest radiograph. Upright posterior-anterior and lateral (the ubiquitous "PA and Lat") imaging is superior to supine chest imaging (the "portable AP") for diagnostic purposes; however, portable imaging is typically adequate for evaluation of supportive tube and line placement (Figure 17.2). Many portable X-ray units will have a digital screen on the unit. Such screens allow the technician to determine the adequacy of their technique with respect to exposure and anatomy imaged; as these screens do not contain the resolution necessary to fully identify important abnormalities, they are not intended for use for full diagnostic interpretation. Entities such as small pneumothoraces may be missed when using these monitors for interpretation. The concern over aspiration pneumonitis during a procedure is often raised and typically demonstrates increased lung density in the mid to upper lungs on supine images as the triggering event typically occurs in the supine position leading to involvement of the superior segments of the lower lobes or inferior portions of the upper lobes.[4]

Fluoroscopy and Interventional Radiology

Fluoroscopy and interventional radiology (IR) are not typically available in most austere environments in the absence of higher-level resources. If available, the X-ray source will be a mobile "C-arm" unit. These units are familiar to most anesthesiologists from their operating room experience. In brief, an X-ray source is placed on one end of a rotating, open C-shaped arm with the more bulky image intensifier on the opposite open arm of the "C" (Figure 17.3), typically above the patient. The arm is rotated to the desired position in order to fluoroscopically evaluate relevant anatomy. In non-shielded operating suites where fluoroscopy is utilized, proper shielding may not be in place and

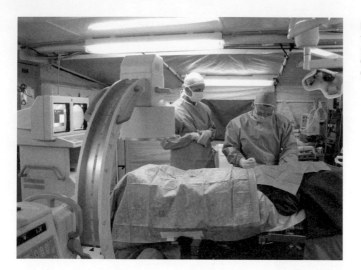

Figure 17.3 Standard C-arm at the ready for an interventional procedure (image courtesy of Captain Steven Ferrara, Medical Corps, US Navy (Flight Surgeon)).

additional caution should be exercised with radiation protection in adjacent rooms or the local area. Interventional radiology procedures performed in austere environments may occur in the context of operating theatres that are not specifically designed for fluoro-scopic imaging.[5] The patient care table may not be radiolucent, resulting in the need for unconventional C-arm positioning and potentially non-standard patient positioning in order to successfully complete a fluoroscopically guided procedure. In most IR proce-dures, above average dose is required to ensure the proper diagnosis and treatment for appropriate patient care (especially during digital subtraction angiography, or DSA). During instances when DSA is performed, the anesthesiologist and assisting personnel should step out of the immediate area whenever possible. To elect to stay at the bedside may result in a significant radiation dose exposure.

Ultrasound

Ultrasound (US) is similarly a familiar entity to most anesthesiologists, often being employed at the point of care for its facilitation of vascular access or nerve blocks, and may be the most advanced radiologic modality available in an austere or disaster environ-ment. Once charged, most small units can be used for several hours without the need for an external power source. Advances in US technology have made diagnostic examinations with highly portable systems able to be performed by individuals with only a modest amount of experience.[6] In some cases, the anesthesiologist may have the greatest degree of familiarity with the operation and use of a US unit. A full discussion of ultrasound physics is beyond the scope of this text, but the following general information and imaging tips will likely be of utility to the anesthesiologist primarily through familiarization of ultrasound use for vascular access or image-guided procedures.

As with any procedure, the proper tool is critical for success. In the performance of any US exam, use of the correct US probe should be a priority. Anesthesiologists are generally familiar with high-frequency linear probes that are of greatest utility in evaluation of superficial structures and performance of vascular access procedures. Unfortunately, the utility of such probes in imaging deeper structures is limited, as high-frequency sound waves are rapidly attenuated by soft tissues, especially in the presence of reflective interfaces that occur in the chest and abdomen. A lower frequency (3–6 MHz) curved or vector probe is of greater utility in diagnostic examinations of the chest and abdomen. At interfaces of air and soft tissue, sound waves are highly attenuated, resulting in extensive shadowing and non-visualization of target tissues.[7] If US is to be used, a coupling gel of some kind between the probe and the skin surface is a necessity. This coupling gel may be dedicated US gel, surgical lubricant, saline, or even blood.

Once a coupling gel is acquired and the correct probe is available, the next consideration should be the depth of the target anatomy. The depth setting should be adequate to fully visualize the relevant anatomy, but not extend a great degree beyond it. If available, the US beam should be "focused" at the target level. This is typically performed by a specific knob on the unit that toggles a marker along the side of the imaging screen indicating the focal zone of the US beam. Even in the absence of focal zone selection capability, most modern portable US units have a button known as the "time-gain compensation" or more simply the "TGC," which will automatically adjust image gain (i.e. brightness) across the entire depth of the image to give a more homogeneous gray-scale appearance.

In a disaster scenario, a common indication for sonographic imaging is trauma. As a potential trauma team caregiver, anesthesiologists should have basic familiarity with a FAST (Focused Abdominal Sonography for Trauma) exam. Variations of the FAST exam are in use and have further demonstrated the use of US in various clinical scenarios.[8] The exam is readily performed by non-radiologists.[9] The determination of clinical competency across specialties is variable based on the professional society in question, and some have very modest requirements.[10] Of note, if significant hemoperitoneum is present, some literature supports that the hepatorenal fossa or "Morison's pouch" view alone is of greatest utility.[11]

Computed Tomography

Computed tomography (CT) is unlikely to be available in most disaster environments short of established facilities with reliable sources of power, or possibly aboard advanced floating platforms (e.g. hospital ships). If a hardened structure and a standard CT suite are present, the typical issues and limitations will likely parallel those found in most modern hospitals.

In some cases, a CT may be deployed into an austere environment within a freestanding isoshelter (Figure 17.4). The primary concern to the anesthesiologist in this situation is a severe limitation on physical space (Figure 17.5) while acting as the primary caregiver for a critically ill or injured patient. In this cramped space, personnel should be limited to those absolutely necessary to the care of the patient during imaging. Close proximity to the CT scanner demands attention to the many buttons on the face of the gantry cover that could impact functioning of the scanner. Emergency stop buttons and CT couch alignment sensors are the most easily triggered by the anesthesiologist during airway management. Awareness of these impact points is imperative so as not to impact CT function and delay potentially critical imaging exams. Portable ventilator and suction capability may be available in these spaces, and should be evaluated by the anesthesiologist prior to their use to ensure proper function. The limited space of such "remote" locations typically also means a dearth of readily available supplies or life-saving medications beyond what is brought by the anesthesiologists themselves.

When a large number of patients are to be imaged with a CT scanner in an isoshelter, the ambient temperature in which the scanner is placed is an important consideration.

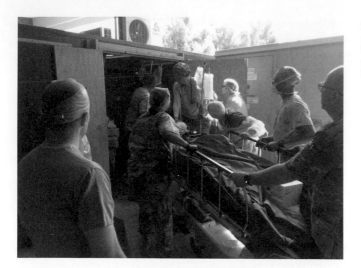

Figure 17.4 A patient being moved to an external isoshelter for CT scanning (image courtesy of Commander David Besachio, Medical Corps, US Navy).

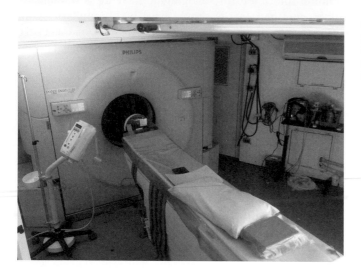

Figure 17.5 The cramped space in austere CT scanners will complicate anesthetic care (image courtesy of Commander David Besachio, Medical Corps, US Navy).

Excessive heat will rapidly render a CT scanner inoperable. Therefore, patient movement in and out of an isoshelter when ambient temperatures are elevated should be practiced routinely, with the goal of minimizing temperature elevations around the CT scanner. Once temperature limits are exceeded, modern scanners will not allow continued scanning.

Magnetic Resonance Imaging

As with CT, MRI will likely not be available in the disaster environment in the absence of higher-level resources. Nevertheless, issues surrounding MRI in the disaster setting will likely mirror those familiar to most anesthesiologists in the tertiary care setting with respect to the need for patient compliance, sedation, or paralysis, limitations on patient access, and consideration of types of anesthesia equipment that can be used near an MRI.

References

1. Amis SE, Butler PF, Applegate KE, et al. American College of Radiology white paper on radiation dose in medicine. *J Am Coll Radiol* 2007;**4**:272–284.

2. World Nuclear Association. Nuclear Radiation and Health Effects. www.world-nuclear.org/info/Safety-and-Security/Radiation-and-Health/Nuclear-Radiation-and-Health-Effects (accessed September 2019).

3. Domino D. Court transcripts don't resolve questions in Mad River CT case. AuntMinnie. 10 July 2010. www.auntminnie.com/index.aspx?sec=sup&sub=cto&pag=dis&ItemID=91193 (accessed September 2019).

4. Franquet T, Gimenez A, Roson N, et. al. Aspiration disease: findings, pitfalls, and differential diagnosis. *RadioGraphics* 2000;**20**:673–685.

5. Ferrara S. Interventional radiology in the austere environment. *Semin Intervent Radiol* 2010;**27**(1):3–13.

6. Andersen GN, Graven T, Skjetne K, et. al. Diagnostic influence of routine point-of-care pocket-size ultrasound examinations performed by medical residents. *J Ultrasound Med* 2015;**34**:627–636.

7. Feldman MK, Sanjeev K, Blackwood MS. US artifacts. *RadioGraphics* 2009;**29**:1179–1189.

8. Brook OR, Beck-Razi N, Abadi S, et al. Sonographic detection of pneumothorax by radiology residents as part of extended focused assessment with sonography for trauma. *J Ultra Med* 2009;**28**:749–755.

9. Shackford SR, Rogers FB, Osler TM, et al. Focused abdominal sonogram for trauma: the learning curve of nonradiologist clinicians in detecting hemoperitoneum. *J Trauma* 1999;**46**:553–562.

10. ACEP Emergency Ultrasound Imaging Criteria Compendium. www.acep.org/patient-care/policy-statements/Emergency-Ultrasound-Imaging-Criteria-Compendium (accessed September 2019).

11. McGahan JP. Richards JR. Blunt abdominal trauma: the role of emergent sonography and a review of the literature. *AJR* 2000;**172**:897–903.

Chapter 18

Communications

Marina Zuetell

Executive Summary

Hospitals and the healthcare systems are dependent upon reliable and redundant communication systems. Communications is the most common failure complaint following a disaster. When these systems fail, as they often do during a disaster or other event that puts an overload on normal ways of conducting business, there needs to be an ultimate, reliable fall-back solution. Volunteer communications experts, known as Amateur Radio operators can provide communications and hold things together until the commercial phones and radio systems can recover.

What is Amateur Radio?

Amateur Radio is a technical hobby that teaches people how to use two-way radio to communicate. Many people use the hobby to acquire new friends, contest, talk to the space shuttle, bounce signals off the moon, and experiment with radio and other technical aspects of the hobby. The Federal Communications Commission (FCC) has granted the Amateur Radio Service access to a wide variety of the radio spectrum, with the stipulation that it be used to develop new radio technologies and provide emergency communications (www.access.gpo.gov/nara/cfr/waisidx_04/47cfr97_04.html). The term "amateur" denotes that the operators are unpaid volunteers, not that they are unprofessional or unskilled. They are also called "hams," although the derivation of that term is lost to history.

There is one aspect of the hobby that serves a more serious mission – that of emergency communications. Amateur radio operators use their hobby to provide backup and emergency communications during disaster situations, and when normal communications fail. They like to communicate, and they volunteer their skills and interest by helping the agencies and organizations who rely on communications to fill the gap when things go wrong. Hurricanes, floods, earthquakes, tsunamis, and other geological events can cause complete or partial failure of the normal phone, cell phone, and commercial radio systems. So do man-made events such as the collapse of the World Trade Center towers or a large terrorism or bioterrorism event, where regular communication systems are overloaded or compromised.

There are two commonly known groups who provide these emergency communications. One of these is sponsored by the ARRL (Amateur Radio Relay League) (www.arrl.org) – the national organization for amateur radio; and the other is sponsored by the federal and local governments, an offshoot of the old Civil Defense system. Different operating requirements and restrictions apply to each:

- ARES®: Amateur Radio Emergency Service – Public service communications have been a traditional responsibility of the Amateur Radio Service since 1913. In those early days, such disaster work was spontaneous and without previous organization of any kind. In today's amateur radio, disaster work is a highly organized and worthwhile part of day-to-day operation, implemented principally by the Amateur Radio Emergency Service (ARES) and the National Traffic System (NTS), both sponsored by ARRL (www.arrl.org).
- RACES: Radio Amateur Civil Emergency Service is no longer referenced or supported by FEMA, although individual teams still exist within some local jurisdictions. Their primary mission is to provide communications support for local government jurisdictions. Other communications support activities are left to the ARES and ACS (Auxiliary Communications Service) groups.

Emergency service is one of the basics of the Amateur Radio Service and there is sometimes confusion about ARES, the ARRL branch of emergency services, and RACES, the government arm of amateur emergency services. ARES is activated before, during, and after an emergency. Generally, ARES handles all emergency messages, including those between government emergency management officials. As an example, the ARRL recruited ARES team members from all over the country to provide communications in response to the Katrina and Rita hurricanes. They supported field kitchens, mobile meal delivery, shelters, and wherever else they were needed, around the clock, for about six weeks. RACES, on the other hand, almost never starts before an emergency and is active only during the emergency and during the immediate aftermath, if government emergency management offices need communications support. RACES is normally shut down shortly after the emergency has cleared. Radio operations are limited to one hour of training per month, and team members can only be called upon by a government agency when there is a formal emergency declaration.

What Motivates "Hams" to Volunteer Their Time, Skills, and Equipment?

It is significant that Part 97 of the Federal Communications Commission's (FCC) Rules and Regulations states, as the first principle under "Basis and Purpose," the following: "Recognition and enhancement of the value of the amateur service to the public as a voluntary non-commercial communication service, particularly with respect to providing emergency communications." (www.access.gpo.gov/nara/cfr/waisidx_04/47cf r97_04.html). Amateur radio operators are encouraged to provide community and public service responses to various agencies and organizations, in return for the use of the radio spectrum they utilize.

There are only about 15–20% of licensed amateur radio operators who take this to heart and volunteer their time and belong to and participate in the activities of the ARES and RACES teams in their communities. Those who do usually spend a lot of time training and preparing for that big event when their services are really needed. The recent hurricanes on the East Coast are a perfect example of this. Amateur radio operators came from all over the country, at their own personal expense, to provide communications for the beleaguered government and non-government organizations.

External Hospital Communications

Hospitals need to be able to communicate with a variety of organizations and agencies without interruption. When these communication systems fail or are over-loaded, it places a huge stress on the facility's ability to serve its patients and provide safe and effective healthcare. During a routine business day, hospitals have a variety of means for communicating internally and with other hospitals, emergency medical systems (EMS), vendors, suppliers, and health departments, as well as patients and their families. If this is disrupted, because of a large mass casualty incident, a natural or man-made disaster, or even just a technological failure, communications become a huge problem. Building communication redundancy and flexibility into the hospital response system is a vital necessity. There are a variety of ways to do this:

1. Most hospitals already have a variety of radio communication systems, in addition to the normal land-line and cellular telephone systems. Sometimes these radio systems can take up the slack, but often they become overloaded as well. The HEAR (Hospital Emergency Administrative Radio) system is relatively common across the United States in hospitals and EMS units. It is often used for EMS units to notify hospitals that there are incoming casualties or patients. This system was developed in the 1960s and not much has been done to modify it, although there is some newer equipment available, which has improved the operations and ease of use. The technology is old enough that it is unlikely that it can ever be brought up to current inter-operability standards (APCO-25).

2. Other radio systems, in addition to, or replacement of, the HEAR system include UHF, VHF, 800 MHz, and others commonly used by public safety agencies (fire, EMS, police). These are used day-to-day to communicate with the hospitals, but often become overloaded when some unanticipated large-scale event occurs. Many facilities have satellite phones as well.

UHF/VHF/HF – These terms indicate various bands of the radio spectrum, each with its own characteristics for distance, penetration, and inter-agency communication. Ultra-high frequency (UHF: 300–3000 MHz) has shorter wavelengths, but greater penetration within a building; very-high frequency (VHF: 30–300 MHz) has somewhat longer wavelengths and distances, but works less well within the facility compound. High-frequency (HF: 1.8–30.0 MHz) is used for long-distance communications – across state or national boundaries, depending on the frequency band and antenna used (www.ntia.doc.gov/osmhome/allochrt.html).

The Amateur Radio Service has multiple segments of all of these bands, which allows it to be more versatile and responsive to various communication needs than many of the public safety radio systems.

HF system issues– there are a number of technological challenges to be aware of when using HF frequencies in the healthcare environment. Radios which transmit on these frequencies are often higher-powered than those on the UHF and VHF bands, and the antennas often have a stronger radiation pattern, which have the potential to interfere with medical telemetry and other biomedical equipment. Careful location and polarization of the antenna in or above patient-care areas need to be taken into consideration when installing HF radios in a hospital setting.

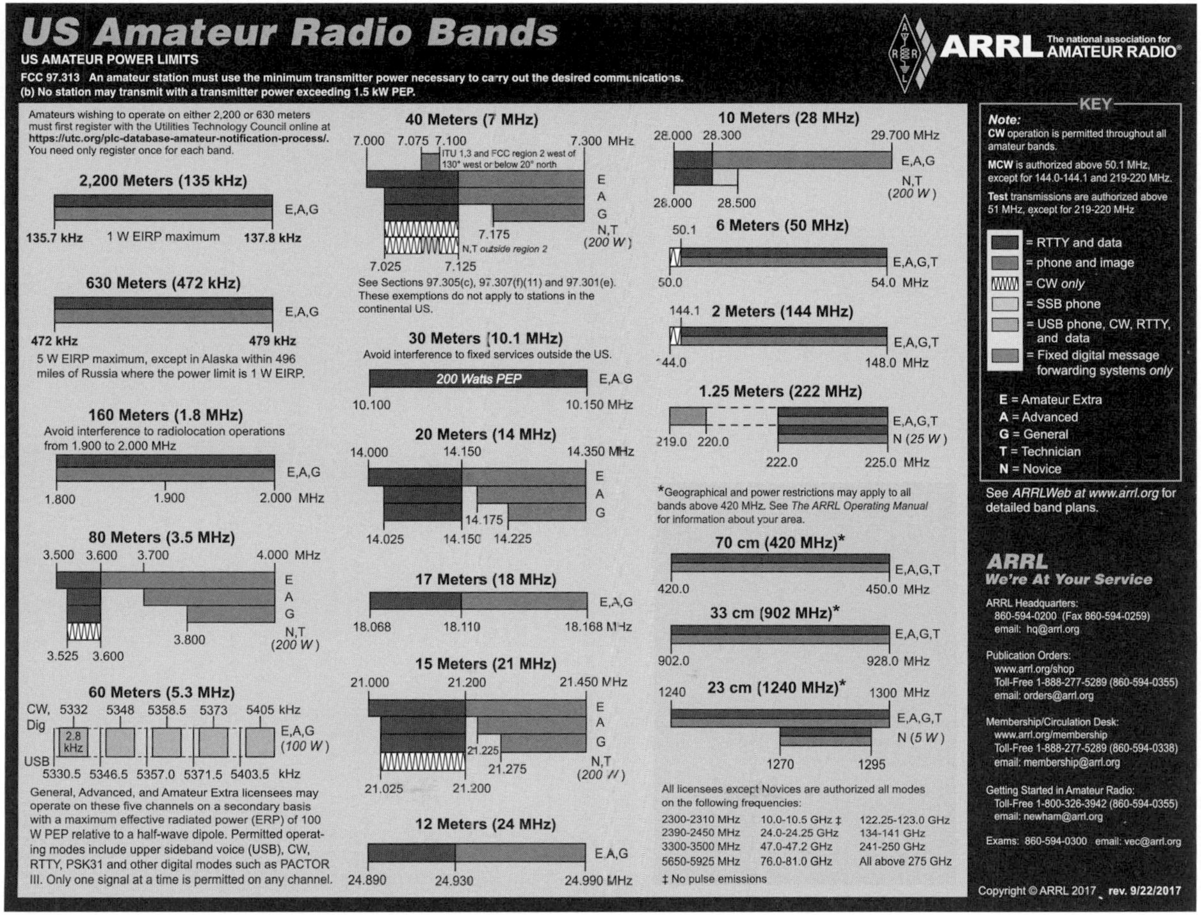

Figure 18.1 Amateur *Radio Spectrum Chart* showing band allocations (www.arrl.org/of/files/Fle/Regulatory/Band%20Chart/Hambands_grayscale.pdf)

Communication systems for hospitals, and other health care entities, depend on reliability, constancy, and redundancy. Systems need to be reliable; they need to be there all the time and they need to be redundant. It is strongly recommended that hospitals have a minimum of three redundant communication systems, in addition to the day-to-day landline and cellular phones, and data networks.

There are multiple anecdotal examples of how systems can fail, what other systems can replace or supplement them, and, when all else fails, who comes to the rescue:

- King County, WA –December 1998 – A large metropolitan hospital suffered a failure of a co-generation electrical system. A routine test of the cutover from commercial power to a new $5.9 million hospital co-generation system, with the failure of a $10.00 part, caused the evacuation of an entire hospital, potentially life-threatening patient care events, and huge loss of revenue. Most of the patients transferred out were not returned to the hospital after power was restored. This power failure lasted over eight hours.

- Clallam County, WA – February 2004 – A Port Angeles hospital reported that the entire community had lost Internet, 800, long distance, and Metro call paging as well as cell phone coverage. The call came via wireless cell phone from a cell tower on Vancouver Island, BC. This single Verizon cell phone was apparently the only means of communications outside of Port Angeles that the hospital was aware of. Their contingency plan, should they need aero-medical evacuation or other assistance would be to use this phone or someone would go to the nearby Coast Guard Station which had communication with Seattle Coast Guard. Due to topography (Olympic Mountains) there is no line of sight communications from Seattle to Port Angeles. Apparently a second cable failed at about 15:00 which caused a more significant loss of communication. Reasons for the failure of fiber-optic cables is still unknown.

- Lewis County, WA – February 2004 – Approximately 8:40 AM, the hospital's internal phone system went dead. Investigation identified that the UPS (uninterruptible power supply) failed, which shorted out the ability to turn on the backup battery function. The hospital's emergency fail-safe phones were turned on manually and were also affected. Some did not have dial tones. Some could make calls out of the facility, but could not get calls in. Additionally, staff members reported that they could not call out on their cell phones. Power was returned to the telephone system about 9:55 AM by re-wiring around the UPS. Hospital communications were limited for 2–3 hours.[1]

- Snohomish Co, WA – November 2013 – A fire in the main electrical room of a 217 bed hospital completely destroyed 95% of the electrical circuits in the hospital, which also took out all communications that depended on electricity – phones, radios, etc. The diesel generators that were in place to provide backup power never fired, because the electricity was gone. The fire was caused by a leaking water pump for a 3000 gallon water tank on the floor above the electrical vault – an engineering flaw from the 1960s. It was seven days before full power was restored.

Redundant Systems and Pathways

Every hospital communication system should have multiple routes for incoming and outgoing messages. Phone and electrical systems should have multiple access points to the facility, and multiple central office connections. Single-point access paths are bound to fail eventually. In addition to multiple access points, there should be a variety of systems to perform similar functions. Reliance on any single communication system could result in serious adverse events for the hospital. The capacity to do this depends on the telecommunications and information technology departments within the facility. Technology is expensive and complex, but lack of communications can be even more expensive in the long run.

Amateur radio can contribute significantly to recovery from a communications failure by providing backup emergency communications until normal systems are restored. In each of the above-mentioned events, amateur radio operators were called in to provide communications to support the hospital mission. Depending on the facility, these resources were used to greater or lesser degree. But each facility learned that the amateur radio operators could provide the necessary links to keep life-safety and basic, essential communication functioning. Amateur radio has the advantage of being frequency-agile (meaning the ability to change frequencies and bands readily, which most public-safety and commercial radios cannot do), communications-savvy, and knowledgeable as to what services operate on which frequency bands. They can usually contact the necessary agencies, or route information to them, using the assigned amateur radio frequencies, or by linking the radio to a telephone-patch (see Figure 18.1).

Amateur radio operators commonly support many different communication activities. These include hospital–hospital, hospital–emergency operation center (EOC), hospital-field sites (usually mass casualty incidents), internal inter-departmental communications, and hospital–medical suppliers. Wherever portable communications are needed, amateur radio operators can usually go.

Where Can a Hospital or Health Care System Find Amateur Radio Resources?

Often the best recruiting source is within the staff of the facility, or within the ranks of hospital volunteers, or even patient populations. Recruitment ads in hospital newsletters, employee and patient bulletin boards, etc. often produce immediate results. However, often times staff members will be required to perform their professional assignments during a disaster, and won't be available for "radio" duty. They can be useful for making that initial call, or serving until outside volunteers can arrive.

If internal recruiting doesn't work, then contacting the local ARES Emergency Coordinator and requesting their assistance is the next step. Usually, the local emergency management agency will know who that is; or you can access the ARRL web page to find out who to contact (www.arrl.org/sections). Once you have identified some radio operators, then the task is to form them into a hospital-focused team. This is the job of the emergency coordinator, but he or she will need help from the health care providers, for they need some orientation to hospital culture, operations, and hierarchy. In many locations, there may not be enough operators to dedicate to a specific mission, and they will be shared with emergency management, search and rescue, and other mission-oriented tasks. There are some hams who choose not to support these other government-focused groups, but would be really enthusiastic about supporting "their" hospital, so it is definitely worth asking the question, or sending out a special invitation.

The operators will need some training to familiarize them with how the hospital works, and special needs and concerns when working in this environment. Some suggested topics include:

- Orientation to hospital environment and culture
- HIPAA Awareness – (Health Insurance Portability and Accountability Act)
- HICS – (Hospital Incident Command System) last revised in 2014
- Medical radio systems
- First aid, CPR, and blood-borne pathogens
- Working in a professional/business environment
- NIMS Awareness – (National Incident Management System) IS-700.A and IS-100.HC.

(The last two classes are ones that are required of many hospital personnel if they are recipients of Homeland Security or Health and Human Services grants.)

Most ham radio operators have their own radios, and are well prepared to bring their kits with them; however, an appropriate antenna installed on the hospital roof will vastly improve the signal strength and distance that the operator can reach, when talking to facilities or agencies outside the hospital. This will also lessen the effect of any radio signals within the hospital environment. To go one step further, installing amateur radios in a secure location within the building will speed up the process of getting communications up and running when they are needed. It takes time to bring in equipment, set it up, test it, and then start operations.

It is important that radio operators be given regular access to the installed radio equipment. They need to be familiar with the operation of it, and also to verify that it is operational when needed. There have been frequent instances where roofers have taken down antennas, or someone has cut the coaxial feed line, or the radios become inoperable for some other reason. Without regular testing, they might not be available when really needed. Additionally, it is beneficial for the radio operators to train and interact with the hospital staff, so that they become comfortable with the hospital environment. Incorporating radio operators into the twice-yearly required disaster exercises familiarizes both sides with how each functions in an event.

In the event of a switchboard or power failure situation, internal communications can be carried out within the hospital campus using portable radios between departments or floors. The UHF band usually works best because of the wavelength and penetration characteristics. This usage can be combined with external-to-the-hospital communications, using the amateur radio antenna installed on the roof. If this is a localized emergency, the outside antenna can be used to stay in contact with public safety or other hospitals, and the portables can be used to communicate and coordinate between hospital departments. There are a few areas of the buildings where radio waves don't penetrate well, such as shielded radiology suites, basement areas, etc., but for a limited time this support should be adequate.

Amateur radio is not limited to purely voice transmission. There are a number of digital forms of communications that allow the conversion of computer digital information to radio analog signals which can be sent over the airwaves, and then converted back to computer format at the receiving end. This facilitates the sending of large amounts of data, such as lists of supplies, damage assessment reports, or even email. Higher transmission speeds and bandwidth will allow diagrams, photos, maps, etc.

Additionally, there is another protocol that incorporates the use of amateur television to send live video feeds from the field, such as a mass casualty incident, back to the hospital or emergency operations center. While not used widely as yet, this format has tremendous potential for keeping the emergency managers or Emergency Department personnel apprised of what the scene looks like. It also has the capability of providing damage assessment information via either portable cameras in so-called "windshield" surveys, or through fixed camera sites in key areas.

Hospital Disaster Plan

Make sure that the hospital's disaster plan incorporates using amateur radio for backup communications, and that there is a slot on the organization chart for communications, (which is different from the liaison–public information officer position). Often, the technical communications position falls under logistics, but not always. Also make sure that you invite the volunteers to practice and train with the hospital when it conducts drills and exercises. The ham radio person should have a vest, and a job action sheet, like every other member in the HICS plan of action (Figure 18.2).

Expeditionary Medical Operations

Amateur Radio is also an essential communication mode when deploying to a disaster-stricken area. The inclusion of at least one dedicated communications operator and several other licensed personnel will guarantee the ability to communicate regardless of the degree of infrastructure degradation. A careful consideration of equipment portability, power needs, and bandwidth requirements will help to delineate the level of communications support needed.

Summary and Conclusions

Hospitals depend on reliable and redundant communications to provide safe and effective health care to patients. Most of the time, wired and wireless telephone systems provide the majority of the communication "transactions," and some use of public safety or commercial radio systems is used to augment this. Treatment orders, tests, information requests, supplies, and pharmaceutical orders are all relayed by some form of telephone, radio, or computer system. Patients are delivered or discharged using phones, radios, etc. What would happen if, suddenly, all these communication systems failed?

Hospital disaster plans should include alternative and redundant communication methods, and they should be trained on and practiced right along with other elements of an exercise or drill.

Amateur radio operators, also known as hams, are experienced, trained emergency communicators who are volunteers. Their services are free; they really enjoy performing their special service and using their skills. They usually bring their own equipment, although having equipment in the hospital ready to go will speed up the response time. They can provide both internal and external communications, and they have use of a wide variety of radio frequencies and modes. They can free up hospital personnel to perform patient care, and leave the monitoring of radios, and sending and receiving messages to those who really like to do that.

Amateur radio is an excellent resource that should be included in every hospital's planning for response and recovery.

Hospital Incident Command System
Job Description
AMATEUR RADIO OPERATOR

Date: _____ Start: _____ End: _____Position Assigned To: _____ Init: _____

TAC ID: _____ (Radio Title)

Position Reports To: _____ (Logistics Officer or Designated Contact) Sign _____
Hospital Command Center Locations: _____
Telephone: _____ Fax: _____ Other Contact Info: _____

Mission: **To provide communication either external or internal during times when normal hospital communications have failed or been disrupted.**

Immediate (Operational Period 0-2 Hours)	Time	Initial
Put on emergency medical team identification.		
Check in at Incident Command Center (ICC).		
Receive Section package with Job Action Sheet, etc.		
Read this entire Job Action Sheet.		
Obtain briefing from Designated Contact or Incident Commander (IC).		
Begin documenting your actions on an Activity Log & Action Plan Log.		
Turn these forms into Documentation Supervisor at the end of incident.		
Set up radio in designated location and assure functioning.		
Check in with Net Control (NC) via amateur radio and follow any instructions given.		
If NC not available, check in with the local emergency operations net and follow any instructions given.		
Communicate directly with Logistics Officer, or designee, about any urgent communications.		

Intermediate (Operational Period 2-12 Hours)	Time	Init.
Obtain situation status report from NC.		
Relay hospital status to net control as required.		
Log all relevant communication including messages sent or received.		
Ensure messages requiring action are followed up according to message precedence.		
Do not leave amateur radio without coordination with net control.		
Request a runner from the Personnel Pool – request runner to stop at scheduled intervals.		
Post all messages where a runner can take them to the ICC.		
Communicate directly with Designated Contact or IC in urgent communications.		

Figure 18.2 – Amateur radio job action sheet for Hospital Incident Command System (HICS).

Hospital Incident Command System
Job Description
AMATEUR RADIO OPERATOR

	Time	Init.
Respond to external requests by NC for additional information on hospital status. Hospital status is obtained from the ICC via Designated Contact or IC		

Extended (Operational Period Beyond 12 Hours)	**Time**	**Init.**
Do not leave your post until released by Incident Commander.		
Request relief operator from NC if prior arrangements have not been made.		
Turn in all documentation in to Documentation Supervisor.		
Secondary operators may be used in the following ways:		
• To provide internal communications within hospital with assignment to specific location or with specified people.		
• Assist with other communications (i.e. HEAR, 800MHz, telephone).		
Radio operator's relief checklist. When a new operator arrives to relieve, the following steps are taken:		
• Identify new operator to current operator		
• Obtain briefing from current operator including any pending actions		
• Ensure new operator is familiar with radio equipment including frequencies in use.		
• Identify new operator to Logistics Officer or Designated Contact or IC.		
• New operator checks in with NC		
• Log the change of shift and any significant pending issues.		

Figure 18.2 (cont.)

Author

Marina H. Zuetell, N7LSL, is President of Western Washington Medical Services Communications and Assistant Section Emergency Coordinator for Medical Services Communications for the W. WA. Section of ARES. She has been a Communications Technology Specialist contractor for the Washington State Department of Health from 2004 to 2015, and private communications consultant for health care, as MHz Consulting Services, in 2015. Further information can be obtained by contacting the author at N7LSL@ARRL.NET.

References

1. Zuetell M. Providing efficient healthcare when the phones fail. *Washington Family Physician*, 2004;**31**(2):30–32.

Further Reading

ARRL – Amateur Radio Relay League – www .arrl.org/ (accessed September 2019)

ARRL – www.arrl.org/emergency-communi cations-training (accessed September 2019)

FEMA Emergency Management Institute – https://training.fema.gov/emi.aspx (accessed September 2019)

Hospital Disaster Support Communications System – www.hdscs.org (accessed September 2019)

Western Washington Medical Services Communications – www.ww7mst.org (accessed September 2019)

Zuetell M, Mariotti D. Ham system helps hospitals in disasters. *Public Safety Communications*, 2006 March, pp. 38–39.

Chapter 19

Security in Disaster Anesthesia

Martin Graves and Corry Kucik

A disaster may occur through natural or man-made events. It can be the result of war, terrorist events, or through so-called acts of god such as floods, tsunamis, earthquakes, and droughts. The international anesthetist may be called upon to serve in these areas in surgical teams as part of a medical response, or may simply be passing through. Whilst the "disaster zone" will be inherently more dangerous than your operating theatre at home there are things you can do to mitigate the risk.

What is the Threat?

When responding to a disaster you now have the same risks as the population that you are there to help. In addition, whether a disaster is man-made or caused by nature, the population will now be struggling to survive and you may be seen as a way of improving their financial or ideological situation.

In 2012, 176 acts of violence were carried out against aid workers resulting in 274 aid workers being killed, kidnapped, or seriously wounded, and the rate of kidnapping of aid workers has been rising over the last 10 years.[1] International medical workers are targeted more in kidnapping compared to local medical staff.

Risk to medical staff in disaster zones can be divided into non-violent and violent or criminal risks.

Non-Violent Risks

In the immediate aftermath of a natural disaster the population having survived the initial risk are now at risk from a further set of problems. Following an earthquake or flood, buildings will be damaged and therefore unsafe. They may collapse at any moment, or they may have dangers inside such as live electricity, jagged and rusty metal, or broken glass.

When setting up your treatment area, if you use existing buildings you should ensure that they are safe prior to allowing your team to enter. Many Non-Government Organisations (NGOs) have engineers, plumbers, or electricians attached to them performing other roles such as provision of clean water. These personnel will prove vital in the assessment of suitable accommodation and working areas for your medical team.

There may still be a requirement to enter unsafe areas to extract or treat casualties of the natural disaster. In these cases you should make a quick risk assessment of the situation before rushing in to help, as if you are injured there is now one more casualty and one less responder. Ensure you have adequate protective equipment. This equipment may be in short supply, and so it may be best to deploy with it. A non-exhaustive list includes:

1. Overalls or coveralls
2. Sturdy boots
3. Safety helmet
4. Thick gloves
5. Eye protection
6. Disposable treatment gloves
7. High visibility jacket.

Whilst it is tempting in a tropical area to wear flip-flops and board shorts, comfort from the heat may place you at risk from a preventable accident.

Infectious Diseases

The disaster will have disrupted local infrastructure such as sewerage, plumbing, and electricity. Much of the local population will have no shelter and there may be a large proportion of refugees. These factors all lead to an increase in the threat of infectious diseases such as malaria, dengue fever, and diarrheal disease. In order to provide the best care for the population you must ensure your and your team's health. This is best done through preventive measures as follows.

Preventing Vector-Borne Diseases

1. Regular use of insect repellant (containing DEET)
2. Impregnating clothing with permethrin
3. Wearing long sleeves and pants at night
4. Sleeping under a mosquito net or dome
5. Removing potential mosquito breeding sites such as water buckets and coconut shells
6. Regular fogging and spraying of insecticide
7. Malarial preventative medication (doxycycline, mefloquine, or chloroquine in non-resistant areas).

Preventing Diarrheal Disease

1. Use of safe water for drinking, cooking, and brushing teeth
2. Washing hands regularly and after toileting (e.g. with personal alcohol-based cleaner)
3. Setting up a cleaning station for food utensils
4. Avoiding local food that is not piping hot
5. Proper siting of toilets.

Treatment of Drinking Water

Water may be treated by filtering, boiling, or by addition of chlorine or iodine. If planning for a group you should estimate the requirement of 10 liters of water per person per day.

There are many commercial filters available through camping stores. They are reasonably cheap and easy to use. Most will remove protozoa and bacteria, but often the size of the filter pores are such that they don't filter out viruses such as hepatitis A. Such a filter will require the added use of chlorine- or iodine-based treatments. The filters will last longer if larger particles are removed first. This can be done by filtering through clean cloth or coffee filters.

Boiling will kill most protozoa, viruses, and bacteria. To be effective the treated water needs to be kept at 80° for greater than 60 seconds. The best way to ensure this is to bring the water to boil for 10 seconds prior to allowing it to slowly cool.

Chlorine treatments are available in tablet form, with each tablet normally treating one liter of water. The process takes 20 minutes to effectively treat all infective organisms in the water, however its effectiveness is reduced by the presence of semi-solids in the water. Cloudy water should be filtered before adding the chlorine. If treating large quantities pool chlorine or household bleach is as effective and may be more convenient. The bleach must be simple unscented bleach. Twenty liters of water requires half a teaspoon of granulated pool chlorine or 1 ml of 6% hypochlorite bleach. Two drops of iodine will treat one liter of drinking water. This is readily available to surgical teams in the form of betadine.

Road Traffic Accident

One of the biggest risk to travelers in the Third World is being involved in a road traffic accident (RTA). Many Third World cities have congested roads filled with unsafe vehicles. Road rules are often different to those in the travelers' home countries and cars may be driven on the opposite side of the road too. Locals may use a different form of indication. In many nations rather than using an indicator, honking the horn signals an intention to do something. This can lead to an increased incidence of RTAs. On the upside most traffic is traveling at a reduced speed compared with First World nations, which may reduce the chances of being seriously injured if involved in an RTA.

Drivers should avoid distractions such as radios or talking on the phone, along with driving under the influence of drugs or alcohol. They should plan a route and study it prior to embarking on a road trip. As the risk from an impact is likely to be greater than the risk of entrapment, driver and passengers should wear seatbelts. The driver should avoid speeding and always allow a safe distance between their vehicle and the one in front. This will depend upon road conditions.

In RTAs, there may be an issue of compensation. If the medical aid worker is perceived as being wealthy it may lead to a situation where compensation is demanded. Local police may also see this as an opportunity to obtain money by way of a bribe through charging the aid worker with an offence. If it appears that the situation is starting to become dangerous for you after being involved in an RTA it may be prudent to move to a safe area such as your work place or a local embassy.

Vehicle Issues

You should ensure the vehicle is always fueled. It should be refilled when it gets to below half a tank to prevent running out in an emergency situation. A spare container of fuel is a good idea, but must be stored properly as petrol and diesel are dangerous goods. Fuel may be in short supply in a disaster and people may try to siphon fuel from your vehicle for use in their own vehicle or for use in a generator, for cooking etc. You can minimize the risk of this by ensuring the vehicle is parked in a secure area, and by using a locking fuel cap.

The vehicle should always be prepared for an emergency. There should be stores inside including drinking water, emergency food rations, first aid equipment, a torch, and communications equipment.

Vehicles should be parked in a well-lit area if possible and facing front out, this avoids reversing in an emergency. Before leaving a vehicle the driver should ensure that all windows are up, doors are locked, and there are no attractive items on display.

You should avoid posting stickers or signs on the vehicle that may upset or inflame situations. Whilst you may be proud of your nation there may be individuals in the country that you are in that have pre-conceived attitudes towards your country and its government. Medical stickers and signs may garner good will from some people; however, this must be balanced by the fact that certain criminal organizations may perceive that there are medical goods inside that will be of value to them on the black market.

Vehicles should be checked regularly to ensure they are road worthy. Daily checks should include:

1. Tyre condition and pressure, including spare
2. Brake and indicator lights
3. Head lights and tail lights
4. Fuel level
5. Oil and windscreen washing fluid
6. Horn
7. Cleaning of windscreen and windows if dirty.

Violent Risks

Criminal Activity

Following disaster situations there is often a breakdown of law enforcement. There may be looting, which may in turn lead to violence. You may be perceived as being a soft target and viewed as a wealthy Westerner. You should avoid wearing jewelry or carrying expensive items (remember that what you perceive to be a cheap camera or watch may be an attractive item and even costume jewelry may look to be expensive).

Your most valuable items in the disaster situation are your passport, money (particularly US dollars), credit cards, and phone, if functioning. You can protect these items with the use of money belts or neck wallets. It is a good idea to have a photocopy of your passport and travel documents which can secured in your hotel room safe. Copies can also be saved using an internet cloud-based storage or by emailing yourself a copy.

Credit cards may have limited use in a disaster situation; however, they are easy to carry and the use of a travel debit card will reduce the risk of your personal bank accounts being drained by cyber criminals. Cash is always reliable, especially an internationally recognized currency like US dollars or Euros. It is wise to carry some of these types of currency separately to your wallet in case you are the victim of a hold-up. Carrying a small amount of local currency for this possible event may appease an opportunistic petty criminal. It is better to give up a small amount of money than be the victim of violence.

If you have a large amount of money, for example to pay local hospital workers or to purchase supplies, it may be safer to leave this at a hotel if you have one. Placing it in the hotel safe as apposed to the room safe places the hotel liable for any loss.

You may be carrying a significant amount of medical stores that could be vital to your mission. These stores and equipment (especially drugs of addiction) may be very attractive to thieves and black marketeers. Your medical team should be vigilant to theft of these stores, particularly when in transit. You may be able to deploy with a small safe or obtain one locally that you can use to store restricted medications. This may also provide a place to secure your team's passports and money.

Security of Your Accommodation

Staying in a more secure part of town will increase your security. You can enhance the security of your hotel room by:

1. Not opening the door to persons you do not know
2. Use of the door chain when you are in the room
3. Placing your foot up against the door so it can not be forced open if answering the door
4. Carrying a rubber window wedge that you can jam under the door to reduce the risk of it being forced open while you are in the room
5. Sleeping with your clothes ready to be put on and your important documents in a bag ready if you need to move suddenly
6. You should attempt to accommodate all team members in the same area of the hotel. It may be safer for team members to share a room rather than be alone.

Vital Documents

1. Passport
2. Money (local, US dollars, Euros)
3. Credit cards
4. Mobile phone
5. List of contact numbers
6. Local area maps.

Terrorism

Kidnapping

Caregivers in a disaster zone are at risk of being taken hostage by a number of different groups for a host of different motives. The group may be a criminal organization with a monetary aim, demanding a ransom from your national government, family, or the organization that you work for, or a militant group who will use you to achieve political goals such as overthrowing the local government, demanding release of prisoners, or gaining publicity. In general, foreign aid workers are more likely to be taken for political gains than financial ones. It is possible that once taken hostage the aid worker might be sold on from one criminal group or terrorist organization to another for financial or some other gain. In the past decade 80% of foreign aid workers taken hostage have eventually been released.

Kidnapping can occur in any situation whilst in a disaster zone. It could occur at the hotel, at your medical facility, outside in the street, or in your vehicle moving from your hotel to the medical facility.

Being away from your work or living area will be when you are most vulnerable. The threat is likely to have been planned and you may have been under surveillance for some time.

You should make every effort to ensure planning an attack against you is difficult. To do this:

1. Ensure you and your group are properly briefed by your organization's security advisor for local threats
2. Plan safe routes when driving
3. Avoid always traveling by the same route and at the same time
4. Inform other members of the team of your movements and when to expect your return. Brief them on what to do if you do not return by the expected time
5. Watch out for individuals or vehicles that appear to be following or watching you
6. Be alert to ruses that may be used to hijack you while driving, such as an accident, fake detours, road blocks, or your vehicle being deliberately run into by another large vehicle or van
7. Be aware of unusual absence of the local population
8. Allow enough distance between your vehicle and the one in front when stopped so you can pull around it and not be boxed in by other vehicles should a threat eventuate
9. Coast slowly to a red light to avoid stopping completely
10. If stopped at traffic lights or stop signs leave the vehicle in gear to allow a quick get away.
11. Have your phone loaded with an emergency number that you can call in the event of a threat. The phone may be able to be set up so that this number is called automatically when you press the call button
12. Ensure your phone is always fully charged
13. Keep windows and doors locked, in a hot environment this may require an air conditioner
14. Park rear to curb so you don't have to reverse out in an emergency
15. When approaching your vehicle have your keys ready and only open your door rather than using central locking as this may give an attacker access to your vehicle
16. Before getting in the vehicle perform a quick once over to ensure no one has tampered with it. Leaving sticky tape surreptitiously on part of the door can identify if someone has opened it in your absence.

You should rehearse in your mind what you are going to do and the route to a safe place if you are placed in a car-hijacking situation. Should it occur, sounding your horn will attract attention and possibly place the attackers off guard. The use of high beams may temporarily blind your attackers at night, allowing you to take evasive action and get away.

Escape maneuvers include:

1. Swerving and driving past the attackers
2. Reversing away from the blockage
3. Turning your vehicle around and driving off in the opposite direction
4. Ramming the other vehicle or obstruction out of the way.

A vehicle will jump the gutter if hit at a 45° angle traveling at a speed of 40 to 50 km per hour. The best place to ram the attackers' vehicle is adjacent to the rear wheels at an angle of 45°. This gives the best chance of spinning the attackers' vehicle, as the engine makes the front heavier than the rear. If the roadblock consists of two cars you should aim your vehicle at the gap between the two cars. Be aware that any impact may cause injury to yourself, your passengers, or innocent bystanders. An impact may also result in the vehicle being disabled foiling your getaway, and if your vehicle is fitted with airbags they may deploy, which could impair your vision.

Hostage Situation

In the event of being taken hostage, your chance of escape is likely be best at the start; however, this time may also be the most dangerous as your attackers will be armed and possibly inexperienced with the use of weapons. The hostage-takers will have planned this and so will try to catch you off guard to improve their success. Your immediate actions can include:

1. Screaming, yelling, and attracting attention to yourself
2. Use of violence may deter your attacker, however it may also result in you being injured, but you may be fighting for your life
3. Simple methods of keeping your attacker at bay like punching while holding a set of keys in your hand. Other defense techniques to help you in hostage situations can be learned through attending a self-defense class.

If you are taken hostage try to remain calm. You will still have adrenaline circulating from the fight or flight response so you must actively work to regain your composure.

Be observant of your attackers and your surroundings, you will almost certainly have a bag placed over your head to obstruct your vision and your arms and legs may be bound or zip tied; however, you should try to make mental notes of:

1. Your attackers:
   a. How many of them are there?
   b. What do they look like?
   c. How old are they?
   d. What are they wearing?
   e. What weapons are they carrying?
   f. Do they appear well prepared or amateurish?
   g. Are they using names?
2. The route:
   a. How long does it take to get where you are going?
   b. What direction are you heading?
   c. What sounds can you hear?
3. Yourself:
   a. Have you been injured?
   b. How secure are your restraints?

Remember that the hostage-takers want you for a reason and so will most likely try to keep you safe. You will be flooded with emotions such as fear, guilt about worrying loved ones, and anger at your attackers and at yourself for letting yourself get into such a situation. You will improve your chances of getting through the event by remaining calm and keeping yourself as healthy as possible.

Your government will be trying to get you home safely through negotiation and rescue. There will be professional experts in hostage rescue preparing to get you home safely. You can make help them by preparing yourself for when the time comes.

1. Keep yourself healthy:
   a. Make sure you eat and drink
   b. Try to maintain your hygiene as best as you can
   c. If you have any injuries or wounds try to get your attackers to have them treated, or treat them yourself with whatever you have available
   d. Try to exercise. Simple things like walking round the room regularly and stretching will help to maintain your strength for rescue or an escape attempt and will help you psychologically
2. Try to hold onto your possessions. These may be useful for:
   a. Bartering with guards
   b. Maintaining protection against the elements (particularly cold and insect bites)
   c. Give you a psychological lift
3. Take anything that your captors offer. Even if you do not smoke, a cigarette may be used to barter with another guard
4. Try to have your captors view you as a human and build rapport with them. Engaging the guards with conversation about their family may result in more favorable treatment. Try to give your captor a reason to view you with respect.
5. If there are other hostages try to stay in contact with them. If they are panicking or overtly hostile towards your captors attempt to calm them as this may inflame the situation.

When security forces make a rescue do not panic, as you will be at risk of injury from your captors as well as the rescuers. If you have been a while in captivity, your appearance may have changed and you may look very similar to your captors. Follow your rescuers' instructions and answer their questions. You may be handled roughly or even be restrained by your rescuers. Remember they are doing this for your safety so do not fight or resist them.

Following the safe return of a hostage there is often a requirement for further medical or psychological support. It is worthwhile finding out from your organization what level of insurance cover they have for you if you are abducted while deployed.

Improvised Explosive Devices

Improvised explosive devices (IEDs) are home-made bombs using conventional military explosives or a mixture of chemicals. They have become the weapon of choice for terrorists as they are cheap, easy to manufacture, and can cause significant injury. In the second Iraq war, 63% of coalition deaths were caused by IEDs.[1] They may be set up to cause injury to a pedestrian or designed to take out a car or armored vehicle. Often they contain home-made shrapnel such as nails or ball bearings to increase their lethality. They will normally be placed in an area of high use by the terrorists' targets and may be placed well in advance of an attack. They may be detonated by a simple pressure device or from a distance using a switch connected to the device by a wire or an electronic remote control.

Paying attention to your surroundings is the best way to protect yourself against these devices. Signs of possible IEDs include:

1. Avoidance of an area by locals
2. Rubbish normally scavenged by locals stacked by the roadside
3. Signs of recent digging adjacent to the road

4. Visible wires
5. Marking by locals, such as rocks stacked on one another.

If the device is remotely detonated you may observe the perpetrator watching your movement or reporting on it via a mobile device. There may also be a simple sighting system for the device such as two rocks that are aligned between the firing point and the device.

In the event of being around an IED attack, be aware that terrorists sometimes plant a secondary device, detonating it when first responders arrive to treat the injured.

Devices have been planted on injured patients being taken into medical facilities with the intent of injuring the medical personnel working there. While government and military facilities are more likely to be the object of attack it is possible that an NGO surgical team responding to a disaster situation may be targeted.

A Final Word on Preparation

Serving on a disaster response mission can benefit the anesthetist, both professionally and personally. Your experience will be all the more rewarding if you stay safe by preparing yourself physically and mentally for the challenges ahead. Time spent researching the security situation before deploying, while other preparations might appear to be of higher importance, is a must for the international anesthetist.

References

1.   Harmer A, Stoddard A, Toth K. Aid Worker Security Report 2013: Humanitarian Outcomes. https://aidworkersecurity.org/sites/default/files/AidWorkerSecurityReport_2013_web.pdf (accessed September 2019).

Further Reading

EASO Afghanistan country of origin information report. Insurgent strategies: intimidation and targeted violence against Afghans. www.ecoi.net/en/file/local/1314553/90_1354794367_easo-2012-12-afghanistan-insurgents.pdf (accessed September 2019).

Elgafi S. Medical liability in humanitarian missions. *J Humanitar Assist* 11 Nov 2014.

IFRC. Volunteers, stay safe! A security guide for volunteers. https://media.ifrc.org/ifrc/wp-content/uploads/sites/5/2018/03/Volunteer-Security-manualENGLISH.pdf (accessed September 2019).

Saferworld. Issue paper 3: Addressing conflict and violence from 2015. November 24 2012. www.saferworld.org.uk (accessed September 2019).

Stoddard A, Harmer A, Haver K. Providing aid in insecure environments: trends in policy and operations. Humanitarian Policy Group Sept 2006; Briefing Paper 24.

US Department of Agriculture. Kidnapping and Hostage Survival Guidelines. www.wrc.noaa.gov/wrso/security_guide/kidnap.htm (accessed September 2019).

US Department of Agriculture. Defensive Driving Overseas. www.wrc.noaa.gov/wrso/security_guide/driving.htm#Driving (accessed September 2019).

US Department of Agriculture. Security and Safety Recommendations. www.wrc.noaa.gov/wrso/security_guide/safety.htm (accessed September 2019).

UNODC. Statistics on crime: kidnapping. www.unodc.org/unodc/en/data-and-analysis/statistics/crime.html (accessed September 2019).

Chapter 20

International Humanitarian Law

Christopher M. Burkle

Introduction

Sadly, war has perhaps been one of the few constants throughout the history of humanity.[1] This has in turn necessitated rules and law that place boundaries on these hostilities. International humanitarian law is applicable in times of armed conflict, while human rights law provides protection during both war and peacetime. The present basis for international humanitarian law (IHL) rests with international treaties and customary international law (CIL).[2,3]

Treaty-Based IHL

As a jurist and diplomat, Grotius is known as the father of the "law of nations."[2,4] Yet it was not until Henry Dunant in the nineteenth century that contemporary international humanitarian law took shape.[2] Dunant with other founders of the International Committee of the Red Cross (ICRC) prompted the Swiss government to convene a meeting of sixteen States who ultimately adopted the Geneva Convention for the Amelioration of the Condition of the Wounded in Armies in the Field.[2,4] The 1864 Geneva Convention (GC), in addition to other facets, helped to ensure respect for medical personnel and equipment, along with the protections implied to these with markings of a red cross with a white background.[4] The GC was revised over the years since 1864 and has resulted in the four GCs of 1949:

- GGC for the Amelioration of the Condition of the Wounded and Sick in Armed Forces in the Field
- GC for the Amelioration of the Condition of the Wounded, Sick, and Shipwrecked Members of Armed Forces at Sea
- GC relative to the Treatment of Prisoners of War
- GC relative to the Protection of Civilian Persons in Time of War

The necessity of four GCs evolved from the changing environment of modern warfare. Since enactment, new wars and hostilities continue to challenge and pierce the boundaries of prior protective clauses as is reflected in individual State governments adopting their own treaties regulating conflicts.[2] Two Additional Protocols to the GC of 1949 were added in 1977 to help mesh these bodies of humanitarian law in a changing war time environment. These Additional Protocols were implemented in large part as a response to increases in guerrilla warfare developments and weapon technology leading to greater civilian harm.[5] Additional Protocol I affords protections in times of international conflict, while Additional Protocol II tackles those concerns occurring during non-international hostilities. These two Additional

Protocols, along with the Four GCs of 1949, form the basis for treaty-based rules governing protections during conflicts.[2] Since the GC of 1949 and the Additional Protocols set in place in 1977, States themselves have added additional treaties to assist in managing unique aspects of protections due during times of hostility.[2] These needed additions speak to the fluid nature involved with trying to adjust provided protections through treaty-based IHL following constant advances in conventional and unconventional tactics of war.

Customary International Law (CIL)-Based IHL

Jacob Kellenberger, the former President of the ICRC, has suggested the continued importance of CIL as an addition to treaty-based IHL.[2] First, CIL can help interpret treaty-based IHL.[2] Second, treaty-based IHL is best suited to protect during internationally based conflicts, but less comprehensive in protections associated with non-internationally based hostilities.[2] CIL agreements of States often provide rules applicable to all conflicts without reference to their international or non-international status.[3] Lastly, the Four GCs are abided to by all States, yet the two Additional Protocols and other treaties are applicable to only those States that have ratified them. CIL is considered "general" international law and therefore requires all States and parties to a conflict to adhere to its tenets.[2]

Protection of Humanitarian-Based Medical Services

Articles 55 and 56 of the Fourth GC places a duty on States to provide to the fullest extent possible, medical care and public health services to the population during times of armed conflict.[6,7] As a means of ensuring this important need, together the Four GCs of 1949, the two Additional Protocols approved in 1977, along with CIL form the basis of protection for humanitarian efforts directed to medical care during times of international and non-international hostilities throughout the world. The discussion below provides excerpts from these IHL sources that relate directly and indirectly to medical-based humanitarian protection.

International Conflict Protection

Medical Personnel

Medical personnel that are "exclusively engaged" in medical duties are to be both protected and respected under the First GC and the Fourth GC. Article 15 in Additional Protocol I has extended these protections to civilian medical personnel in addition to military medical personnel.[2,7,8] The International Criminal Court (ICC) considers it a war crime to intentionally direct attacks against personnel with the emblems of the GC such as those carrying out medical duties.[2] In addition to these general protections, Article 16 of Additional Protocol I protects medical personnel from "punishing a person for performing medical duties compatible with medical ethics" or requiring them to "act contrary to medical ethics."[7,8]

The drafting committee for the Additional Protocols to the GC are said to have necessitated that any aid organization other than the Red Cross must be located "within the territory of the State where armed conflict is taking place" so that they are not viewed as an "obscure private group from outside the country establishing itself as an aid society within the territory and being recognized by the rebels."[2]

While protections afforded to medical personnel cease if they act in a hostile manner outside their humanitarian purpose, Article 13 of Additional Protocol I allows for civilian medical personnel to protect themselves or those they are caring for from attacks with "light individual weapons."[2,7]

Medical Units

Article 19 of the First GC and Article 18 of the Fourth GC ensures that medical units and civilian hospitals may not be attacked and shall be protected and respected. Article 19 of Additional Protocol I helps offer the same protections to civilian medical units as afforded to military medical units.[2] As with medical personnel, the ICC considers it a war crime to intentionally direct attacks against medical units flying the emblems of the GC.[2]

Medical Transports

Article 35 and Article 21 of the First and Fourth GCs respectively spell out the requirement for protection and respect for medical transports. As is seen with medical personnel and units, Article 21 of Additional Protocol I ensures these same protections are offered to both civilian and military medical transport vehicles and vessels.[2] Article 36 of Additional Protocol I also protects aircraft carrying the wounded or medical supplies to be protected from attack when flying at altitudes and times agreed upon by the fighting party.[8] Attacks against medical transports are also considered war crimes under statutes of the ICC.[2]

Medical Emblem

The Fourth GC Articles 18, 20, 21 state that the emblem (e.g. Red Cross, Red Crescent, Red Star of David [recognized only by Israel and the USA]) signifying medical activities shall be present on civilian hospitals, medical personnel, and medical transports.
The only entities that may use the emblems are:
1. Medical staff and services of the armed forces
2. Volunteers to the ICRC of National Red Cross or Red Crescent Society members from the International Federation of Red Cross and Red Crescent Societies (IFRC), after duly being authorized by the State
3. Non-medical staff of the ICRC and the IFRC.[1]

Attack on any personnel or property using these emblems is considered a war crime by the ICC.[2] Deceitful use of these emblems for non-medical service needs is forbidden under Article 38 of Additional Protocol I.[8] Unfortunately, the number of cases of misuse of the emblem are reported to be high.[9] Furthermore, the protection provided by the emblem within the Articles of the GC has been diluted by the many entities (e.g. ambulances, hospitals, ancillary commercial health companies) using the emblem during peacetime.[9]

Additional Protocol III was introduced in 2005 to allow the additional use of the Red Crystal as an emblem of protection.[7] Concerns had arisen that the prior emblems were perceived by some as having a political or religious inference.[7] Both a lack of respect due to these emblems as well as some relief societies refusing to display them was thought to diminish the protections afforded by their use.[7]

Non-International Conflict Protection

Medical Personnel

Common to Article 3 among all four GCs states that the "wounded and sick shall be collected and cared for."[7] Because this task requires personnel, those personnel in turn are required protection.[2] More specifically, Article 9 of Additional Protocol II spells out that "medical...personnel shall be respected and protected" as they carry out their tasks.[7,8] As with hostilities in international arenas, the ICC considers it a war crime to intentionally direct attacks against personnel wearing the emblems of the GC such as those carrying out medical duties.[2] Additional Protocol II, Article 10 protects medical personnel from being either punished for practicing in line with medical ethics or requiring them to perform against the edicts set forth in medical ethics.

Interestingly, while medical humanitarian personnel working in international venues of hostility may carry light weapons for their protection (see International Conflict Protection, above), this has not been formally approved through either the GC or Additional Protocol II for those working in non-international environments of conflict. However, many State officials and military manuals suggest these protections would be allowable as they do not pose a true threat to the enemy.[2]

Medical Units

As with medical personnel, Article 3 common to all four GCs indirectly affords protections to medical units in their pursuit of caring and collecting for the sick and wounded.[2] Article 11 of Additional Protocol II more clearly states that medical units "shall be respected and protected at all times and shall not be the object of attack."[7]

Medical Transports

Consistent with the protections afforded to both medical personnel and units, Article 3 of all four of the GCs is also applied to medical transports. More clearly this protection is contained in Article 11 of Additional Protocol II.[2]

Medical Emblem

Article 2 of Protocol II states that the distinctive emblem signifying medical services (e.g. Red Cross, Red Crescent, Red Crystal, Red Star of David [recognized only by Israel and the USA]) shall be displayed on medical personnel, medical units, and medical transports, and shall be respected and not improperly used.[2]

Discussion

Despite implementation of the GCs, Additional Protocols and CIL, IHL remains fluid. Just as centuries of armed conflict help mold IHL as we know it now, today's hostilities around the globe offer new challenges to the law, requiring adjustments to better ensure the continued safety of citizens, peace workers, and humanitarian personnel.[2,8] Today, we have seen the highest rate of mortality among NGOs, adding to an increase in concern for the safety of health care workers.[10]

This changing wartime environment has in turn caused some to question the relevance of the GCs and their two Additional Protocols in offering protection to these entities.[11] One recent example of this is criticism that they are structured for protections in States with hostilities between armed forces rather than the growing number of conflicts involving militant groups often referred to as "unconventional warfare."[11] In a 2009 survey commissioned by the ICRC, less than half of the 4000 people polled across eight countries experiencing conflict at that time knew that the GC helped place limits on war activities among fighting parties.[5] Furthermore, only 56% felt that the GCs were effective in curbing the suffering among civilians living in hostile war environments.[5] In October 2014, representatives from 16 African countries came together to discuss current ratification and implementation of the IHL across their region.[12] They acknowledged that there has been a transition from primarily cross-border inter-state battles of years past to the complex intra-state conflicts of today where parties to the conflict may claim sovereignty and object to any outside interference.[12] They went on to suggest that while the GCs remained relevant, both development and implementation of this body of law were required to continue their value.[12] In an attempt to curb some of the concerns regarding the efficacy of the GCs of late, the ICRC has attempted to identify and support application of the rules of customary humanitarian law that exist regardless of the incomplete implementation record of treaty law. However, it's also acknowledged that customary law alone cannot replace the legal security gained by treaty implementation.[5]

Recently, independent groups have also looked for ways to better ensure protection of civilians suffering from the ailments of war. All humanitarian activities are guided by the four humanitarian principles: humanity, neutrality, impartiality, and independence derived from the ICRC/IFRC, which provide the "foundations for humanitarian action to establish and maintain access to affected populations whether in a natural disaster or armed conflict" and are considered essential elements of effective humanitarian coordination.[13]

Over the last 20 years, international NGOs have developed several inter-agency projects with a goal to improve accountability and quality in humanitarian efforts.[14] Some of these are being used as legal or pseudo-legal guidelines for humanitarian care, such as the Sphere Project, which lacks any binding legal status, but serves as a source of "persuasive authority" and is used by NGOs, ICRC/IFRC personnel, and military health providers.[6] By coming together on these projects, the knowledge and resources borrowed from multiple organizations has resulted in agreement of common standards or tools for improving both accountability and quality in humanitarian care efforts:[14]

Initiatives	Began
The Emergency Capacity Building Project (ECB)	2005
Synergie Qualité	2003
Humanitarian Accountability Partnership (HAP)	2003
The Inter-Agency Network for Education in Emergencies (INEE)	2000
Quality COMPAS	1999

(cont.)

Initiatives	Began
The Sphere Project (Humanitarian Charter and Minimum Standards in Disaster Response)	1997
The Active Learning Network for Accountability and Performance in Humanitarian Action (ALNAP)	1997
People In Aid	1995

Certain humanitarian groups have also worked to establish standards within specific areas of medical care being provided to civilians impacted by humanitarian emergencies.[15] Best practice guidelines have been employed in the past by humanitarian workers to ensure appropriate patient care during disasters, including those instigated by hostilities between parties to the conflict.[15] These standards help to establish quality and accountability of medical care in these often chaotic and difficult environments.[15] Legal experts also emphasize that standards of care protocols for resource-poor or constrained settings in crises are crucial in protecting the legal, ethical, and moral rights of the victims and the providers of care. Largely as a result of deficits in medical care provided during the Haitian earthquake in 2010, during their summit in 2011 the Humanitarian Space Working Group proposed a set of guidelines for the surgical and anesthesia care provided during humanitarian relief efforts.[15,16] The goal of these guidelines was to define scope of practice along with helping to facilitate collaboration, cooperation, and coordination between health care workers, as well as helping to work towards consensus-driven surgery and anesthesia best practice standards within the humanitarian community.[15,16] While the standards set forth in these guidelines have not yet been tested from a legal obligation perspective, they may be used in the future as a template for expected care provided in these challenging environments.

The struggles that have ensued with implementation of and compliance with IHL are well known. While the basic foundation of IHL may continue, the need to implement change in order to effectively address changing wartime environments will likely result in a much different set of laws in the future.

References

1. ICRC. War surgery: working with limited resources in armed conflict and other situations of violence. Vol I. 2009. www.icrc.org/en/publication/0973-war-surgery-working-limited-resources-armed-conflict-and-other-situations-violence (accessed September, 2019).

2. ICRC. Customary International Humanitarian Law Volume 1: Rules. 2009. www.icrc.org/en/doc/assets/files/other/customary-international-humanitarian-law-i-icrc-eng.pdf (accessed September, 2019).

3. Footer KHA, Rubenstein LS. A human rights approach to health care in conflict. 2013. www.jhsph.edu/research/centers-and-institutes/center-for-public-health-and-human-rights/_pdf/human%20rights%20approach%20health%20care%20in%20conflict.pdf (accessed September 2019).

4. ICRC. International Humanitarian Law: answers to your questions. www.icrc.org/en/doc/assets/files/other/icrc_002_0703.pdf (accessed September 2019).

5. ICRC. The Geneva Conventions of 1949: origins and current significance. 2009. www.icrc.org/eng/resources/docu

ments/statement/geneva-conventions-s
tatement-120809.htm (accessed
September 2019).

6. Burkle FM, Jr. Military-civic action and
    the 4th Geneva Convention: lessons
    learned or ignored? *Prehosp Disaster Med*
    2006;**21**:139–140.

7. International Committee of the Red
    Cross: Geneva Conventions. www.icrc.or
    g/en/war-and-law/treaties-customary-la
    w/geneva-conventions (accessed
    September 2019).

8. Goniewicz M, Goniewicz K. Protection of
    medical personnel in armed conflicts: case
    study, Afghanistan. *Eur J Trauma Emerg
    Surg* 2013;**39**:107–112.

9. Hospitals for War-Wounded. 1998.
    www.icrc.org/eng/assets/files/other/icr
    c_002_0714.pdf (accessed
    September 2019).

10. Humanitarian Outcomes. Aid Worker
    Security Report – Unsafe Passage: Road
    attacks and their impact on humanitarian
    operations. 2014. https://aidworkersecur
    ity.org/sites/default/files/Aid%20Worker
    %20Security%20Report%202014.pdf
    (accessed September 2019).

11. RFE/RL. Sixty years later, how relevant are
    the Geneva Conventions? 2009. www.rfer
    l.mobi/a/Sixty_Years_Later_How_Releva
    nt_Are_The_Geneva_Conventions/17981
    77.html (accessed September 2019).

12. ICRC. The Geneva Conventions 150 years
    later. . . still relevant? 2014. www.icrc.org/
    en/document/geneva-conventions-150-ye
    ars-later-still-relevant (accessed
    September 2019).

13. OCHA. OCHA on message: humanitarian
    principles. 2012. https://docs.unocha.org/
    sites/dms/Documents/OOM-humanitaria
    nprinciples_eng_June12.pdf (accessed
    September 2019).

14. Ouyang H, VanRooyen M, Gruskin S. The
    Sphere Project: next steps in moving
    toward a rights-based approach to
    humanitarian assistance. *Prehosp Disaster
    Med* 2009;**24**(3):147–152.

15. Chackungal S, Nickerson JW,
    Knowlton LM, et al. Best practice
    guidelines on surgical response in
    disasters and humanitarian
    emergencies: report of the 2011
    Humanitarian Action Summit Working
    Group on Surgical Issues within the
    Humanitarian Space. *Prehosp Disaster
    Med* 2011;**26**:429–437.

16. Knowlton LM, Gosney JE, Chackungal S,
    et al. Consensus statements regarding the
    multidisciplinary care of limb amputation
    patients in disasters or humanitarian
    emergencies: report of the 2011
    Humanitarian Action Summit Surgical
    Working Group on amputations
    following disasters or conflict. *Prehosp
    Disaster Med* 2011;**26**:438–448.

Chapter 21

Operation Tomodachi: Anesthetic Implications

Jeffrey M. Carness and Mark J. Lenart

Introduction

On March 11, 2011, at 2:46 PM Japanese Standard Time, an earthquake registering 9.0 on the Richter scale occurred with an epicenter located approximately 43 miles east of the Tohoku region along the eastern coast of Japan. The effects of the earthquake were largely felt on the island of Honshu (Figure 21.1), Japan's largest island. From its epicenter, the earthquake generated a reported 124–133 ft tsunami wave which inflicted devastating damage, striking Miyagi, Iwate, Fukushima, and Ibaraki Prefectures (Figure 21.2).[1] Final tallies report at least 15 000 fatalities (with ranges from 15 188 to 20 000+), 8742 missing persons, 5314 injuries, and 130 927 displaced persons. [2,3,4]

In addition, the Congressional Research Service reported the destruction of 432 047 homes, 3700 roads, and 27 019 additional buildings.[2] The majority of casualties and damage were likely secondary to the tsunami and not the result of the earthquake itself. The United States Geologic Survey reported a total economic loss in Japan estimated at $309 billion with disruption of electricity, gas, water, telecommunications, and railway service. A devastating consequence of the tsunami was a loss of electricity at the Fukushima Daiichi Nuclear Power Plant in the Fukushima Prefecture, which led to a loss of cooling capacity, resulting in a nuclear accident. This nuclear event was declared at the highest level on the International Nuclear Event Scale and contributed to the suffering of the Japanese people as a result of a "triple disaster" (i.e. the combination of earthquake, tsunami, and nuclear disaster).[5,6]

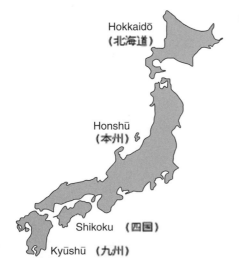

Figure 21.1 The island of Honshu.

Hokkaidō
(北海道)

Honshū
(本州)

Shikoku （四国）

Kyūshū （九州）

191

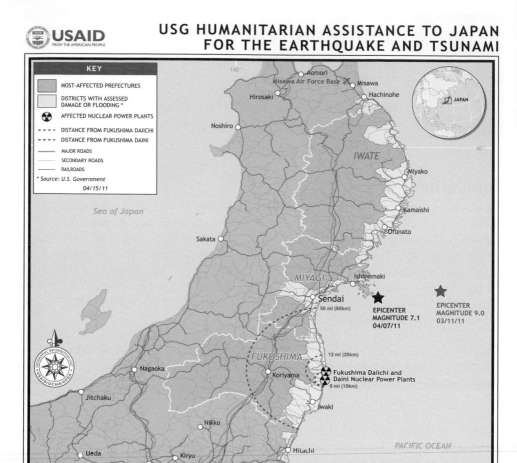

Figure 21.2 USG humanitarian assistance to Japan for the earthquake and tsunami.

A comprehensive understanding of this post-triple-disaster environment will establish a foundation of knowledge that will assist anesthesia providers in synchronizing health care delivery with aspects of disaster response in the future. This introduction to the Great East Japan Earthquake and Fukushima Daiichi Nuclear Disaster sets the stage upon which an understanding of the response may be appreciated. The aspects of the Japanese response to this triple disaster include: (1) The initial response during the immediate aftermath of the event, (2) the available methods of communication, (3) the magnitude and anticipated casualty load, (both acutely and chronically in the setting of ongoing inpatient care delivery), (4) the available medical resources, (5) the available facility resources, (6) facility activity/limitations (patients, water, electricity, personnel, logistics, etc.), and (7) the ability to transport patients, establish hardened supply lines, and record actions for process improvements in the future.

Immediate Aftermath:Initial Response with Focus on Force Protection and Threat Neutralization

In the aftermath of the earthquake and tsunami, Prime Minister Kan established an Emergency Response headquarters in the Ministry of Defense. A state of emergency was not declared since the National Diet of Japan was in session and was capable of coordinating legal action with the Cabinet in response to the disaster. Japanese Disaster Response Basic Law was enacted dictating the delivery of care coordinated through prefectural and municipal governments.[7] Foreign Minister Matsumoto formally requested the assistance of United States Forces Japan via the United States Ambassador to Japan (John V. Roos) on the evening of 11 March 2011. As the evening progressed, Prime Minister Kan subsequently declared a nuclear state of emergency and directed the evacuation of residents within 3 km of the nuclear power plant. Within 24 hours, residents within 20 km were ordered to evacuate. By March 15, residents living within 20–30 km were ordered to remain indoors (Figure 21.3).[8] By March 17, the United States Department of State had authorized the voluntary evacuation of between 9000 and 10 000 family members and dependents. This scale of personnel evacuation/sequestration must be considered with regard to force protection, and employee assignment in the aftermath of such a disaster.[2]

Establish Communication

As response forces activated, it became imperative to establish and maintain communication and logistical support. The Japanese Emergency Disaster Response Headquarters coordinated with the Ministry of Defense in the dispatch of Self-Defense Forces, police emergency units, firefighters, and emergency medical teams. With the deployment of up to 107 000 personnel, this was the largest operation since the establishment of the Japanese Self-Defense Forces.[9] Logistical coordination occurred via a relief hub at Sendai airport.[2] The United States Air Force Base, Misawa, located in the Aomori Prefecture, escaped the disaster with minimal damage and was identified as a forward operating base for United States Forces and Japanese Self-Defense Forces.[2] Furthermore, the Yamagata airport was identified as the base for a Marine Expeditionary Force (MEF) command and control (C2) headquarters/forward refueling point.[2] The 31st Marine Expeditionary Unit (MEU), consisting of ground, aviation, control, and logistics personnel, established a headquarters in Matsushiman after disembarking from the USS Essex.[2] The United States, through the State Department's Agency for International Development (USAID), also dispatched a Disaster Assistance Response Team (DART), which included urban search and rescue (USAR) capabilities. Author H. Fukunaga reported the establishment of communication with the Prefectural Health Division Representative, thereby enabling coordination with surrounding hospitals, pharmacies, and medical associations. With the closure of private medical practices in the aftermath of the earthquake, H. Fukunaga also describes the establishment

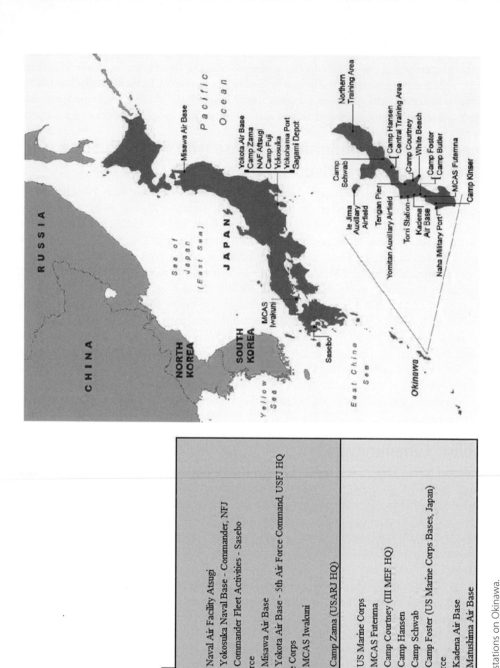

Figure 21.3 US Military stations on Okinawa.

of communication and collaboration of government and military physicians with private practice physicians at evacuation shelters to assist with delivery of patient care.[10]

Nakagawa describes the challenges of in-hospital communication, given the loss of power in the immediate aftermath of the disaster.[11] Regardless of the role that a provider may have in normal day-to-day hospital activities, it is easy to appreciate, given the magnitude of this disaster response, the possibility that medical personnel will be required to communicate for the first time with surrounding units with which they may be unaccustomed. Establishing internal and external lines of communication must, therefore, be considered of primary importance.

Anticipate Casualty Load and Types of Casualties

In 2013, an article by Missair et al. focused on traumatic injury patterns and anesthesia techniques implemented after major earthquakes.[12] They reviewed 31 articles which reported on the aftermath of 15 separate earthquakes over a 30-year span between 1980 and 2010. This review did not include the Great East Japan Earthquake, but did discuss several applicable points regarding the administration of anesthesia post-disaster. They noted that the vast majority of patients that die do so in the midst of the event. These deaths are associated with traumatic brain and spinal cord injury. A separate subset will die in the immediate aftermath of the disaster, often secondary to splenic and hepatic lacerations, subdural hematomas, and pelvic fractures. Of the remaining injuries, >50% are limb injuries, with lower limb involvement exceeding upper limb involvement in >90%. This patient population has injuries amenable to regional anesthetic techniques. However, of the 31 studies reviewed by Missair et al., only eight reported on the type of anesthetic provided; 50%, or four studies, reported on the utilization of general anesthesia and 50% on the use of regional techniques.[12] Concerning the Great East Japan Earthquake, K. Iinuma reported that the majority of mortality resulted from the tsunami and not from the earthquake. Thus, injuries were mostly of low acuity. Of note, however, is that the Ishinomaki Hospital received 99 casualties on the day of the earthquake, but 1251 patients on the day after, with 63 patient helicopter transfers completed on the third day.[13]

In a separate report published in the journal *Disaster Medicine and Public Health Preparedness* in 2014, Kodama et al. discussed the challenges they faced at Minamisōma Municipal General Hospital. They reported caring for 39 patients who were injured in the earthquake/tsunami, and 22 patients who were suffering from environmental exposure. Much as Missair et al. reported, one patient succumbed to shock/crush injury, two suffered pelvic fractures, two had lower extremity fractures, and two others sustained "other" fractures.[14]

Concerning the provision of general anesthesia to these patients, several reports (both following this disaster and previous disasters) have discussed the utilization of ketamine anesthesia as a sole anesthetic agent in the setting of austere devastated environments. Remarkably, the majority of patients that present for emergency care do so in the near aftermath (two to five days) following a disaster. During this time, medical services are often interrupted with shortages of electricity, water, transportation, and personnel. As such, ketamine, with its unique, beneficial properties, including disassociation, NMDA-receptor-associated analgesia, absence of respiratory depression to slight respiratory stimulation, and absence of significant vasodilation and hypotension, may serve as an ideal anesthetic agent. In a separate report by Missair et al. in 2010, they report on the utilization of ketamine-based monitored anesthetic care (MAC) in combination with a peripheral nerve block in >500 surgical procedures following the earthquake in Haiti.[15] Unfortunately this type of detailed anesthesiology reporting in English is not readily available. However, it is easy to see that, in a patient population impacted by triple disaster, there are likely to be many benefits of regional anesthesia. The required equipment is minimal and easily portable. The technique provides significant post-operative benefits (including improved cardiopulmonary function, decreased post-operative opioid consumption, faster return of bowel function, and minimal post-operative monitoring requirements). Missair et al. in their report from 2013, address the utilization of continuous peripheral nerve catheters. Again, while providing significant and continued post-operative analgesia, these catheters ultimately require more nursing care (dressing management/oversight), as well as the utilization of specially trained personnel (both of which may be in short supply in the immediate aftermath of a disaster). It is important to note that the employment of neuraxial anesthetic techniques should be performed cautiously, with special attention to hemodynamic status. Many of these patients are dehydrated and hypovolemic due to blood loss. A neuraxial technique, with associated sympathectomy, may be ill advised.

Regarding the anticipated casualty load, it is important to consider surrounding environmental factors and operating facilities. The Great East Japan Earthquake was unique because it was the first large-scale earthquake to occur during normal business hours on a normal weekday in modern Japan.[16] Furthermore, while the earthquake was associated with significant destruction, the mortality associated with the triple disaster was mainly attributed to the drownings associated with the tsunami. Other deaths were attributed to the several fires that began, including a petrochemical plant in Sendai, and a portion of the city in Kesennuma (a city to the northeast of Sendai). A fire at the Cosmo Oil Company refinery in Ichihara city remained ablaze for several days despite multiple attempts to extinguish the fire. There was also widespread destruction of homes and damage to power lines, water systems, roads, and railways. When considering the patient population in this disaster, the anesthesiologist must be prepared to assist with delivery of care to burn patients, blast and crush injuries, and patients exposed to radiation. Furthermore, emergency protocols must be developed in preparation for patients including pediatric and geriatric. In the Tohoku region of Japan most damaged by the triple disaster, approximately one-third of the patients were over the age of 65. [17]

Undoubtedly, patient care delivery was impacted by the post-disaster environment, including the potential for dehydration (as water sources were disrupted and affected by the release of radioactive materials) and malnutrition (the food supply was similarly affected). Hypothermia was another factor impacting the care of the wounded from this disaster, as many were affected by the cold tsunami water. The timing of this disaster also compounded the disaster because it occurred when temperature often remained below 0 °C (32 °F). Amidst reports of snow in the region, it is easy to appreciate the tragic combination of cold temperatures, cold tsunami water, absent electricity, and destroyed homes. Therefore, the potential for hypothermia and its consequences must also be considered in preparation plans.[11]

Understand the Resources: Personnel and Facilities

Personnel

Because of the significant number of organizations activated in response to the crisis, and the number/types of casualties that can be expected, it is important to recognize the type of responders with which you may have to interact. Since the treaty of Mutual Cooperation and Security was ratified in January of 1960, nearly 40 000 US troops have been stationed in Japan. For this crisis, the Japanese Self-Defense Forces and United States Armed Forces were activated and deployed to the affected region within 24 hours of the earthquake. At the peak, nearly 24 000 US personnel, 189 US aircraft, and 24 US Navy vessels were located within the region in response to the disaster.[2] In addition, the Japanese Self-Defense Forces mobilized 106 200 personnel, 200 rotary aircraft, 322 fixed-wing aircraft, and 60 ships.[2]

Several medical facilities within the Fukushima Prefecture have reported on their experiences responding to the crisis and these are discussed further in this chapter. These institutions include the Aizu General Hospital, the Fukushima Medical University Hospital, the Minamisōma Municipal General Hospital, the Red Cross Ishinomaki Hospital, and the Tohoku University Hospital. Undoubtedly, additional facilities were activated and assisted with the response to the significant casualty load (though their experiences with the delivery of anesthetic care are not easily readily identifiable in English print). Of the 170 reported hospitals in the region, 145 were fully functional in the aftermath of the disaster. Furthermore, according to a USAID report, 552 Japanese Disaster Medical Assistance Teams were activated and provided care for individuals affected by the natural disaster.[18]

US State Department/USAID

With a state of emergency and disaster declaration from John V. Roos, the USAID activated a Response Management Team in Washington DC and created a Disaster Assistance Response Team for deployment to Japan. They further facilitated the deployment of two urban search and rescue teams, as part of the Disaster Assistance Response Team.[18]

Non-Governmental Organization (NGO) Medical Support Staff

Both the Japanese Red Cross and the American Red Cross were actively engaged in disaster aftermath assistance. The Japanese Red Cross reportedly mobilized 900 medical teams with more than 161 000 volunteers. They report treating more than 87 000 patients.

Facilities

The United States Department of Defense maintains military members on a total of 85 different installations in Japan. They maintain seven military installations on mainland Japan and eight installations on the island of Okinawa. There are also four US military hospitals in Japan (Misawa, Yokosuka, Yokota, and Okinawa).

Japanese Hospitals

Several hospitals reported on their experiences during the aftermath of the Great East Japan Earthquake. Minamisōma Municipal General Hospital is the closest general hospital to the Fukushima Daiichi Nuclear Power plant. It is a 16 department, 4 ward, 230 bed hospital located 23 km north of the power plant. Due to its proximity, the power plant employees were directly impacted by the orders to evacuate and sequester indoors.

The Fukushima Medical University Hospital, located in Fukushima in the Nakanido region of Fukushima Prefecture (Figure 21.4), is a 778 bed/30 department facility associated with the medical school. It is an emergency medical center, located 57 km from the Fukushima Daiichi Nuclear Power Plant and maintains a helicopter landing site. It operates 12 surgical suites and maintains 8 active intensive care unit beds. By report it is capable of accommodating 600 critically ill patients per year and performing 5500 surgeries annually.[16]

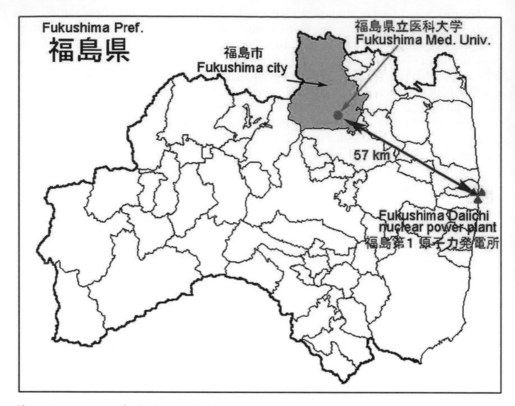

Figure 21.4 Location of Fukushima Medical University Hospital.

Tohoku University Hospital is a 1308 bed, level I trauma center and public academic medical facility with 57 departments located 80 km (49 mi) away from the Fukushima Daiichi Nuclear Plant.[11]

Aizu General Hospital, located in Aizuwakamatsu city in Fukushima Prefecture, is a 300 bed mid-level facility with 6 floors and 17 departments. It is located approximately 100 km from the Fukushima Daiichi Nuclear Plant.[1]

Facility Activity

Immediate Action

Upon notification of a seismic event, the initial response by staff inside a nearby hospital must focus on the evacuation of all personnel (inpatient and outpatient) from the building until it is certified as structurally sound. A report by Irisawa would suggest this to be a reasonable course of action[1] that can begin by evacuating all outpatients initially to the building entrance, with subsequent release.

In contrast, mobilization of inpatients presents a greater challenge. Murakawa reported on the concern for ongoing aftershocks necessitating inpatient transport.[16] When elevators are secured (a routine precaution in many facilities when there is seismic activity of magnitude 5.0 or greater), patient transport becomes increasingly difficult and necessitates stretcher movement up and down stairwells. Ultimately the movement of inpatients proved too difficult and all inpatients were returned to their rooms.

Simultaneously, a central command structure must be created, much like the disaster countermeasures office, which was established under the leadership of the university president in the office of the director of the hospital at Fukushima Medical Center. It was from this central office that commands were issued and reports recieved from each department.[16] Nakagawa et al. similarly reported on the establishment of a central authority within the hospital (i.e. a disaster control headquarters).[11]

Facility Preparation for Casualties

Ironically, while coordinating inpatient and outpatient evacuation, facility providers may also be engaged in preparation to receive casualties. Disaster plans should be executed with appropriate first responders. Triage areas should be established with a focus on separating surgical and medical casualties. The maximum effective number of operating rooms must be calculated based on staffing and resources. All personnel must be recalled. Murakawa describes the events at Fukushima Medical Center in a similar nature. Hospital beds were assembled at the entrance of the facility to receive casualties. Triage occurred at the entrance, and primary, secondary, and tertiary priority cases were triaged to the orthopedic clinic, internal medicine clinic, and the emergency center, respectively. In the operating theatre, five rows of operating rooms were prepared and staffed with appropriate anesthesia and surgical staff. Also, two clinical engineers were employed to maintain uninterrupted operating theatre function.

Operating Room

Intra-operative Management

Based on his experience in the Great East Japan Earthquake, Murakawa provides an algorithmic approach to providing appropriate patient care in the event of an earthquake.[16] He recommends the removal of all surgical lights over the patient to avoid contamination of the surgical field or injury to the patient. Simultaneously he recommends a drape be placed over the surgical equipment to prevent contamination by falling dust and debris. The OR staff should consider possible routes of evacuation from the operating room. Attention should be given to the operating room doors to ensure that they are not obstructed, to enable appropriate egress. If the earthquake occurs while patients are in the OR, discussion with the surgeon should focus on early completion of the procedure, if possible. The individual identified as the director of anesthesia services should ensure adequate bag valve masks are distributed, along with oxygen and appropriate sedation medications transport. All electrical surgical equipment and anesthesia machines should be checked for continuing and appropriate function. Each case should be individually evaluated, depending on the patient and type of procedure. Murakawa describes continued aftershocks during the Great East Japan Earthquake, which required ongoing decision-making.

Cessation of Further Surgical Activity

If the anesthesia provider finds themselves in the operating room at the time of the event with a surgical procedure underway, they should discuss with the surgeon the most expedient and appropriate means of completing the procedure. One of the few anesthesiology reports written in English, published after the Great East Japan Earthquake, describes nine patients who were in the operating room. They report that all surgeries were concluded appropriately, secondary to the strong shaking in the operating room (including those performed under local anesthesia).[16] Additionally, Nakagawa noted a lack of information in the aftermath of the earthquake which led to difficulties in deciding to terminate ongoing operations.

Patient Evacuation/Transport

Finally, the potential for building evacuation and preparation for receipt of casualties necessitates a comprehensive understanding of the local and regional medical environment to enable appropriate patient transport. In the Fukushima area, more than 1300 inpatients from multiple institutions were ordered to evacuate. Initial transfers were distributed throughout western Fukushima Prefecture, but eventually the number of patients exceeded the region's capacity, and patients were transported outside the Prefecture. Patients were moved by helicopter, ambulance, or Japanese Self-Defense Force buses. Of note, some facilities in the Fukushima Prefecture were unable to accommodate additional patients due to the disruption of water and electricity. In this case, they served as a transit point for relay inside and outside the prefecture.[16]

Limitations (Patients, Water, Electricity, Personnel, Logistics, etc.)

Supply

Water?

In the aftermath of the disaster, supply and logistics assumed an even more prominent role in healthcare delivery. Irisawa describes disruption of the water supply to the 5th and 6th floors of Aizu General Hospital which resulted in an inability to use those spaces for several months.[1] At Fukushima Medical Center, a restricted water supply resulted in cancellation of endoscopic procedures. Water supply failure for eight days resulted in water conservation efforts to include cancellation of outpatient clinic, cancellation of elective surgeries, and optimization of patient discharge to decrease the hospital census to about 70% of normal. Murakawa describes the water wagon supply of more than 100 tons of water daily. This too was insufficient, and the water supply was exhausted after a period of around one week.[16] In Tohoku, water, gas, and electricity supplies were stopped immediately after the earthquake. This created a challenge as the private diesel generator had only enough diesel fuel for approximately 72 hours of operation. Additionally, water leaks caused the closure of several wards. Sterilization limitations occurred due to a prohibition on entry into the building where instrument sterilization was performed. As Nakagawa reports, many sterilized medical items had to be obtained from neighboring prefectures after that.[11]

Oxygen?

At Fukushima Medical Center, there was reportedly a sufficient liquefied oxygen store ($8600 \, \text{m}^3$) for about ten days without interruption and an anticipated replenishment after one week. Small oxygen cylinders were used without difficulty.[16] Red Cross Ishinomaki Hospital continued operations without interruption.[13] Other hospitals in the area, however, were not as fortunate and reported oxygen shortages.[10] Anesthesia providers should be aware of the potential for this shortfall and have a backup plan of action.

Food?

Food supply was also a source of concern. Supply shortages were variable. For example, Fukushima Medical Center possessed three days of reserved food stores and seven days of medication and test reagent reserves. Modifications to the food production process were subsequently enacted to maintain patient safety and prolong food stores (i.e. cooking rice with bottled water and covering the counters with cling wrap to decrease cleaning requirements).[16] Minamisōma Municipal General Hospital was less fortunate in that supply of food and medical goods within the 30 km radius from the Fukushima Daiichi Reactor was suspended. This resulted in dependency upon goods delivered by the Japanese Self-Defense Forces (i.e. water, food, medicines, fuel oil, and oxygen cylinders). The first delivery occurred on 16 March, five days after the initial disaster. Nurses prepared meals using available ingredients.[14] Of note, several towns and villages reported contamination of drinking water, milk, and leafy vegetables with ^{131}I. Subsequently, "additional food sources were measured and other foods, in particular mushrooms and sand lances (small eel-like fish), were also found to be contaminated with ^{131}I, ^{134}Cs, and ^{137}Cs at levels exceeding their respective limits."[8]

Electricity Disruption?

The loss of electricity generates many more challenges. Nakagawa describes the maintenance of emergency backup electrical power at Tohoku University Hospital based on a backup generator. This backup generator, however, was not tied into the cooling system for the computer room, so even though the computers were functioning, there was no way to cool the server, which led to a shutdown of computer systems. This resulted in the absence of computer charting and laboratory testing to exclude bedside testing. Disruption of power also resulted in damage to the circuit boards associated with in-hospital communication systems and a shutdown of elevator systems. This shutdown necessitated the transport of six patients up and down the stairwells. As Nakagawa describes, this created space limitation in the lower floors of the 17-story hospital building.[11]

Personnel?

In the immediate aftermath of this disaster, as noted by Iinuma, the majority of casualties were not seriously injured. Murakawa reiterated this fact. As such, though instinctively an immediate recall of anesthesia providers would be considered, this was not performed at the Fukushima Medical Center. However, a means of immediate communication should be established. This course of action is in line with consideration of the potential disruption and congestion of roadways. The utilization of anesthesia providers for triage and appropriate patient disposition may also be considered. Dispatch of anesthesia providers to surrounding facilities to assist with surgical care delivery (i.e. triage of patients with larger medical centers focusing on the performance of high-level surgical intervention) should be considered. However, gasoline shortages may also contribute to personnel difficulties in commuting to and from facilities in the affected regions.[16] Ultimately, as was the case at Tohoku University Hospital, many personnel were inadequately resourced due to the challenge in communication and lack of information regarding the severity and complexity of the disaster.[11]

Personnel evacuation must also be considered in the aftermath of the disaster. Kodama describes the course of action for personnel at the Minamisōma Municipal General Hospital. Of the 254 employees, one nurse died in the earthquake, and six lost their families. Additionally, with the explosion of the Fukushima Daiichi Nuclear Power Plant on 14 March, an evacuation order was given, and medical personnel were given the option to evacuate. In making this decision, six doctors, 80 nurses, and 96 staff members, or 70% of hospital personnel chose to evacuate.[14] It is important to recognize that, in the event of a natural disaster, though a recall may be initiated, only a fraction of health care employees may choose to, or be in a condition to, respond.

Nuclear Contamination

Recap History of Nuclear Disaster

On March 11, 2011 the Fukushima Daiichi nuclear power plant was severely damaged as a result of the Great East Japan Earthquake and follow-on tsunami. Similar to other surrounding nuclear power facilities in the coastal Tohoku region (Sanriku), the Fukushima Daiichi nuclear power plant subsequently underwent an emergency cooling shut down. At Fukushima Daiichi, only units 1–3 were operating at the time of the earthquake (while units 4–6 were offline). Although successful in initial shutdown associated with the earthquake itself (with insertion of a control rod into the reactor core), the units required continued cooling (facilitated by external electrically driven cooling equipment). With the ensuing tsunami, the protective seawall was breached and seawater subsequently incapacitated all six external power generators and subsequently rendered inoperable the onsite backup diesel emergency power generators. With continued heat generation, associated with heat production from the reactor cores and spent fuel, and no ability to cool the reactors, increasing pressures within the reactors led to venting of steam, radioactive gases, and hydrogen into the environment. Subsequently, on the afternoons of March 12 (15:36 JST), March 14, and March 15, separate hydrogen gas explosions occurred in units 1, 3, and 2, respectively (thus releasing additional radioactivity into the surrounding environment).[8] Irisawa described it as an explosion in which "the sidewalls of the upper level were blown away, leaving in place only the vertical steel-framed grid works."[1] The ongoing release of radioactivity led to the evacuation order for the surrounding 30 km by March 15, 2011.[16] Subsequent evacuation of over 200 000 inhabitants from the vicinity of the site and areas occurred early in the emergency. Monitoring of food and water and placement of radiation limits on such foodstuffs was initiated. Evacuees were scanned for exposure and given potassium iodide.

Contamination of the Air Handling Systems

Consideration in advance should be given to the potential for adherence of radioactive substances to materials within the air filtration system. In the report by Murakawa the air handling system absorbed and filtered out the majority of radioactive substances such that the concentration that reached the hospital rooms was <0.1 mSv/h.[16]

Preparation for this Type of Catastrophe?

Institutional preparation for response to a nuclear accident can be facilitated by accreditation. As Murakawa explained in his after-action review of the nuclear disaster and their response at the Fukushima Medical University Hospital, "Our hospital is accredited as a medical institution for secondary radiation medicine and accepted exposed sick and injured patients associated with the nuclear power plant accident from the day following the earthquake."[16]

It is further suggested that simulation training for large-scale nuclear disasters be performed in facilities in close proximity to a nuclear facility to expedite the response to a nuclear incident. Discussion of both the methods for preparing the operating rooms for receipt of contaminated patients and the methods for screening patients upon presentation to determine the necessity of decontamination procedures should occur.[1,16] An example of operating room preparation is shown in Figure 21.5.

Additionally, disaster prevention drills should be discussed and performed routinely throughout the operating room spaces to facilitate expedited response in the event of a natural disaster. To this end Nakagawa et al. reported on the speed with which they were able to create a disaster control headquarters at their facility. They reported that this task had consumed greater than one hour when initially drilled, but took less than 15 minutes after the onset of the earthquake under the leadership of the chair of the hospital during repetitive subsequent drills.[11]

Finally, Kodama reported on the exposure of patients and personnel to radiation at Minamisōma Municipal General Hospital. The difference in external and internal radiation levels demonstrated a benefit to keeping patients and personnel inside the hospital, purportedly due to the thickness of concrete used in the construction, which decreased the radiation dose. Furthermore, active and expedient distribution of radiation spatial

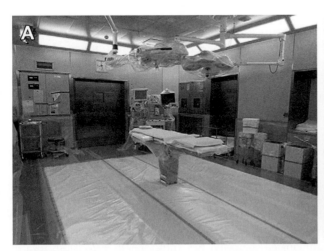
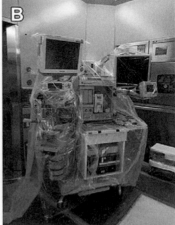

Figure 21.5 Operating room preparation for radiation contaminated patient. (Reprinted from M. Murakawa, Anesthesia department preparedness for a multiple-casualty incident: lessons learned from the Fukushima earthquake and the Japanese nuclear power disaster. *Anesthesiology Clinics* 31:117-125, Copyright 2013, with permission from Elsevier.)

dose forecasts may help in considering the best route of patient evacuation and transportation.[14]

Methods for Sustained Delivery in the Future/Lessons Learned

Many lessons have been learned throughout history regarding the medical response in the aftermath of an earthquake. The triple disaster nature makes the Great East Japan Earthquake notable. Murakawa discusses his recommendations with regard to lessons learned in a paper published in *Anesthesiology Clinics* in 2013. The highlights of his discussion are recapped here. Some of these items have been discussed previously and are repeated for completeness. It is certainly important to verify initial safety of the patients under your care. Ideally, a patient safety system will be employed to ensure their direct safety from falling debris and from overturned hospital beds/operating room tables. As mentioned previously, overhead lights and overhead hanging objects should be removed from the proximity of the anesthetized patient during an earthquake. Prophylactically, shelves should be replaced with cabinets and those items that appear likely to fall reinforced appropriately. The anesthesia machine and anesthesia cart wheels should be locked firmly in place.

Secondary priorities will include ensuring an adequate supply of oxygen for continuation of surgery and for patient care over the following days to weeks. Further provisions must be made for maintenance of an adequate water delivery system, as efforts to conserve water may lead to insufficient personnel hygiene and incomplete surgical instrument sterilization. Electricity may also be a limited resource. Many facilities rely on backup power generators powered with a limited amount of fuel. In the absence of electricity, air handling systems will be unavailable and floating dust increases. As such it is important to minimize foot traffic in and out of the operating room as much as possible. Surgical procedures should be completed in an expedient manner and patients transported from the operating room as expeditiously as possible. Ideally, operating rooms will be on the same floor as the intensive care unit, enabling easy transport from the operating room. One cannot forget that patient transport will become increasingly difficult without electricity to power elevators. Transport of pharmaceuticals and food throughout the hospital, in the absence of electricity for elevator function, will also be increasingly difficult. For all of these reasons it is intuitive to cancel all elective procedures and conserve resources appropriately. Staffing should also be considered and appropriately anticipated to ensure adequate food and provision of long-term staff quarters.[16]

Conclusion

The Great East Japan Earthquake, tsunami, and Fukushima Daiichi Nuclear Power Plant explosion created a unique and devastating triple disaster with tragic loss of life. In the aftermath of such a disaster, anesthesia providers have a responsibility for the intraoperative management of patients and may well be tasked to contribute to any number of other recovery objectives. The establishment of internal and external communication and the sharing of information is imperative. Casualty types will depend on the type of disaster and in this case, they reflect largely unanticipated characteristics. Intra-operative decisions regarding procedure termination and immediate post-operative patient placement may be challenging. Anesthesia providers may anticipate a potential shortage of patient food, medication, water, oxygen, and electricity affecting sterilization, lab testing, pharmacy, computer documentation, and other ancillary services. Personnel challenges may include direct injury from the disaster, exposure to radiation, gasoline shortages, road damage, and lack of food/ personal hygiene supplies when reporting to the hospital. Dispatch to surrounding facilities to aid in care delivery, dependent upon facility capability in the aftermath of the disaster, may be anticipated. Preparation and disaster response drills should be executed routinely to stream-line and facilitate a rehearsed and well-executed emergency medical response.

References

1. Irisawa A. The 2011 Great East Japan earthquake: a report of a regional hospital in Fukushima Prefecture coping with the Fukushima nuclear disaster. *Dig Endosc* 2012;24(Suppl 1):3–7.

2. Feickert A, Chanlett-Avery E. Japan 2011 Earthquake: US Department of Defense (DOD) Response. (CRS Report No. R41690; 2 June 2011). https://fas.org/sgp/c rs/row/R41690.pdf (accessed October 2019).

3. Cyranoski D. Japan faces up to failure of its earthquake preparations. *Nature* 2011;471:556–557.

4. Nakahara S, Ichikawa M. Mortality in the 2011 Tsunami in Japan. *J Epidemiol* 2013;23(1):70–73.

5. USGS. M 9.1 – 2011 Great Tohoku Earthquake, Japan. https://earthquake .usgs.gov/earthquakes/eventpage/offi cial20110311054624120_30/impact (accessed October 2019).

6. Nanto DK, Cooper WH, Donnelly JM, et al. Japan's 2011 Earthquake and Tsunami: Economic Effects and Implications for the United States. (CRS Report No. R41702; 6 April 2011). https://fas.org/sgp/crs/row/ R41702.pdf (accessed October 2019).

7. Umeda S. Japan: Legal Responses to the Great East Japan Earthquake of 2011. The Law Library of Congress. September 2013. Web. 10 October 2019. www.loc.gov/law/h elp/japan-earthquake/index (accessed October 2019).

8. Dauer LT, Zanzonico P, Tuttle RM, Quinn DM, Strauss HW. The Japanese tsunami and resulting nuclear emergency at the Fukushima Daiichi power facility: technical, radiologic, and response perspectives. *J Nucl Med* 2011;52 (9):1423–1432.

9. Public Affairs Division, Ministry of Defense, Japan. Great East Japan Earthquake and SDF's activities. *Japan Defense Focus.* 2012. www.mod.go.jp/e/jd f/pdf/jdf_sp.pdf (accessed October 2019).

10. Fukunaga H, Kumakawa H. Disaster management at Soma General Hospital in response to the Great East Japan Earthquake. *Japan Med Assoc J* 2014;57 (5–6):331–334.

11. Nakagawa A, Furukawa H, Konishi R, et al. The Great East Japan Earthquake: lessons learned at Tohoku University Hospital during the first 72 hours. *IEEE Pulse* 2013;4(3):20–27.

12. Missair A, Pretto EA, Visan A, et al. A matter of life or limb? A review of traumatic injury patterns and anesthesia techniques for disaster relief after major earthquakes. *Anesth Analg* 2013;117 (4):934–941.

13. Iinuma K. Lessons from "the 2011 off the Pacific coast of Tohoku Earthquake" through activity of Japanese Red Cross Ishinomaki Hospital (JRCIH). *Brain Dev* 2013;35(3):190–192.

14. Kodama Y, Oikawa T, Hayashi K et al. Impact of natural disaster combined with nuclear power plant accidents on local medical services: a case study of Minamisōma Municipal General Hospital after the Great East Japan Earthquake. *Disaster Med Public Health Prep* 2014;8 (6):471–476.

15. Missair A, Gebhard R, Pierre E, et al. Surgery under extreme conditions in the aftermath of the 2010 Haiti earthquake: the importance of regional anesthesia. *Prehosp Disaster Med* 2010;25(6):487–493.

16. Murakawa M. Anesthesia department preparedness for a multiple-casualty incident: lessons learned from the Fukushima earthquake and the Japanese

nuclear power disaster. *Anesthesiol Clin* 2013;**31**(1):117–125.

17. Harney, A. Japan's earthquake and the hazards of an aging population. *The Atlantic*. 23 March 2011. www .theatlantic.com/international/archive/ 2011/03/japans-earthquake-and-the-hazards-of-an-aging-population/ 72892/ (accessed October 2019).

18. United States Agency for International Development. Bureau for Democracy, Conflict, and Humanitarian Assistance. Japan Earthquake and Tsunami. Fact Sheet #4, Fiscal Year (FY) 2011. www .cidi.org/wp-content/uploads/03.14.11%2 0-%20USAID-DCHA%20Japan%20Earth quake%20and%20Tsunami%20Fact%20S heet%20%234%20-%20FY%202011.pdf (accessed October 2019).

Austere Obstetric Anesthesia

Johanna de Haan, Kristin Falce, and Nadia Hernandez

Situations of disaster, whether due to natural disaster or man-made disaster, are non-discriminatory. All individuals are affected equally, whether male or female, young or old. Persons who are providing medical care in an area affected by disaster may come across patients who are pregnant and in need of urgent care. Obstetric care along with injury-related care is considered among the forefront of necessary surgical services in disaster situations. The need for anesthetic care is recognized as an integral component of these hospital services.[1] In the United States, 99% of all births occur in a hospital or clinical setting, which may be inaccessible and severely damaged during the inciting disaster. During times of stress, women experience increased risk of health complications associated with pregnancy, including stress-induced premature labor and birth, low birth weight infants, and neonatal and infant death.[1]

In a disaster setting, in many facets and not just medically, focus shifts from the care of individuals to care for the greater good. Finite resources should be distributed to the largest number of patients, prioritizing those with the greatest potential benefit. Medical practitioners providing care during a disaster need to be more aware of the fact that they are not functioning within a vacuum and their decisions for care of one patient may impact several others. If a provider is faced with an overwhelming number of patients and has limited supplies for placement of epidural or spinal anesthesia and analgesia, we would recommend prioritizing more critical laboring patients (Table 22.1). Conditions which may signify priority may include: patients undergoing trial

Table 22.1 Risks for laboring patients

Type of risk	Possible condition
Risk of fetal demise	Placental abruption, abdominal injuries during trauma, late decelerations
Risk of postpartum hemorrhage	Placenta previa, placenta accreta, prior cesarean section, uterine window, obesity, fetal macrosomia
Risk of infection	Active herpes simplex lesions, HIV, known Group B strep (GBS) without available antibiotics
Risk of difficult airway	Pregnancy, obesity, prolonged labor, cervical spinal instrumentation, anatomical airway abnormailities

of labor after cesarean (TOLAC), patients with known difficult airways, and patients with pre-eclampsia.

This list is by no means all-inclusive, and the situation should be gauged by the practitioner at the bedside. However, these situations represent cases where a rapid anesthetic delivery option may be advantageous due to propensity for obstetric emergencies.

Personnel also need to ensure that they continue to be able to provide care to as many patients as possible, meaning that practitioners need to provide adequate self-care. For example, during Hurricane Harvey in Houston, Texas, practitioners attempting to arrive at their hospitals flooded their vehicles and waded to their workplaces.

As a general rule, in obstetric anesthesia, general anesthesia is to be avoided due to worsening of airway concerns in the parturient and its effects on the neonate. [Editor's note: Ketamine has been found to be useful in low-resource countries.] However, in disaster circumstances, additional consideration will need to be made for placement of a neuraxial anesthetic. Unless there is a situation which necessitates spinal or epidural anesthesia, it is good for the practitioner to remember that ultimately, labor epidurals are elective procedures and may not be necessary in an austere circumstance. Advocating for natural birthing may be warranted if there are not sufficient supplies for all patients to receive epidurals, or if there is a shortage of available skilled staff for neuraxial anesthesia or analgesia.

In a disaster setting, there will be multiple ways in which stress is placed on medical providers and hospitals in general. There may be situations in which some hospitals must evacuate their patients to a hospital in a safer location. This will place a strain on the receiving location's supply of manpower, equipment, and medications. The incoming supply will hopefully not be limited or strained due to the safe location presumed to not be affected by disaster. This was evident in Louisiana during Hurricane Katrina, where roughly 30 hospitals were made to evacuate their patients to hospitals in safer locations. Receiving hospitals required additional staff and additional supplies to function and handle the unusual load of patients.

Other hospitals may not be able to evacuate and may be required to shelter in place. This was the situation for many hospitals in Texas during Hurricane Harvey. This created a scenario in which supply of medications, manpower, food, and medications were strained and had to be conserved. In Houston, Texas, supplies of preferred local anesthetics for spinal anesthesia dwindled, and care coordination with obstetricians was necessary. Only emergent or urgent surgeries were able to be performed, so that medications were not used and potentially wasted for elective cases.

During Hurricane Katrina, Keesler Medical Center offered shelter in the hospital to patients who were 36 weeks pregnant or greater. Parturients at earlier weeks of gestation were also admitted if they were defined as a high-risk pregnancy: cases of placenta previa, pre-term labor, or hypertensive disorders. The increase in admitted patients placed strain on medical staff and supplies. It also required obstetricians and anesthesiologists to shelter in place at the hospital. Space may be a limitation in this scenario, and has been experienced by many hospital staff in locations prone to natural disasters such as hurricanes.

In Corpus Christi, Texas, during Hurricane Harvey, patients were transferred from a hospital with a labor and delivery unit to another hospital further from the floodplain, which did not have a labor and delivery unit. Anesthesia staff who were relocating to the safer hospital transported as many supplies as they could in their private vehicles. This included a supply of emergency medications, spinal and epidural trays, intubating equipment, and bag-mask ventilation equipment. At night, as the storm hit the city, cesarean sections were performed in cardiac operating rooms with generator power.

There may be multiple shortages which lead to a provider's inability to place an epidural for a laboring patient in a disaster situation. They could be shortages in personnel, supplies, or medications. Personnel may need to work in shifts and provide each other with significant moral support to endure the experience. Medications may need to be substituted as availability of preferred agents dwindles. Attention will need to be paid closely to multidose vials and sterile technique to ensure preservation of medications.

Due to the current conditions of local anesthetic shortages in the United States, the Society for Obstetric Anesthesia and Perinatology (SOAP) has issued recommendations for next-line therapy when hyperbaric bupivacaine hydrochloride 0.75% in a volume of 1.5 to 2 ml is not available. Lower doses should be used if one is able to also administer neuraxial opioids:.

- Isobaric bupivacaine hydrochloride preservative-free 0.5% for a dose between 12 and 15 mg.
- Tetracaine can also be used for spinals, in a concentration of 1% with a dose of 7 to 9 mg depending on the patient's height. Attention should be paid to the increased duration of tetracaine, to possibly 3 hours or more.
- Lidocaine can be used, if anesthesia is not required for more than about one hour. The concentration recommended by SOAP[2] would be 5%, with a dose of 50 to 75 mg, once again depending on the patient's height.
- Mepivacaine is not recommended in the obstetric patient due to a long half life in the neonate.
- Prilocaine is also not recommended due to the risk of methemoglobinemia.
- The ED50 for spinal hyperbaric bupivacaine was found in one study to be 1.58 mg.[3]
- If using hyperbaric ropivacaine for spinal anesthesia, the ED50 of this has been shown to be 14.22 mg.[3]

In the case of a labor epidural, the preferred agent would be isobaric preservative-free bupivacaine hydrochloride 0.25% in an appropriate volume for the clinical situation; lower volumes for epidural bolusing, higher volumes for initiation of neuraxial analgesia. SOAP states in their advisory statement that ropivacaine is also able to be used for epidural labor analgesia, but that it is 40% less potent than bupivacaine.[4]

If surgical anesthesia is needed through an epidural route, both preservative-free lidocaine 2% with or without preservative-free epinephrine and chloroprocaine can be used if the surgery is emergent. If there is time available to allow for the slower onset of bupivacaine or ropivacaine, these could be used instead to provide surgical anesthesia through the epidural. Keep in mind that with continued usage of lidocaine over a prolonged period of time, tachyphylaxis can develop. Combined spinal epidural techniques or dural puncture epidural techniques may also allow for a reduction in required doses of local anesthetic and less bolusing by providers.[5]

Continuous spinals for labor analgesia may be an interesting option for practitioners attempting to conserve resources, as the volume of local anesthetic needed to provide anesthesia or analgesia will be decreased. Requiring smaller volumes of local anesthetic may be ideal in a situation of limited medication supply. However, increased incidences of hypotension and post-dural puncture headache (PDPH) may ultimately require greater time and attention from the practitioner. However, if used appropriately and with appropriately monitored patients, this could be a viable option. The situation would need to be evaluated closely by the practitioner providing care at the time. If an intrathecal catheter is placed, it needs to be very thoroughly labeled as such. Consequences of bolusing an intrathecal catheter with epidural doses could be catastrophic: this could result in total spinal anesthesia, need for endotracheal intubation, or need for immediate cesarean delivery of the fetus.

There are some reports of using transversus abdominus plane (TAP) blocks for surgical anesthesia in cases where patients cannot tolerate either a neuraxial or a general anesthetic. The TAP blocks reported were performed with 20 to 30 ml of local anesthetic on each side; choice of local anesthetic was determined by the attending anesthesiologist. Two patients reported received 20 ml of 0.25% bupivacaine hydrochloride, and a third patient received an equal mixture of 1% lidocaine and 0.25% ropivacaine.[6] Another report describes a cesarean section performed with local anesthesia for a patient in whom a neuraxial was inappropriate and general anesthesia would not have been tolerated; 8 ml of 0.5% bupivacaine were injected into the skin at the location of incision, and 6 ml were injected into the rectus sheath for abdominal closure. The surgeons were mindful not to use any retractors or packing, because of the lack of visceral anesthesia. The patient received only a total of 30 µg of fentanyl during the 45 minute procedure.[7] The American College of Obstetricians and Gynecologists (ACOG) has stated that infiltration of local anesthesia can be used for cesarean delivery if there is a situation where general anesthesia or neuraxial anesthesia is not available.[8]

Ability to treat PDPH and potentially perform epidural blood patches may need to be prepared for in the case of disaster. The incidence of PDPH will likely not decrease during the time of disaster, and practitioners will need to be prepared to treat it. It would be unacceptable to allow patients to suffer with this condition, placing them in a situation where they may not be able to care for their newborn infant in a disaster. Allowing PDPH to continue and develop sequelae would also not be ideal in a situation of limited resources. Conservative measures that can be used to treat PDPH include: acetaminophen alone, a combination of acetaminophen, butalbital, aspirin, and caffeine, increased fluid intake, flat positioning, and sphenopalatine ganglion block. Sphenopalatine ganglion block can be easily performed if the practitioner can obtain concentrated lidocaine, either 2% or 4%, and cotton swabs. The cotton swabs are soaked in lidocaine, and then advanced to the back of the nose above the middle turbinate until they meet the posterior wall of the nasal cavity. This is left in place for 10 minutes on each side and then repeated with an additional lidocaine-soaked cotton swab bilaterally.[9,10] If none of these conservative measures result in resolution of PDPH, the practitioner may need to perform an epidural blood patch. The decision for this procedure would depend on the clinical condition of the affected patient, and availability of supplies. The risks and benefits of the procedure would need to be weighed against using an epidural kit for placement of a blood patch, which another laboring patient may need for neuraxial anesthesia.

Laboratory values may not be able to be obtained at all or may be significantly delayed, so laboratory evaluation of coagulation may not be possible before placing neuraxial anesthetic. During Hurricane Harvey in Houston, Texas, Ben Taub Hospital experienced flooding of its basement laboratory, making lab tests unobtainable for practitioners. Discretion of the anesthesiologist had to be used. Trauma or another disaster scenario could have resulted in significant blood loss or development of coagulopathy. The American Society of Anesthesiologists (ASA) practice guidelines issued in 2016 indicate that an intra-partum platelet count is not required in the healthy parturient, but the decision to obtain a platelet count should be left to the discretion of the anesthesiologist based on the patient's medical history.[11]

Elective cesarean sections should be postponed as long as possible to allow the disaster circumstance to abate. Discharge of patients after care may be difficult during this time, thus reducing patient volume will be advantageous for staff and others who may need emergency care. Patients being discharged home will have a newborn to care for, and this may be less than ideal in the setting of a natural disaster or other traumatic circumstance. However, postponing patients may result in development of obstetric emergencies, such as uterine rupture during labor after previous cesarean, or shoulder dystocia of large birth-weight infants. Providers will need to be prepared for emergency circumstances and the potential for patients to present in extremis. Labor and neuraxial placement may be occurring in atypical areas, such as emergency departments or in triage settings. Postponing cesarean sections may require implementation of additional monitoring of the mother. If equipment is in short supply, these may be simple monitors such as fetal movement and fetal heart rate Doppler, if standard fetal heart rate and uterine tone tracings are not available.

Equipment may also in short supply during these circumstances. Epidural pumps for continuous infusions may not be available. Epidurals may need to be bolused intermittently to provide analgesia. This will allow for greater spread and less use of local anesthetic, as well. The required volume for intermittent bolusing without a continuous infusion would likely be between 10 and 20 ml, depending on the height of the patient, and higher concentrations will be needed for more dense blocks, depending on the clinical scenario. For labor analgesia, 10 to 20 ml of 0.1% ropivacaine or 0.125% bupivacaine with or without opioids would likely be sufficient for most patients. One study to obtain the EC50 for labor analgesia was 0.065% for bupivacaine with a volume of 20 ml, and 0.37% for lidocaine in a volume of 20 ml.[12] This technique will require more time and attention from the practitioner, but may be the only option, if there is a shortage of pumps or if they are unable to be operated due to lack of battery power or electricity. Generators in the basement or ground levels of hospitals may be easily affected by natural or man-made disasters.

Peripheral nerve block techniques may also be useful during a time of reduced supply of equipment and pain medications. Pudendal or perineal blocks may be performed by obstetricians before delivery, and may alleviate the need for neuraxial placement by anesthesiologists, who may be spread thin due to non-obstetric surgical emergencies or staffing intensive care units. The pudendal block is performed trans-vaginally and with the patient in lithotomy position. The physician palpates the ischial spine and introduces a needle about half an inch to pierce the sacrospinous ligament. After negative aspiration, a 10 ml volume of local anesthetic is injected. This process is repeated on the opposite side.

Alternative therapies for laboring mothers may also be helpful to reduce the need for anesthesia care of the laboring patient. The standard breathing exercises, massage, and white noise that are standard in current labor and delivery care should continue to be employed as available, as they may help alleviate further strain on anesthesia care for analgesia.

The knowledge of anesthesia staff is indispensable during time of disaster, even when caring specifically for the obstetric patient. Our specialty is known for its ability to care for patients who need definitive line placement, resuscitation with blood products or fluids, or acute airway management. Recent studies have shown that use of tranexamic acid for prevention of obstetric hemorrhage is beneficial.[13] Not only would this be useful for individual patients, but would also be helpful in the setting of disaster or mass casualties, where blood products must be conserved. The obstetric patient in a disaster scenario may be more likely to require this type of attention than the usual obstetric patient encountered in our standard day-to-day practice.

Allocation of staff may need to be considered during the disaster. Anesthesiologists may need to fulfill other roles as needed: replenishing supplies as a technician, performing secretarial duties, transporting patients, or performing administrative tasks. Reasonable standards of care and training should not be ignored, but during times of stress and decreased availability of the aforementioned facets of care, mid-level providers will naturally be relied upon to extend the care of the physicians whose direction they are functioning under. This will include delegation of tasks to nurse anesthetists, anesthesiologist assistants, nurses, and anesthesia technicians.[14]

References

1. Abdullah F, Troedsson H, Cherian M. The World Health Organization program for emergency surgical, obstetric, and anesthetic care: from Mongolia to the future. *Arch Surg* 2011;**146**(5):620–623.

2. SOAP. Society for Obstetric Anesthesia and Perinatology (SOAP) advisory in response to shortages of local anesthetics in North America. https://soap.org/2018-bupivacaine-shortage-statement.pdf (accessed September 2019).

3. Parpaglioni R, Frigo MG, Lemma A, et al. Minimum local anaesthetic dose (MLAD) of intrathecal levobupivacaine and ropivacaine for Cesarean section. *Anaesthesia* 2006;**61**:110–115.

4. Polley LS, Columb MO, Naughton NN, Wagner DS, van de Ven CJ. Relative analgesic potencies of ropivacaine and bupivacaine for epidural analgesia in labor: implications for therapeutic indexes. *Anesthesiology* 1999;**90**(4):944–950.

5. Chau A, Bibbo C, Huang CC, et al. Dural puncture epidural technique improves labor analgesia quality with fewer side effects compared with epidural and compared spinal epidural techniques: a randomized clinical trial. *Anesth Analg* 2017;**124**(2):560–569.

6. Vuong, JT, McQuillan PM, Messaris E, Adhikary SD. Transversus abdominus plane block as the primary anesthetic for laparotomy. *J Anaesthesiol Clin Pharmacol* 2014;**30**(3): 419–421.

7. Mahawar B, Baduni N, Bansal P. Cesarean section under local anesthesia: a step forward or backward? *J Anaesthesiol Clin Pharmacol* 2014;**30**(4):578–579.

8. ACOG. Obstetric analgesia and anesthesia. ACOG Practice Bulletin No. 36. July 2002.

9. Kent S, Mehaffey G. Transnasal sphenopalatine ganglion block for the treatment of postdural puncture headache in obstetric patients. *J Clin Anesth* 2016;**34**:194–196.

10. Cohen S, Sakr A, Katyal S, Chopra D. Sphenopalatine ganglion block for postdural puncture headache. *Anaesthesia* 2009;**64**:570–579.

11. ASA/SOAP. Practice guidelines for obstetric anesthesia: an updated report by the American Society of Anesthesiologists Task Force on Obstetric Anesthesia and the Society for Obstetric Anesthesia and Perinatology. *Anesthesiology* 2015;**124** (2):1–31.

12. Columb M, Lyons G. Determination of the minimum local anesthetic concentrations of epidural bupivacaine and lidocaine in labor. *Anesth Analg* 1995;**81**:833–837.

13. Franchini M, Mengoli C, Cruciani M, et al. Safety and efficacy of tranexamic acid for prevention of obstetric haemorrhage: an updated systematic review and meta-analysis. *Blood Transfus* 2018;**16**:329–337.

14. Daniels K, Oakeson AM, Hilton G. Steps toward a national disaster plan for obstetrics. *Obstet Gynecol* 2014;**124**:154–158.

Chapter 23

Pharmacy in Disaster Anesthesia

Robert Bishop and Ashlee Klevens Hayes

Introduction

In September 2017 Hurricane Maria made landfall in Puerto Rico. The Category 4 hurricane destroyed the power grid, communication networks, and caused significant flooding that left 3.4 million residents in the dark, unable to communicate, and with a contaminated water supply.

The evolving humanitarian crisis required a large-scale coordinated response and involved government and non-government humanitarian organizations. On arrival, aid workers were confronted with a large, heterogeneous population needing assistance with both acute and chronic medical issues.

Variables in the Disaster Response

A number of factors need to be considered when implementing an anesthetic pharmacy in an austere environment. They can be summarized as follows:

1. Location – weather extremes, travel time, departure time
2. Organization and regulation – procuring, transporting, and storing scheduled drugs
3. Population – likelihood of pediatric, obstetric patients, endemic disease
4. Duration – expected time on site, resupply likelihood, and supply chain method.

Considerations for an Anesthetic Pharmacy

The components of an ideal anesthetic pharmacy would be as follows:

1. Adequate inventory of anesthetic drugs and ancillary medications (fluids, antibiotics, vaccines, etc.)
2. Obtaining a reliable source for procuring and storing medications
3. Mechanisms to ensure safe and secure handling of medications.

The austere environment that results from a natural or a man-made disaster presents a number of challenges to this ideal.

The most obvious challenge is a disruption to the supply chain. For example, in the aftermath of Hurricane Maria only 29% of local pharmacies were open.[1] Resupply was initially via an "air-bridge" of shuttle flights from the US mainland co-ordinated by FEMA.[2] The problem of supply disruption is twofold: first, there will be reduced ability to procure drugs from local resources that will be required for acute care, and second, the local population will likely be seeking ongoing treatment for management of pre-existing medical conditions. Often, first-responders and aid organizations are ill-equipped to manage

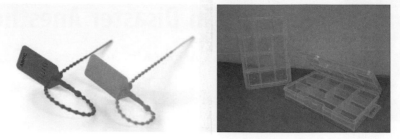

Figure 23.1 Secure pull-tie sealing device and improvised drug storage box.

chronic medical conditions.[3] When arriving on site, it is vital to make contact with local hospitals, pharmacies, and wholesalers that can be used to resupply medications. When making an inventory, ordering or dispensing drugs, the generic or international non-proprietary name of the drug should be used. This allows for more consistent communication between arriving aid teams and local assets.

The absence or interruption of electricity will impact the ability to maintain a constant environment for the storage of drugs. Even with backup generators, the electricity supply cannot be guaranteed. This can be mitigated by selecting drugs that are less prone to degradation in variable temperatures; however, drugs such as insulin, vaccines, and blood products may require a cold chain with temperature data logging and reliable documentation. Small battery-powered monitors with RFID technology are simple to use, easy to transport and can be synced with electronic databases.[4] The World Health Organization (WHO) recommends the use of water-containing ice-packs and filling the refrigerator or cool box with excess water bottles if space permits to give a buffer should power fail. The use of a top-loading refrigerator keeps the cool air in. Less sensitive drugs should be stored in a cool, dark, well-ventilated area.[5]

To minimize the risk of contamination, there should be as minimal handover of medications as possible. However, this needs to be balanced against the risk of the drug becoming unstable and therefore unusable. Where possible pre-drawn syringes should be sought. These are mixed in sterile conditions, are well labeled and are typically a standard concentration of drug.

In the immediate aftermath of a disaster there will likely be a degraded security situation. Often, there are several agencies working together who may have access to common areas. This can present problems with the secure storage of scheduled drugs. In hospitals, electronic dispensaries (e.g. CareFusion Pyxis) may not be functional or may be inaccessible to temporary staff. Portable safes are not always practical, given their weight. A secure area should be located and access controlled.[5] Drugs can be stored in sealed plastic containers such as fishing tackle boxes that can be sealed with labeled, tamper-proof, pull-tie closing devices (Figure 23.1).[6] When staff are required to be mobile, the drugs can be transported and kept on the person inside a fanny pack/bum bag (Figure 23.2).

Specific Anesthetic Pharmaceuticals

The WHO provides a comprehensive list of medications to guide first-responder teams.[7] It provides a detailed list of oral and injectable drugs, as well as non-medication supplies and

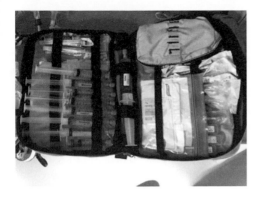

Figure 23.2 Personal bag containing pre-drawn drugs.

equipment. In addition to the above list the following anesthesia-specific drugs are recommended.

Intravenous Fluids

Intravenous fluids will be used in a resuscitative phase, and for maintenance fluids where the oral route is not suitable. The amount that can be taken to a remote site can be limited by the bulk and weight of the fluids. Sodium chloride 0.9% (normal saline or NS) is an intravenous fluid that serves a variety of purposes and is the most suitable. Normal saline can be used to reconstitute other drugs, and can be diluted to hypotonic solutions that may be better suited to pediatric populations. D5NS can be made by adding 10 ml of 50% dextrose to 1 L NS. NS is also suitable in neurotrauma where sodium homeostasis is impaired, and reduces the worsening of cerebral edema. NS is relatively insensitive to variations in temperature and has a long shelf life.[8]

Colloid solutions have a limited role in the early phases of a disaster scenario. They are not superior to crystalloids for resuscitation. They also require more controlled storage conditions.

Blood products are some of the the most impacted drugs in a disaster situation. Transporting blood products to a remote disaster site may not be practicable, given the specific temperature and handling requirements. On site, the blood bank supply may be disrupted or destroyed. Often, the local population will be available and prepared to donate blood, but the necessary laboratory testing would be necessary to ensure ABO compatibility and minimize the risk of disease transmission. Citrated blood collection sets would allow for fresh whole blood transfusion provided there was a suitable donor panel. Freeze-dried plasma, while not FDA approved in the USA yet, is an alternative to fresh frozen plasma. Freeze-dried plasma is stored at room temperature, reconstituted in sterile water, and has been shown to enhance clot formation and inhibit fibrinolysis.[9]

Induction and Maintenance Drugs

The pharmacological properties of induction and maintenance drugs are discussed elsewhere in this book. Ketamine has a well-established history in austere environments as it can be used in a variety of situations across a broad spectrum of the population. Ketamine has a long shelf life, is stable across a broad range of temperatures, and is resistant to degradation after dilution, even in sunlight.[10]

Propofol is less suited to an austere environment as it is more sensitive to changes in temperature, and once open is prone to bacterial contamination, even when an aseptic technique is used.[11]

Volatile anesthetics require additional infrastructure to facilitate their administration. This may be as simple as a draw-over circuit, or a modern plenum anesthetic machine. With a modern machine, the reliable supply of pipeline gas or even bottled gas and electricity is unlikely. Furthermore, volatile anesthetic agents are considered dangerous goods alongside compressed gases, and require extra considerations when shipping via air. If bottled gas is being utilized from an unfamiliar source then an oxygen analyzer is essential to ensure that the contents of the bottle match the label.

Muscle Relaxants

Succinylcholine is typically used for rapid sequence induction given its favorable pharmaco-kinetic profile. The manufacturer recommends storage at 2–8 °C. However, it is relatively stable at room temperature and only undergoes a small amount of degradation resulting in a 10% decrease in potency over five months.[12]

Vecuronium is an intermediate-duration non-depolarizing muscle relaxant that has one of the lowest rates of anaphylaxis. It is available as powder for injection and is stable at room temperature. It can be given as a bolus and also used for infusions at 1μg/kg/min if paralysis is indicated for patient transport. It can be reliably reversed with sugammadex.

The benzylisoquinolines, atracurium and cisatracurium, have similar onset and duration of action as vecuronium. They are advantageous as they undergo Hofmann degradation and will therefore be eliminated regardless of the patient's hepatic and renal function. Their disadvantage is they are more sensitive to ambient temperature and should be refrigerated. When left at room temperature, a longer onset time and shorter duration of action is observed.[13]

Antimicrobials

There are a number of considerations when selecting which antimicrobials will be required for a given scenario. Endemic disease and local resistance to antimicrobial medication will vary from location to location, and local advice or information from the WHO/Center for Disease Control (CDC) or other authority will be required.

The types of surgery being performed in the early phases of a disaster scenario will likely be limited to damage-control surgery for trauma, the main examples being trauma laparotomy and orthopedic limb procedures, including amputation. The scope may broaden once the initial phase of the disaster is over, depending on how long the aid team is on location.

Antibiotic prophylaxis is common when undertaking a surgical procedure. Most of the emergent surgery performed in an austere environment will fall into CDC Categories III or IV, meaning contaminated or dirty. These have the highest likelihood of surgical site infections.

Antibiotic prophylaxis in an austere environment should cover skin and bowel organisms, as these are most likely to be encountered. Table 23.1 summarises some useful antimicrobials and their activity.

Table 23.1 Summary of common antimicrobials used in surgery

Drug	Antimicrobial activity	Suggested use	Instructions, stability and storage
Cefazolin	Gram-positive and Gram-negative aerobes	25 mg/kg Redose in 4 h Laparotomy Orthopedic surgery Urinary tract infection	D5 W, NS, sterile water for mixing Use within 1–2 hours to maintain sterility and stability Store in cool dry place
Ceftriaxone	Gram-positive and Gram-negative aerobes	50–75 mg/kg Crosses blood–brain barrier Use as above, plus CNS infections, early sepsis	D5 W, NS, sterile water for mixing. Should be used within 1–2 hours to maintain efficacy, sterility, and stability. Store in cool dry place
Vancomycin	Gram-positive aerobes Methicillin-resistant *Staphylococcus aureus*	25 mg/kg Give slowly over 60 min Orthopedic surgery	Keep frozen until 1 hour prior to administration. If provided as a powder, D5 W, NS, sterile water for mixing is suffice. Should be administered within 1–2 hours to maintain efficacy, sterility, and stability To prevent adverse events (red man syndrome), administer slowly; at minimum, 30 minutes Administer diphenhydramine if red man syndrome allergy is recognized
Clindamycin	Gram-positive cocci Gram-negative rods	5 mg/kg adult 600–900 mg 90% bioavailable Alternative where allergy to β-lactam or cephalosporin suspected Antimalarial	High likelihood of diarrhea associated with clindamycin Stable in D5 W, NS, sterile water Store at room temperature Infusion rates should not exceed 30 mg per minute
Metronidazole	Anaerobic bacteria and protozoa	15 mg/kg 80% bioavailable Bowel surgery	Store at room temperature Protect from light Incompatibility: metronidazole injection USP should not be mixed with sodium lactate 5% w/v and dextrose 10% w/v injection

Analgesics and Local Anesthetics

The WHO list does not comprehensively cover all options for analgesia and it would be prudent to carry drugs in addition to that list.[7] The local laws concerning transportation and possession of scheduled drugs should be clarified prior to departure to ensure compliance.

A simple opioid pharmacy would cover short- and longer-acting drugs, as well as the oral and intravenous routes of administration. Intravenous fentanyl and intravenous fentanyl plus oral morphine should be able to address most situations encountered in the early phases of an austere environment.

Fentanyl is usually available in ampoules in 50 µg/ml. It is stable at room temperature, stable in solution for infusion, resistant to breakdown in sunlight, and has a long shelf life without the addition of preservative. Fentanyl has a peak effect five minutes after IV injection with its offset of action due initially to redistribution to other tissues. It can be given intranasally at 1.5 µg/kg, which is useful for short painful procedures such as suturing or closed reduction of fractures where IV access may not be indicated.

Morphine is the ubiquitous opioid and has been in use since its discovery in 1827. It has a longer onset and offset time than fentanyl and is used to provide longer-acting potent analgesia. It has an oral to IV ratio of 3:1 that is consistent across the dose spectrum, allowing for easy conversion. It is sensitive to degradation by sunlight, heat, and exposure to air. Any morphine solution that contains preservative should not be used in an epidural or spinal solution.

As discussed elsewhere in this book, it has become more feasible to utilize regional anesthetic techniques in an austere environment. As such it is a requirement to stock long-acting local anesthetics. Ropivacaine is a long-acting amide local anesthetic that can be used to facilitate surgical anesthesia as well as provide post-operative analgesia. It has a lower affinity for cardiac sodium channels and has a greater margin of safety than bupivacaine. Ropivacaine 1% can be diluted 50:50 with 2% lidocaine to facilitate surgical anesthesia and provide post-operative analgesia. At concentrations of 0.2% it will provide analgesia with minimal motor block. It is stable at room temperature. The duration of action can be prolonged with the addition of dexamethasone to the nerve block solution.[14]

Vaccines

Vaccines typically do not make up the core pharmacy of aesthetic drugs, however they are commonly used in a disaster situation. Of all the drugs that will be carried, they are the most sensitive to environmental variations during transport. As such, the handling and storage of vaccines is worth mentioning.

Following are recommendations on how to safely store vaccines:[5]

- Only pack enough vaccines for immediate use. Until administration, keep all vaccines in their original vials or boxes.
- Use an insulated, hard-sided cooler with at least 2-inch thick walls.
- When packing the vaccines in the cooler, always ensure an insulated barrier is stuck between the vaccine and the ice. Never place vaccines directly on an ice pack.
- Make sure to include a label on the outside of the cooler.

References

1. Lavery AM, Patel A, Boehmer TK, et al. Notes from the field: pharmacy needs after a natural disaster – Puerto Rico, September–October 2017. *MMWR Morb Mortal Wkly Rep* 2018;**67**:402–403.

2. FEMA. Hurricane Maria Federal response timeline. https://www.fema.gov/hurricane-maria (accessed October 2019).

3. Jhung MA, Shehab N, Rohr-Allegrini C, et al. Chronic disease and disasters medication demands of Hurricane Katrina evacuees. *Am J Prev Med* 2007;**33**:207–210.

4. Wessel R. DB Schenker uses temperature-logging tags to monitor drug shipments. *RFID J* 2011. https://www.rfidjournal.com/articles/view?8629 (accessed September 2019).

5. World Health Organization. Guidelines for the storage of essential medicines and other health commodities. http://apps.who.int/medicinedocs/en/d/Js4885e/6.6.html (accessed September 2019).

6. B-Sealed. Pull-tight closure product website. www.bsealed.com.au/product/pull tight/ (accessed September 2019).

7. World Health Organization. Disaster response team bags. http://apps.who.int/medicinedocs/documents/s21310en/s21310en.pdf. (accessed September 2019).

8. Puertos, E. Extended stability of intravenous 0.9% sodium chloride solution after prolonged heating or cooling. *Hosp Pharm* 2013;**49**(3):269–272.

9. Huebner, BR, Moore EE, Moore HB, et al. Freeze-dried plasma enhances clot formation and inhibits fibrinolysis in the presence of tissue plasminogen activator similar to pooled liquid plasma. *Transfusion* 2017;**57**(8):2007–2015.

10. Donnelly, RF. Stability of diluted ketamine packaged in glass vials. *Can J Hosp Pharm* 2013;**66**(3):198.

11. Aydin O, Aydin N, Gultekin B, et al. Bacterial contamination of propofol: the effects of temperature and lidocaine. *Eur J Anaesthesiol* 2002;**19**(6):455–458.

12. Adnet, F, Le Moyec L, Smith CE, et al. Stability of succinylcholine solutions stored at room temperature studied by nuclear magnetic resonance spectroscopy. *EMJ* 2007;**24**(3):168–169.

13. Geng Z, Wu X. The effect of different storage temperature on the pharmacodynamic dose-response of cisatracurium besylate: 9AP5-1. *Eur J Anaesthesiol* 2014;**31**:154.

14. Cummings KC, Napierkowski DE, Parra-Sanchez A. Effect of dexamethasone on the duration of interscalene nerve blocks with ropivacaine or bupivacaine. *Br J Anaesth* 2011;**107**(3):446–453.

Chapter 24

Regional Anesthesia in Disaster Circumstances

Nadia Hernandez and Johanna de Haan

Regional anesthesia has undergone a great deal of growth in recent years, due in part to the ability of peripheral nerve blockade to treat pain without the administration of opioids, and the resultant avoidance of their systemic side effects, such as respiratory depression, sedation, nausea, and constipation. In addition to this advantage, adequate control of acute pain as can be achieved with regional techniques prevents the central sensitization that can result in chronic (including phantom limb) pain. Reduced exposure to opioids also decreases the risk of physical dependence and addiction. Regional techniques have also been demonstrated to reduce hospital length of stay.

Regional anesthesiologists in modern urban settings are accustomed to practicing with near-unlimited resources, including high-tech equipment, but in austere settings with limited resources, a few adjustments to practice must be considered.[1–4] Despite limitations, regional anesthetic techniques can still be performed; in fact, in the resource-constrained environment (e.g. no anesthesia machines are available for general anesthesia cases, lack of end-tidal gas monitoring, limited trained nurses for post-anesthesia care, etc.), regional techniques may become preferred. Health care workers in disaster circumstances must preserve precious supplies, and regional anesthesia can vastly extend the ability to respond through the conservation of pain medications and nursing support. Nerve blocks can take seconds to minutes to perform, and if long-acting medications are available, they will be effective for several hours, not only conserving resources, but also reducing complications. For example, in individuals who may have broken ribs, a serratus anterior plane block (or PECS II block) can be performed to alleviate this pain and help to reduce probability of hypoxemia or respiratory failure due to hypoventilation from splinting and poor respiratory mechanics.

In the OR, regional anesthetic techniques allow for decreased turnover time between patients; in the PACU, they shorten time needed to reach discharge criteria by improving pain control pain and obviating opioid side effects of sedation, nausea, and vomiting.

Limitations in the following facets of regional anesthesia performance in a disaster or other low-resource environment will be discussed, along with suggestions for how to perform a nerve block despite them:

- Medications
- Monitors
- Equipment
- Supplies
- Documentation
- Patient information

Limitations in Medications

Local Anesthetics

- We recommend using the smallest volume and most dilute concentration of local anesthetic needed to provide either analgesia or anesthesia, depending on the goals of the anesthesiologist.
- Studies have been performed to identify the minimum effective concentration (MEC) for ropivacaine, bupivacaine, lidocaine, and mepivacaine in various blocks as well as the minimum effective volume (MEV) for various blocks.
- Usage of the MEC and MEV of local anesthetic will help to conserve supply of medication in the resource-constrained environment. This will also reduce the risk of local anesthetic toxicity in patients whose weight is uncertain, in the event of inadvertent intravascular injection, or when rescue medications are not readily available.
- It should be borne in mind that all blocks may not require a "recommended" volume if ultrasound guidance is used to visualize adequate spread of local anesthetic. MEC and MEV which have been published in the literature are shown in Tables 24.1 and 24.2.

Limitations in Monitoring

Vital Signs During Block Placement

- ASA standards for monitoring state that during a regional or local anesthetic without sedation (which is what we recommend), adequacy of ventilation of the patient should be continually observed by qualitative clinical signs. Adequacy of circulation can be assessed by manual observation of a pulse or auscultation of heart sounds, if needed.[21]
- Continual monitoring in the form of constant meaningful communication and assessment of mental status can be used as secondary indicators of adequate circulation and oxygen saturation, as both are required to maintain mental status and phonation.

Table 24.1 Minimum effective concentration

Block type	Type of local	Volume	MEC >90	Citation
Supraclavicular	Ropivacaine	40 ml	0.257%	5
Axillary block	Bupivacaine	20 ml	0.241%	6
Femoral	Lidocaine	15 ml	0.93%	7
Femoral	Ropivacaine	15 ml	0.167%	8
Subgluteal sciatic	Mepivacaine	30 ml	1.12%	9
Popliteal sciatic	Mepivacaine	30 ml	1.98%	9

MEC 90 is the concentration at which >90% of patients underwent a surgical procedure without supplementation of analgesia or anesthesia. All studies were done with ultrasound-guidance.

Table 24.2 Minimum effective volume

Block type	Type of local	Volume	MEV >90	Citation
Interscalene	Ropivacaine	7 ml	0.75%	10
Interscalene	Bupivacaine	0.95 ml	0.5%	11
Infraclavicular	Lidocaine	14 ml	2%	12
Supraclavicular	Mepivacaine	17 ml	1.5%	13
Supraclavicular	1:1 lidocaine levobupivacaine	23 ml	2% 0.5%	14
Supraclavicular (elderly)	1:1 lidocaine levobupivacaine	11.9 ml	2% 0.5%	14
Axillary brachial plexus	Lidocaine	1 ml /nerve	2%	15
Axillary brachial plexus	Bupivacaine	1.56 ml /nerve	0.5%	16
Axillary brachial plexus	Lidocaine	23 ml perivascular	1.5%	17
Popliteal sciatic	Ropivacaine	8.9 ml	0.75%	18
Popliteal sciatic	1:1 bupivacaine lidocaine	13.3 ml	0.25% 1%	19
Popliteal sciatic	Ropivacaine	16 ml	0.5%	20

MEV has been studied with several different ultrasound-guided nerve blocks and local anesthetics at varying concentrations. MEV 90 or greater for surgical anesthesia is summarized in this table.

- Due to the possible limited availability of monitoring equipment such as pulse oximeters, non-invasive blood pressure cuffs (either manual or automatic), and electrocardiography, we recommend that sedation not be administered for the placement of regional anesthetics in circumstances where vital signs cannot be ascertained and the patient cannot be monitored for a length of time sufficient for the sedating medications to resolve.

Limitations in Equipment

- Many articles have been published in the emergency medicine literature about the value of ultrasound-guided regional anesthetic (USGRA) techniques in disaster or combat circumstances. This is readily accepted by health care providers, who can appreciate the value of an anesthetized limb vs the dangers of systemic opioids and other pain medications.
- USGRA will be preferable in this setting, if available. Use of ultrasound has been shown to reduce necessary volume and concentration to achieve a successful nerve block,[22] allowing conservation of local anesthetic in an environment where resupply may be difficult.

- USGRA will also help to avoid toxicity in a patient whose weight may not be known for calculation of a maximum dosage, by allowing the anesthesiologist to use a lower volume and concentration of local anesthetic.
- Ultrasound has also been shown to be associated with a reduced rate of complications, such as vascular puncture and paresthesia.[22]
- In addition, with the availability and usage of USGRA, the practitioner can also utilize point-of-care ultrasound (PoCUS) for diagnostic techniques, including focused cardiac, lung, and abdominal exams. PoCUS can be used to identify contraindications to specific peripheral blocks, such as ruling out contralateral pneumothorax and evaluating excursion of the contralateral lung/diaphragm before performing proximal brachial plexus blocks associated with hemidiaphragmatic paresis. Further discussion of PoCUS is beyond the scope of this chapter, but its potential usefulness in a disaster or other low-resource environment is immense.
    - Proximal brachial plexus blocks are fraught with potential contraindications. Due to risk of phrenic nerve block resulting in hemidiaphragmatic paresis, certain patients with respiratory or neuromuscular disorders may not tolerate the reduction in forced vital capacity. Contraindications to these blocks include severe COPD, severe pulmonary hypertension, myasthenia gravis, contralateral vocal cord paralysis, and contralateral lung or thoracic pathology such as pleural effusion, hemothorax, or pneumothorax. PoCUS can be used to rule out effusions, hemothorax, pneumothorax, and vocal cord paralysis.
- Ultrasound will not always be available, particularly in high-demand, low-resource situations; therefore, facility with a peripheral nerve stimulator can be crucial in localizing nerves and placing peripheral blocks. However, usage of the peripheral nerve stimulator for block placement, especially in fractured extremities, should be done with caution. Not only can this technique be exquisitely painful for the patient, but it can also lead to closed-to-open fracture conversion necessitating debridement.
- Landmark-based techniques can also be used for certain blocks, and can be employed when both forms of guidance are unavailable.
    - For block procedure description, both for ultrasound and landmark-based techniques, please see Table 24.3.

Limitations in Supplies

- In the practice of regional anesthesia, usage of blunt-tip needles is accepted as standard practice to prevent nerve injury in procedures where major nerves are being targeted. Examples of this circumstance include the interscalene (which targets nerve roots), supraclavicular block (which targets the divisions of the brachial plexus), infraclavicular block (which targets the cords of the brachial plexus), the femoral nerve block, and blockade of the sciatic nerve in all locations and from all approaches.

    - Blunt-tip needles have a short bevel which is less likely to pierce the nerve bundles and are able to instead push them away.
    - Blunt needles also allow for the practitioner to appreciate "loss of resistance" in landmark-based block placement, when attempting to identify different tissue planes by haptic feedback.

Table 24.3 Recommended regional anesthetic techniques in trauma or disaster circumstances

Block	Ultrasound (u/s)	Landmark
Head and Neck		
Supraorbital nerve block		Supraorbital notch is palpated along the superior medial orbital bone. Inject 3–5 ml with a 25 g needle.
Greater occipital nerve (GON) block	Occipital protuberance is palpated, 3 cm lateral and 2 cm inferior is the GON. On u/s, pulsation of greater occipital a. should be visible. Perivascular injection 3–5 ml	GON is located 3 cm lateral and 2 cm inferior to the occipital protuberance. Inject 3–5 ml. Aspirate every 3 ml during this block due to greater occipital artery
Superficial cervical plexus SCM: sternocleidomastoid	SCM muscle is identified at the level of C6 (cricoid cartilage). Needle is advanced in-plane until the tip is underneath the SCM. Inject 10–15 ml.	Identify the lateral border of the SCM at the level of cricoid cartilage. Using a 25 g needle, 5ml aliquots are injected in a fan-like distribution: directly perpendicularly at the lateral border of the SCM, directed cephalad and caudad as well.
Inferior alveolar nerve block		Palpate the coronoid notch, and insert a needle at this level into the tissue on the medial surface of the mandible. The needle is inserted ¾ of the anteroposterior distance from the coronoid notch to the deepest part of the pterygo-mandibular raphe. Bone will be contacted at about 20–25 mm of depth. Inject 2–3 ml
Truncal Blocks		
PECS II/ serratus plane block SAM: serratus anterior muscle (Figure 24.2)	Identify the 5th rib in the midaxillary line; SAM over ribs should be visible. Advance a needle in-plane until contact is made with the surface of the rib. Inject 20–30 ml while visualizing hydrodissection over adjacent ribs underneath SAM	Using palpation, identify 5th rib in the midaxillary line, and insert needle through skin. Make contact with the periosteum of the 5th rib and begin to inject 20–30 ml. If injection pressure is tight, may need to retract needle 1–2 mm

Block	Ultrasound-guided technique	Landmark/alternative technique
Transthoracic muscle plane block/parasternal block TTM: transthoracic muscle ICM: intercostal muscle	Linear u/s probe is placed on chest wall in a sagittal plane. Transversus thoracic muscle is identified under intercostal muscles, adjacent to sternum. Needle is advanced in-plane until tip is between TTM and ICM. Spread should cross adjacent rib spaces. 15 ml. Aspirate every 3 ml due to proximity to internal mammary artery	Blind infiltration of the parasternal muscles can be performed in order to anesthetize sternum. Duration will be shorter than TTM plane block with ultrasound. Aspiration every 3 ml due to proximity to internal mammary artery, as well as possible entrance to the thorax.
Posterior transversus abdominis plane (TAP)/quadratus lumborum (QL) 1 EOM: external oblique muscle IOM: internal oblique muscle TAM: transversus abdominis muscle	U/s probe is placed on the abdominal wall in a horizontal manner. The three abdominal wall layers (EOM, IOM, and TAM) are identified and followed posteriorly until the TAM terminates at the QL muscle. Advance needle in-plane until the tip is in the fascia at the end of the TAM. 20 ml	A blunt-tipped needle will be useful for a landmark-based approach to the TAP or QL block for haptic feedback to loss of resistance. The needle entry point for the classic TAP should be at the triangle of Petit (iliac crest inferiorly, EOM anteriorly, latissimus dorsi posteriorly). Two pops will be appreciated as the needle passes the EOM followed by the IOM. Inject 20 ml
Erector spinae block SP: spinous processes TP: transverse processes	Linear u/s transducer is placed on the patient's back in a sagittal plane, and the TP of the spinal column are visualized. Advance a needle in-plane through the erector spinae muscles until contact is made with the TP. Inject 20 ml at T5 (thoracic procedure) or T8 (abdominal/gynecologic procedure)	SP are palpated in order to identify the dermatomal level of interest, and marked. The transverse process is then located 2.5 cm lateral to this point. Needle is advanced perpendicular to the skin until bony contact is made with the TP. Inject 20 ml
Rectus sheath block RAM: rectus abdominis muscle PRS: posterior rectus sheath	U/s is placed on the abdominal wall in a horizontal position. A needle is advanced in-plane until the tip lies between the RAM and the PRS. Inject 20 ml of local anesthetic here. RAM should be lifted off of the connective tissue sheath	Not recommended

Table 24.3 (cont.)

Block	Ultrasound (u/s)	Landmark
Paravertebral block TP: transverse processes SP: spinous processes CTL: costotransverse ligament	U/s probe is placed on the patient's back in a cranial caudal direction. TP are identified. CTL can be seen between the TP, superficial to the shimmering pleura. Advance needle in plane until the tip has pierced the CTL, may feel a "pop," or give. After negative aspiration, LA is administered, and pleura will be seen to sink away from the u/s transducer.	SP are identified in order to locate dermatomal level of interest. TP then identified 2.5 cm lateral to SP on the ipsilateral side. A needle is then advanced perpendicular to the skin until the TP is contacted, and the depth of bony contact is noted. The needle is then walked off of the bone superiorly and advanced an additional 1 cm. Inject 5 ml/level or 20 ml for six dermatomes.
Upper Extremity		
Interscalene ASM: anterior scalene muscle MSM: middle scalene muscle	The nerve roots of the brachial plexus are identified between the ASM and MSM lateral and posterior to the carotid artery at the level of C6 or the cricoid cartilage. Advance needle in-plane from posterior to anterior until the needle tip is carefully placed between the nerve roots. Following negative aspiration, inject 20 ml	Not recommended
Supraclavicular SCA: Subclavian artery	Linear u/s transducer is placed above the clavicle in a horizontal, coronal orientation. The transducer is tilted to aim the beams caudally, underneath the clavicle. The brachial plexus is adjacent and lateral to the SCA, superficial to the first rib. Advance needle in-plane towards the "corner pocket" formed by the SCA and the first rib. Inject 20 ml	Not recommended
Infraclavicular AA: axillary artery PMm: Pectoralis major muscle Pmm: Pectoralis minor muscle	The coracoid process is identified, and a linear u/s transducer is placed on the chest in a sagittal position below the clavicle adjacent to the coracoid process. The AA should be visualized beneath the PMm and Pmm. The three cords of the brachial plexus should be visualized	Not recommended

Axillary brachial plexus AA: Axillary artery MN: median nerve RN: radial nerve UN: ulnar nerve	around the AA. Advance needle in-plane toward the 6 o'clock position on the AA. Inject 20–30 ml perivascularly Near the axilla on the upper arm, a linear u/s transducer is oriented in a sagittal orientation. The AA is identified with the MN, RN, and UN around it. Advance needle in-plane to be near these bundles in the axillary sheath. 15–20 ml perivascular injection or 5 ml at each nerve	Palpate AA. Advance 25 g needle into pulse while aspirating until blood is encountered. Keep advancing through the other side of the artery until blood is no longer aspirated. Inject 10 ml, deep to vessel. Withdraw needle until blood is again aspirated, and continue withdrawing gently until blood is no longer aspirated. Inject 10 ml, superficial to vessel.
Suprascapular nerve (SSN) SSA: suprascapular artery	Place a linear u/s transducer superior to the scapular spine, in a coronal plane. The suprascapular notch should be 2 cm medial to the posterior edge of the acromion and 2 cm superior (cranial) to the scapular spine. Identify the neurovascular bundle running through the notch, and advance a needle in-plane to make contact with the deepest portion. Inject 10–20 ml.	The scapular spine is palpated for the suprascapular notch; it is approximately 2 cm medial from the posterior edge of the acromion, and 2 cm cranial from the scapular spine. Advance 25 g needle until contact is made with the bone. Aspiration should take place every 3 ml due to the proximity of SSA to the SSN
Musculocutaneous nerve (MCN) AA: Axillary artery	Identify the MCN lateral to the AA and brachial plexus, within the coracobrachialis muscle. Advance a needle in-plane towards the nerve, and inject 3–5 ml	Palpate the AA, and the needle is directed lateral to the artery. Inject 5–10 ml into the coracobrachialis muscle.
Intercostobrachial nerve (ICBN)	An u/s probe is placed on the upper arm near the axilla in a horizontal orientation and the AA is identified. The needle is advanced in-plane while injecting into subcutaneous fat tissue from the anteromedial surface of the arm to the posteromedial surface, taking care not to pierce any subcutaneous veins that may be visible on ultrasound.	Near the axilla, a needle is used to make a skin wheal, then advanced under the skin subcutaneously on the medial surface of the upper arm from anterior to posterior. The needle is then slowly withdrawn through the subcutaneous tissue as local anesthetic is deposited. Inject 5–10 ml
Elbow block MN: median nerve	MN: a linear u/s transducer is placed on the coronal plane. The MN lies between the flexor digitorum	MN: palpate the pulse of the brachial artery and insert a 25- or 27-gauge needle 1 cm medial to the pulse to a

Table 24.3 (cont.)

Block	Ultrasound (u/s)	Landmark
UN: ulnar nerve RN: radial nerve MCNF: medial cutaneous nerve of the forearm LCNF: lateral cutaneous nerve of the forearm (Figure 24.3)	superficialis and flexor digitorum profundus, as a hyperechoic honeycombed oval. UN: medial to the ulnar artery in the proximal forearm. RN: identify RN above the elbow joint on the lateral surface of the arm. It lies in a triangle formed by the humerus, biceps, and triceps. Inject 3–5 ml peripherally to each nerve	depth of about 1–2 cm; a loss of resistance may be appreciated as the needle tip passes through the biceps. Inject 5–10 ml, and then withdraw to its insertion and another 5–10 ml subcutaneously along the medial border of the biceps tendon to block the MCNF. UN: identify UN on medial surface of the upper arm, approximately 2 cm proximal to the medial humeral epicondyle. Insert a needle 2 cm proximal to the medial epicondyle and directed 45 degrees cephalad about 2 cm. RN: RN is located lateral to the biceps tendon and medial to the brachioradialis muscle, 2 cm proximal to the elbow crease. Insert needle, advance towards the lateral epicondyle to a depth of 2–4 cm, and deposit local anesthetic. The needle is then withdrawn to its insertion and directed laterally in the subcutaneous tissue lateral to the biceps tendon. Local anesthetic is deposited here to block the LCNF
Wrist block MN: median nerve UN: ulnar nerve RN: radial nerve	MN: linear u/s transducer is placed on the volar surface of the forearm at the wrist crease, and traced 5–10 cm proximally to locate the median nerve proximal to the tendons of the wrist (which can appear similar to nerves). The nerve will have a honeycomb appearance. Inject 3–5 ml. UN: linear transducer is placed on the volar surface of the arm at the wrist crease, UN can be visualized between the hyperechoic ulnar bone and the pulsating ulnar artery.	MN: a 25- or 27-gauge needle is inserted medial or lateral to the flexor palmaris longus tendon and advanced until it contacts bone, taking care not to elicit a paresthesia. UN: a 25- or 27-gauge needle pierces the skin medial and deep to the flexor carpi ulnaris tendon, and is advanced about 1 cm, until the tip is deep to the tendon, without eliciting paresthesia. Inject 3–5 ml. RN: the radial styloid is identified, and a 25- or 27-gauge needle is inserted just proximal to this on the volar surface of the wrist, aiming the needle tip medially. Half

	RN: A field block can be performed at the level of the styloid process on the radius to block the branches of the radial nerve, or the radial nerve can be identified with ultrasound in the forearm. The radial nerve can be identified lateral to the radial artery, superficial to the radius, at the mid forearm.	of the dose of local anesthetic can be deposited here. The needle is then withdrawn to its insertion point and redirected laterally, and the other half of the local anesthetic can be deposited in this location.
Digital Block		Insert a 25- or 27-gauge needle into the web space on the lateral and medial sides of the digit where the digital nerves run. Inject 3–5 ml in each web space.
Lower Extremity		
Femoral	A linear ultrasound probe is placed on the inguinal crease in a coronal plane. The femoral nerve is adjacent and lateral to the femoral artery. Advance a needle in-plane underneath the femoral nerve, towards the femoral artery. Inject 15–30 ml	Not recommended
Fascia iliaca (FI) ASIS: anterior superior iliac spine	Place a linear transducer over the ASIS in a sagittal plane. Tilt the tail of the u/s 5 to 10° medially, and scan medially until the fascial "bow-tie" is seen on the screen, which is formed by the insertion of the sartorius muscle caudally and the internal oblique cranially. The deep fascia of the "bow-tie" is the FI, the iliacus muscle and the ilium. Inject 30 ml between the FI and the iliacus muscle	Palpate the ASIS. Measure 2 cm medial and 2 cm superior. A blunt-tipped needle is then advanced perpendicularly to the skin, looking for two "pops," the first through the fascia lata and the second through the FI. Inject 30 ml. Femoral arterial pulse can be palpated and marked to ensure that the injection point is not near either the femoral artery or nerve
Lateral femoral cutaneous nerve (LFCN)	Identify the ASIS. Place linear u/s probe 2 cm medial and inferior to the ASIS. LFCN runs between the tensor fascia lata muscle and sartorius muscles. Inject 5–10 ml	Identify the ASIS. A point 2 cm inferior and 2 cm medial is marked. A 25- or 27-gauge needle is advanced perpendicular to the skin, until the operator ascertains a loss of resistance or fascial pop, or the patient endorses paresthesia of the lateral thigh. Inject 5–10 ml

Table 24.3 (cont.)

Block	Ultrasound (u/s)	Landmark
Subgluteal sciatic GT: greater trochanter IT: ischial tuberosity QFM: quadrator femoris muscle GM: gluteus maximus	In lateral decubitus position with hip flexed, mark the GT and the IT. Draw a straight line to connect them. Place a curved u/s probe in the midpoint of this line. The GT and IT should be able to be visualized on ultrasound, and just deep to the GM and superficial to the QFM, the sciatic nerve should be visualizec as a hyperechoic structure. Inject 20 ml	Not recommended
Popliteal sciatic TN: tibial nerve PA: popliteal artery CPN: common peroneal nerve (aka common fibular nerve)	A linear u/s transducer is placed on the posterior knee at the popliteal crease. Identify the TN deep to the PA. Trace the TN cranially until the CPN is seen to be joining the TN to form the sciatic nerve. Just below the level of the bifurcation into two discrete nerves, direct a needle in-plane until the tip is between the two nerves and beyond the sheath surrounding the nerves	Not recommended
Adductor canal SFA: superficial femoral artery	At the halfway point between these ASIS and patella, a linear u/s transducer is placed on the thigh in a coronal (cross-sectional) orientation. Increase depth to visualize the femur. Scan medially until the oval or boat-shaped sartorius muscle is seen, with the pulsating SFA beneath it. Advance a needle in-plane towards the 11 o'clock position on the SFA. Inject 10 ml perivascularly	Not recommended
Saphenous nerve (SN) SV: saphenous vein	The SN can be visualized just below the knee at the level of the tibial tuberosity. A linear u/s transducer is placed in a coronal plane on the medial surface of the leg below the knee. The saphenous nerve can be seen adjacent to the saphenous vein. Inject 5 ml	The SN runs with the SV along the medial aspect of the lower leg. Identify the SV 3 cm distal to the tibial tuberosity. Inject anterior and posterior to the SV. Alternatively, the SN can be blocked by palpating the medial femoral condyle and injecting in a fan-like

| Ankle block (Figure 24.1)
TN: tibial nerve
PTA: posterior tibial artery
DPN: deep peroneal nerve
ATA: anterior tibial artery
SPN: superficial peroneal nerve
SN: saphenous nerve
SV: saphenous vein
EHL: extensor hallucis longus | TN: TN runs with the PTA, where the PT pulse s appreciated. Place linear u/s transducer on the ankle at the level of the medial malleolus and identify the PTA. TN should be adjacent to the artery. Inject 3–5 ml

DPN: DPN runs with the ATA at the level of the ankle. A linear u/s probe can be placed on the anterior ankle in a transverse orientation, and the artery and nerve will be seen on the surface of the tibia. Inject 3–5 ml

SPN: SPN can be located just proximal and anterior to the lateral malleolus, as a hyperechoic structure superficial to the fibula. Inject 3–5 ml between the subcutaneous tissue and the periosteum of the lateral malleolus.

Sural nerve: Identify sural nerve posterior to the lateral malleolus on the medial surface of the soleus muscle.

SN: Identify SN on the medial surface of the ankle, adjacent to the SV and slightly anterior. Inject 3–5 ml between the periosteum of the medial malleolus and the skin. | distribution superficial to the periosteum of the medial femoral epicondyle and posterior to it

TN: Palpate for the PTA posterior to the medial malleolus. Insert needle from posterior to anterior towards the arterial pulse until contact with the posterior medial malleolus. The needle is then withdrawn 1-2 mm and after negative aspiration, 5 ml of local anesthetic is injected

DPN: Palpate the groove lateral to the EHL on the anterior surface of the tibia. Inject lateral to the EHL

SPN: Inject 5 ml into the superficial skin from medial to lateral malleolus creating a wheal connected the two

Sural nerve: Inject 5 ml in the subcutaneous tissue posterior to the lateral malleolus and extended towards the Achilles tendon

SN: Insert a needle on the anteromedial surface of the ankle at the level of the medial malleolus next to the SV |

Necessity/availability of ultrasound guidance and any risk/benefit/alternative consideration should be weighed before block performance.

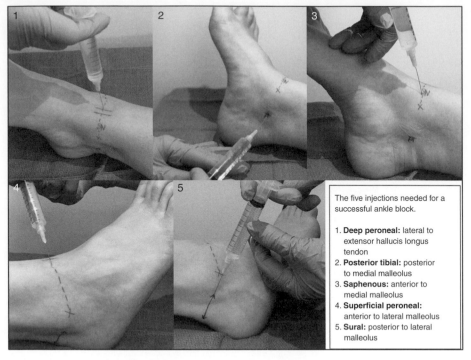

The five injections needed for a successful ankle block.

1. **Deep peroneal:** lateral to extensor hallucis longus tendon
2. **Posterior tibial:** posterior to medial malleolus
3. **Saphenous:** anterior to medial malleolus
4. **Superficial peroneal:** anterior to lateral malleolus
5. **Sural:** posterior to lateral malleolus

Figure 24.1 The five injections needed for a successful ankle block.

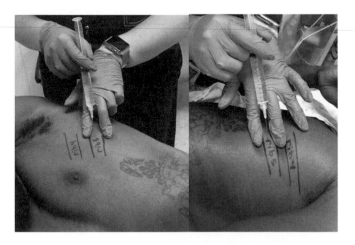

Figure 24.2 Landmark technique for placement of serratus anterior plane block.

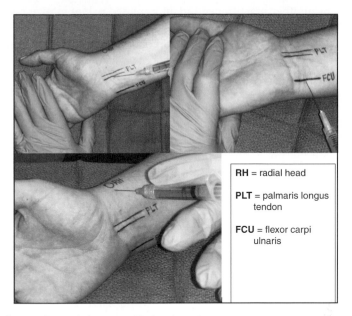

RH = radial head

PLT = palmaris longus
tendon

FCU = flexor carpi
ulnaris

Figure 24.3 Radian, median, and ulnar nerve block at the wrist.

- Short-beveled, blunt needles may be in short supply in a disaster circumstance. If only long-beveled, sharp needles are available, we recommend against regional anesthetic techniques that may place the sharp-tipped needle in the vicinity of a major, large peripheral nerve. Sharp needles *are acceptable* in fascial-plane blocks such as the PECS II, fascia iliaca, transversus abdominis plane (TAP), erector spinae, axillary brachial plexus, isolated suprascapular nerve, isolated axillary nerve, scalp, superficial cervical plexus, ankle, digital, elbow, and wrist blocks.
- Due to the limited availability of specialized short-beveled, blunt-tipped needles in a potentially disastrous environment, we recommend that these needles be reserved for circumstances where a major nerve is being blocked, such as the femoral or sciatic nerves, or the proximal brachial plexus. Obviously, this would also likely limit one to the use of ultrasound-guided regional anesthetics, vs the landmark-based techniques. Careful planning can allow for the use of a single needle for multiple blocks in a single patient (e.g. a sciatic-femoral or sciatic-lumbar plexus combination), and resultant conservation of supplies.

Limitations in Documentation
- Fully developed charting mechanisms will likely be unavailable in an austere environment; practitioners will therefore need to agree on a method for identifying blocked patients. A functioning block could be misinterpreted by other care providers as new-onset weakness or loss of sensation, and could result in injury of the insensate limb, unnecessary diagnostic tests or procedures, and a resultant waste of time and supplies needed elsewhere. Lack of documentation or marking of the patient could also lead to

repeat block by another practitioner and an increased risk of local anesthetic systemic toxicity.

• Any symbol or word that can be placed on the patient to indicate the presence of a block and a dose of long-acting local anesthetic should take into account the training levels of staff as well as any pre-existing language barriers, and should indicate the type, concentration, volume, and time (including date) of local anesthetic used. Patient and environmental factors (skin color, close patterns of wounding, humidity, crowding) can make skin markings difficult to see or easily smudged, and should all be considered in the design of the marking plan to be used.

• In order to limit the amount of required documentation (type, volume, concentration, date/time) and decrease the likelihood of pass-down communication errors, standardization of volume and concentration given for each type of block can lead to improved communication and decreased risk of patient harm.

References

1. Buckenmaier C, Lee EH, Shields CH, Sampson JB, Chiles JH. Regional anesthesia in austere environments. *Reg Anes Pain Med* 2003;**28**(4):321–327.

2. Stojadinovic A, Auton A, Peoples GE, et al. Responding to challenges in modern combat casualty care: innovative use of advanced regional anesthesia. *Pain Med* 2006;**7**(4):330–338.

3. Rice M, Gwertzman A, Finley T, Morey TE. Anesthetic practice in Haiti after the 2010 earthquake. *Anesth Analg* 2010;**111**:1445–1449.

4. Morey T, Rice MJ. Anesthesia in an austere setting: lessons learned from the Haiti relief operation. *Anesthesiology Clin* 2013;**31**:107–115.

5. Fang G, Wan L, Mei W, Yu HH, Luo AL. The minimum effective concentration (MEC90) of ropivacaine for ultrasound-guided supraclavicular brachial plexus block. *Anaesthesia* 2016;**71**(6):700–705.

6. Takeda, A, Ferraro LH, Rezende AH, et al. Minimum effective concentration of bupivacaine for axillary brachial plexus block guided by ultrasound. *Braz J Anesthesiol* 2015;**65**(3):163–169.

7. Taha AM, Abd-Elmaksoud AM. Lidocaine use in ultrasound-guided femoral nerve block: what is the minimum effective anaesthetic concentration (MEAC90)? *Br J Anaesth* 2013;**110**(6):1040–1044.

8. Taha AM, Abd-Elmaksoud AM. Ropivacaine in ultrasound-guided femoral nerve block: what is the minimal effective anaesthetic concentration (EC90)? *Anaesthesia* 2014;**69**:678–682.

9. Cappelleri G, Aldegheri G, Ruggieri F, et al. Minimum effective anesthetic concentration (MEAC) for sciatic nerve block: subgluteus and popliteal approaches. *Can J Anaesth* 2007;**54**(4):283–289.

10. Vadepitte C, Gautier P, Xu D, et al. Effective volume of ropivacaine 0.75% through a catheter required for interscalene brachial plexus blockade. *Anesthesiology* 2013;**118**(4):863–867.

11. Falcão LF, Perez MV, de Castro I, et al. Minimum effective volume of 0.5% bupivacaine with epinephrine in ultrasound-guided interscalene brachial plexus block. *Br J Anaesth* 2013;**110**(3):450–455.

12. Sandhu NS, Maharlouei B, Patel B, et al. Simultaneous bilateral infraclavicular brachial plexus blocks with low-dose lidocaine using ultrasound guidance. *J Ultrasound Med* 2006;**104**(1):199–201.

13. Song JG, Jeon DG, Kang BJ, Park KK. Minimum effective volume of mepivacaine for ultrasound-guided supraclavicular block.

Korean J Anesthesiol 2013;**65**(1):37–41.

14. Pavičić Šarić J, Vidjak V, Tomulić K, Zenko J. Effects of age on minimum effective volume of local anesthetic for ultrasound-guided supraclavicular brachial plexus block. *Acta Anaesthesiol Scand* 2013;**57**(6):761–766.

15. O'Donnell BD, Iohom G. An estimation of the minimum effective anesthetic volume of 2% lidocaine in ultrasound-guided axillary brachial plexus block. *Anesthesiology* 2009;**111**(1):25–29.

16. Ferraro LH, Takeda A, dos Reis Falcão LF, et al. Determination of the minimum effective volume of 0.5% bupivacaine for ultrasound-guided axillary brachial plexus block. *Braz J Anesthesiol* 2014;**64**(1):49–53.

17. González AP, Bernucci F, Pham K, et al. Minimum effective volume of lidocaine for double-injection ultrasound-guided axillary block. *Reg Anesth Pain Med* 2013;**38**(1):16–20.

18. Bang SU Kim DJ, Bae JH, Chung K, Kim Y. Minimum effective local anesthetic volume for surgical anesthesia by subparaneural, ultrasound-guided popliteal sciatic nerve block: a prospective dose-finding study. *Medicine (Baltimore)* 2016;**95**(34):e4652.

19. Techasuk W, Bernucci F, Cupido T, et al. Minimum effective volume of combined lidocaine-bupivacaine for analgesic subparaneural popliteal sciatic nerve block. *Reg Anesth Pain Med* 2014;**39**(2):108–111.

20. Jeong JS, Shim JC, Jeong MA, Lee BC, Sung IH. Minimum effective anaesthetic volume of 0.5% ropivacaine for ultrasound-guided popliteal sciatic nerve block in patients undergoing foot and ankle surgery: determination of ED50 and ED95. *Anaesth Intensive Care* 2015;**43**(1):92–97.

21. American Society of Anesthesiologists. Standards for basic anesthetic monitoring. www.asahq.org/standards-and-guidelines/standards-for-basic-anesthetic-monitoring (accessed September 2019).

22. Lewis SR. Ultrasound guidance for upper and lower limb blocks. *Cochrane Database Syst Rev* 2015;**11**(9): CD006459.

Chapter 25

Power and Light: Impact of Electrical Systems Failure on the Delivery of Anesthetic Care

Frederick W. Burgess and Jordan Anderson

Over the past 50 years, surgery, physiologic monitoring, and the delivery of anesthesia has undergone a high technology revolution. The finger on the pulse, manual blood pressures, and precordial stethoscopes have given way to advances in electrocardiography, automated blood pressure, pulse oximetry, end-tidal capnography, and transesophageal echocardiography, just to name a few of the major advances. As automation has progressed, anesthetic practice and surgery have become extremely dependent upon a reliable power supply for clinical operations. The Joint Commission (TJC) standards require routine testing of the hospital backup power supply (EC.02.05.07.04); 12 times a year, at intervals of not less than 20 days and not more than 40 days, the hospital tests each emergency generator for at least 30 continuous minutes. The completion dates of the tests are documented in the generator and automatic transfer switch (ATS) testing logs by the technicians performing the tests. Additional specifics are addressed in TJC standards on load testing and performance. Despite adherence to these requirements, catastrophic failures still occur with amazing frequency throughout the United States, and routinely throughout the world.[1]

In the United States, a routine search of the Internet will generate numerous news articles describing regional and local power outages on a monthly basis. Causes range from lightning strikes to automobile accidents, and even stray bullets from target practice striking a transformer. The most common cause of power failures in the USA and worldwide are attributable to natural disasters, such as weather, earthquakes, and the like. The most recent example was the impact of "Super Storm" Sandy, which produced major coastal flooding and wind damage along the Northeastern USA. Power outages severely impacted several hospitals in the New York City area, prompting the evacuation of patients and transfer to other healthcare facilities. Although standards were met, the severe flooding compromised the backup electrical power systems, resulting in complete electrical failure. However, even in the absence of catastrophic events, power failures have occurred due to small and seemingly inconsequential events. In 1999, the Rhode Island Hospital experienced a major power outage resulting from a child's helium-filled balloon tangling with power lines and causing a crossed circuit at a power substation, knocking out both feed lines to the hospital complex. The backup electrical systems failed to operate properly, when a transfer switch failed, producing a complete power loss to much of the facility, including life-safety power. Over a span of four years, the facility experienced two more major outages impacting the surgical suite, despite installing additional backup power systems. A systematic literature review on the health impact of power outages produced by extreme events from 2011–2013 was conducted by Klinger et al.[2] During the interval examined, the USA experienced 14 reported power outages, all related to extreme meteorological events. As the national power grid infrastructure ages, the likelihood of more power and light failures will increase. Add to the weather concerns, the risk of computer glitches and computer virus attacks, as was seen in the massive power failure that blacked out the entire Northeast and portions of Canada in 2003, it is essential that anesthesia providers develop plans, policies, and simulation programs to prevent patient harm in the event of a major power outage.[3] This chapter will examine the impact of power and light outages on the delivery of anesthetic care, and recommend steps to avert disastrous consequences.

Impact of Power and Light Outage on Patient Care

In the USA, all hospitals are required to have a backup independent power supply, capable of sensing and responding to external power grid feed-line failures. The backup power supply should assume the workload within 3 minutes, supplying all life-safety essential equipment, which should be plugged into the identified (red) power outlets in critical patient care areas. Most surgical suites should have an ample supply of power lines, but it is important to be aware that not all electrical outlets are powered by the backup generator power lines, and staff should verify that critical equipment, such as monitors, ventilators, anesthesia machines, etc. should be attached to the proper power line circuit. Backup generators should have sufficient fuel to operate for 72 hours at minimal load. Diesel fuel is subject to degradation over time and bacterial growth, and should be subject to monitoring, replacement, or consumption over time to avoid system failures. The National Fire Protection Association (NFPA) has introduced fuel standards to reduce generator failures. As noted above, the NFPA and TJC have specific requirements for regular testing schedules to insure dependability.[1,4]

Although most surgical suites are capable of continuing to operate with reliable backup power systems, the entire hospital may be seriously impacted by power and light outages (see Box 25.1). Emergency lighting is limited in non-patient care areas, and battery backup lighting is only designed to operate for 30 minutes to aide evacuation. Many areas may not have any emergency lighting at all. Elevators may continue to operate under backup power, but the workload may strain the generator capacity and contribute to the loss of essential power. Non-emergent facility activity should be discontinued, including clinic visits, non-emergent (elective) surgery, and even urgent surgeries should be considered for transfer to unaffected healthcare facilities, if feasible. Ongoing surgical cases should be completed as rapidly and as safely as possible.

Areas likely to be adversely effected by a major power outage within the facility include: food service and storage, HVAC operation, temperature regulation, electronic health records (EHR), communications within and outside the facility, transportation within and outside the facility, medication access and storage, blood-banking activity, and lighting. Additional concerns may arise over the impact of the disaster on the surrounding community, regional hospitals, and broader emergency management. In widespread power outages, most hospitals must anticipate a surge in demand on resources, and many patients who receive extensive medical care in their homes, such as the use of oxygen concentrators, home dialysis, and other critical life-sustaining therapies will seek care in the emergency department. Although, the surgical suite may remain operationally capable, supporting elements may be inadequate, making it important to resist the temptation to sustain normal operation.

Box 25.1 Systems Impacted by Power Outage

- Lighting
  - Critical systems will function with backup power supply
  - Total blackout if backup power system fails
- Heating, ventilation, and air conditioning (HVAC)
  - Loss of cooling and heating
  - Lighting
  - Loss of vacuum/suction
  - Loss of anesthesia scavenging system
- Anesthesia critical equipment
  - Ventilators
  - Desflurane vaporizer
  - Physiologic monitors
  - Suction
  - Infusion pumps
  - Patient warming devices
  - Cardiopulmonary bypass pumps and intra-aortic balloon pump
- Communication
  - Fire and patient bedside alarms
- Transportation
- Laboratory and blood-banking support
- Food (storage and cooking)

Anesthetic-Specific Considerations in Power and Light Outages

To address the impact of power outages on the delivery of anesthetic care, it may be helpful to examine the anesthesia clinical care pathway from start to recovery. As outlined in Figure 25.1, loss of power and light will depend on the degree to which the power resources have been compromised. The loss of outside feed power will often be barely perceptible in most modern surgical suites, as the backup power supply switches on. However, in complete failure, a catastrophic loss of power may occur in the operating room (OR) and the impact on normal delivery of anesthetic care would be devastating. To assess your facility's readiness, conducting a live simulation can be very illuminating in identifying unrecognized and potentially fatal flaws. The following discussion will focus on the worst case scenario, loss of the backup power supply.

Pre-Operative Considerations

Increasingly, healthcare facilities and physician practices have converted to electronic health records (EHR). During complete power failure, access to EHR will not be possible; this may extend to include laboratory testing and other clinical data access. Notification of laboratory results may depend on runners to carry information from the lab to the bedside care setting. Some access to battery-operated hemoglobin and blood glucose bedside testing is highly desirable in the surgical suite. Anesthesia notes and records should be recorded on paper records for hand-off to subsequent providers and eventual scanning into the permanent record. As noted above, elective cases should not be started during a power-outage

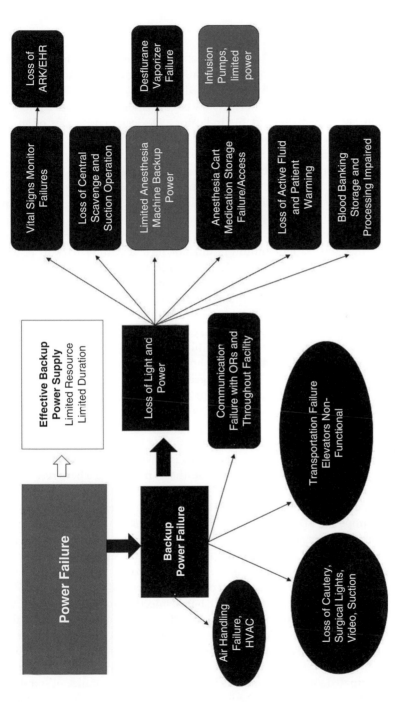

Figure 25.1 Power and light.

emergency. The elective schedule should be held or cancelled, and urgent cases transferred, if possible, to an unaffected facility

Intra-Operative Considerations

During a complete power outage, any ongoing surgical cases should be terminated in the most expedient and safe conclusion possible. As identified in Figure 25.1, many routine monitoring systems may fail, or be available on a limited timeline with battery backup. It is important to note that while many medical devices now have a battery backup, there are still several devices that do not have battery status indicators. Devices that do can often be difficult to assess exactly how much run time is left on the battery under the current conditions. Device manufacturer instructions should be followed regarding device storage (e.g. "Store plugged in") to ensure the battery is at full capacity when needed. Also, a robust facility battery replacement program is imperative to maintain battery capacities and prevent issues such as deformation, swelling, overheating, catching fire, giving off a sulfur odor, or even explosion.

During a recent "stress test" at our institution, it was surprising to many of our providers to discover that our patient monitors did not have a battery backup power source. Attempts to plug the monitors into the auxiliary outlets on the anesthesia machine also failed, as the outlets are not active when external power fails and the machine is operating on battery backup. This included the desflurane vaporizer, which is connected to an auxiliary electrical circuit on the anesthesia machine. Individual patient monitor and anesthesia machine configurations will vary, so it pays dividends to simulate a complete loss of power to determine what will or will not function under worst case scenario conditions. Transport monitors are an alternative should the room monitors fail.[5] Most modern anesthesia machines operate with a rechargeable backup uninterruptible power supply (UPS), capable of operating the electronics for at least 30 minutes, and depending on the electrical load and life cycle of the batteries, considerably longer. Mechanical ventilation will tax the batteries, particularly with piston-driven ventilators, and when feasible, manual ventilation or spontaneous ventilation should be implemented. Regional anesthesia, particularly subarachnoid anesthesia, total intravenous anesthesia (TIVA), and deep sedation are great alternatives to general anesthesia in settings where resources, including electricity, are scarce.

TIVA is a reasonable alternative to inhalation anesthesia; however, the availability of intravenous infusion pumps and inadequate residual battery life may hamper this approach. Propofol infusion pumps operating on disposable C-cell batteries are a great option, but are rapidly disappearing from practice. Most infusion pumps are now operated with rechargeable batteries, which often fail to hold their charge as they approach the end of their life cycle. Gravity-drip intravenous infusion sets are an option, but they will not provide reliable delivery during evacuation transport. Intermittent bolus injection may be a worst case option. Draw-over vaporizer anesthesia machines are viable options for delivering inhalational anesthesia in military and Third World settings, but are not FDA approved for use in the USA. The chief advantage to the draw-over vaporizer is that it does not require a power source to function.

Dependence on automated vital sign monitors has led to the disappearance of standard monitoring devices, such as precordial stethoscopes, manual sphygmomanometers, and battery-operated pulse oximeters from OR anesthesia supplies. Due to infrequent use, they

Table 25.1 Anesthesia blackout/evacuation kit

Anesthesia blackout kit	Add-ins taken from OR room supplies for transport/evacuation
Disposable laryngoscope and blades	Fluids
LED flashlight (AA batteries)	Syringes
LED headlamp (AA batteries)	Medications
Additional AA batteries	Endotracheal tubes
Sphygmomanometer	Stylets
Stethoscope	Tape
Carry bag with shoulder strap to store items	Portable suction unit
Paper anesthesia records and controlled substance inventory	Oxygen bottle with regulator for transport
Portable pulse oximeter	Transport monitor

are often removed and not replaced or checked on a regular basis. During our blackout "stress-test," it was discovered that the flashlight had been removed, and there was no basic monitoring equipment in the room. A handy laryngoscope or cell phone may serve as a critical flashlight until proper supplies can be located. Many operating rooms are constructed with no outside windows, and can be extremely dark as the battery-operated emergency lights fail. Battery-operated headlamps should be stored in conveniently secured locations, to prevent removal for other purposes, and a regular program to replace the battery supplies at least annually should be implemented. Batteries should not be stored in the flashlights or headlamps to prevent corrosion and damage. Selecting headlamps and flashlights with bright LED lamps and capable of sharing the same battery type simplifies procurement and storage. Rechargeable batteries are not recommended, due to the infrequent likelihood of use, and their gradual failure to hold their charge over time. At our institution, we have developed anesthesia "go" bags, which are stored with dated zip-lock closures (see Table 25.1). These bags are designed to be brought to the active anesthesia sites in the event of an emergency evacuation or blackout. Blood pressure cuffs, laryngoscopes, stethoscopes, headlamps, flashlights, portable pulse oximeters, paper records, controlled substance inventory forms and room to carry medication supplies and fluids for transport are included. Portable suction, bag-valve mask assemblies, medications, endotracheal tubes, and portable oxygen supplies are stored in the surgical suite and may be accessed if needed and added to the bag for evacuation. The advantage of using this system is that the needed items are less likely to be misplaced, and periodic battery exchanges can be conveniently accomplished on an annual basis.

Fluid warmers and patient warming systems will not be operational during complete power failures. The inability to rapidly warm and infuse blood products should be taken into consideration when planning surgery under power outage conditions. The concept of second-look surgery should be considered, as it may be better to return and complete the surgery at a later time than risk the consequences of hypothermia, coagulopathy, and acidosis.

Medication Access

At many hospitals, the traditional anesthesia cart has been replaced by some form of medication inventory control system. Most of these medication carts have direct communication with the pharmacy to assess inventory and log the use of individual medications and identify access to controlled substances. Battery backup power supplies attached to these carts may have very limited power supply, providing only 20 minutes of function. In power failure conditions, the cart may remain unlocked, if the provider has logged in and opened the cart. Access to most drawers will remain open; however, once the power pack fails, a key kept in the pharmacy must be brought to the OR to unlock the cart and to access the controlled substances.[5] It will be necessary to keep the key in the individual room to provide security for the controlled substance medications, should the provider leave the area, or to open a previously locked cart. Management of the carts, keys, and records should be identified in a power failure policy or standard operating procedure document.

HVAC Failure

During complete power failures, air-handling capability, heating, cooling, waste gas scavenging systems, and vacuum (suction) may be adversely effected. Positive-pressure airflow may be compromised, increasing the risk of contamination of the surgical field, making all but essential surgery inadvisable. External environmental conditions, if adverse, will influence temperatures within the facility. In glass and steel modern buildings, the ability to open a window to provide ventilation may not be an option. The loss of vacuum systems will compromise suction on the surgical field, and may impact the evacuation of inhalational anesthetics, leading to contamination of the OR. Switching to TIVA may be the best alternative in this situation.

Gas Supplies

In most cases, power outages do not impact critical gas supplies; however, power loss may impact alarm systems. Backup oxygen supplies should be available at all times, in the event of a catastrophic failure of the gas supply. Battery-operated oxygen monitors are found on all anesthesia machines. In the event of a gas supply failure, self-inflating bag-valve mask assemblies should be maintained on the anesthesia cart or machine for emergency use.

Evacuation Transport

Transport within high-rise buildings will be hampered. The used of elevators may be possible in partial power outages, but will not be viable in complete outages. Patient movement to and from hospital wards will require carry transport up and down stairways. Under temporary conditions, the post-anesthesia care unit (PACU) may serve as the recovery and continuous-care delivery location. Evacuation from one level to another may require the use of hand-carry stretchers or other type of carry device. Critical care patients are probably best served by recovering in the PACU and bringing needed nursing staff and equipment to the patient. In the event an evacuation from the location or facility becomes necessary, plans should be made to move to a staging point on the ground floor, such as the emergency department. Documentation of any patient movement or transfers should be carefully registered through patient administration for tracking purposes.

Planning and Training

As alluded to above, conducting realistic power and light failure simulations are very helpful in creating a sense of awareness, and an action plan in the event of a catastrophic failure. Going through the action steps of simulating a surgical procedure in no-light conditions reduces panic, promotes a sense of confidence in the steps to be taken, and provides experience with creative thinking. Many will forget that their cell phone or a laryngoscope can serve as an immediate light source in a power failure. Equally important, a blackout stress test can aid in identifying existing deficiencies, unanticipated equipment failures, or the lack of vital basic monitoring equipment. It also helps to conduct these blackout drills in different rooms and anesthetizing locations with the entire surgical team, as the anesthesia team may be able to function well, but the surgeons and OR nursing staff may be unprepared.

Summary

Limited power failures occur with surprising regularity in the United States, and are often a way of life in the underdeveloped world. Major climatological events have been associated with large-scale power and lighting failures, impacting multiple regional medical centers simultaneously (e.g. Hurricane Katrina), and making patient transfers exceedingly difficult, if not impossible.[2] Anesthesia providers must be prepared to provide limited basic monitoring and anesthetic delivery capability to provide safe care to patients in the surgery during power and lighting failures.[6] Taking steps to develop and test power failure response measures can be lifesaving when the lights go out.

References

1. The Joint Commission. *Sentinel Event Alert: Preventing Adverse Events Caused by Emergency Electrical Power Systems Failures.* Oakbrook Terrace, IL: The Joint Commission on Accreditation of Healthcare Organizations; 2006.

2. Klinger C, Landeg O, Murray V. Power outages, extreme events and health: a systematic review of the literature from 2011–12. *PLOS Curr* 2014;**6**: ecurrents. dis.04eb1dc5e73dd1377e05a10e9edde673.

3. Klein KR, Rosenthal MS, Klausner HA. Blackout 2003: preparedness and lessons learned from the perspectives of four hospitals. *Prehosp Disast Med* 2005;**20** (5):343–349.

4. NFPA. *NFPA 110 Standards for Emergency and Standby Power Systems,* Quincy, MA: NFPA; 2002.

5. Carpenter T, Robinson ST. Response to a partial power faliure in the operating room. *Anesth Analg* 2010;**110** (6):1644–1646.

6. Eichhorn JH, Hessel EA II. Electrical power failure in the operating room: a neglected topic in anesthesia safety. *Anesth Analg* 2010;**110**(6):1519–1521.

Appendix 1

Strategic Packing v13.2
NDMS Gear Guide/Personal Equipment List

Jonathan Malloch, TN-1 DMAT

Greetings motivated and prepared team members: Hopefully here you will find some assistance in putting together your deployment kit with the least amount of time and money wasted as well as reducing the chaos some experience when deployment orders are issued.

When Alert Status is issued, simply print out the checklist of choice and check it off as you pack. Drop it in your bag and zip it up. You will know you are packed and ready.

Seasoned team members know the best time to pack is after you return, that's when you really know what you need and what you don't. Some find it helpful to print off the list when they return and they pack then and zip the list into their kit with any notes for missing items or things that need to be packed at the time of deployment.

For new team members: Depending on your background and experience, this may be a lot of information to absorb. Relax. Read the document at your leisure then focus your build on the Fast Pack list. Build your kit from there.

Whatever you choose to deploy with, you alone must be able to carry. With that in mind, build your kit from the Fast Pack and develop it to suit your needs. The purpose of the comprehensive list is only to stimulate thought based on past experience. All things are not important to all people, so choose what you need and forget the rest.

As always, take from the knowledge of your teammates and leadership. Never hesitate to ask questions. As well, share your knowledge. This is a living document; dynamic and always improving. Feedback is welcomed and encouraged.

Disclaimer: No list or gear guide is 100% comprehensive. All deployments, both national and international require consideration of items and issues not listed here. Additionally, new and better products are being released often and have not yet been tested. I have no personal, professional, or commercial affiliation with any of the products discussed herein.

Feel free to email with comments/considerations and product reviews. jrmalloch@yahoo.com

This Guide Contains:

- **Section 1: "Fast Pack" List: The Essential Gear Checklist.** This "Fast Pack" is the essential basic kit and includes a checklist of the essential gear you will need for a deployment. Print it off and throw it in your bag. Several on the team carry this entire list plus extra gear in one 2600 cubic inch (medium) backpack like the Camelbak BFM or similar. Obviously they are light and fast and have no problem with minimal comfort. This is not a goal for the weak of wallet, as going this light and fast with quality gear requires a serious investment.

- **Section 2: Objectives/Bag and Gear Selection.**This is a general discussion of luggage size and design requirements, and the rationale for such.
- **Section 3: Personal Equipment Checklist: Comprehensive Print Out.**This is a comprehensive list, essentially a compendium of extensive feedback and personal and team experience. While it is lengthy, and perhaps excessive, it is only a guideline for the development of your personal deployment kit. Choose what works for you and ignore the rest.
- **Section 4: Personal Equipment Issues and Considerations**. This is a discussion of particular items on the list and the rationale for why selections are made. It is also part of an effort to help you select the best product for the conditions and obtain the best value for your money.

Section 1: Fast Pack List

Minimum Essential Gear Checklist

Main Bag
- Clothing:
  - Uniforms – 2 sets: (2 BDU blouses, 2 BDU pants, 2 team shirts – name-tagged and labeled). (Depending on travel orders, you may be wearing one full uniform)
  - Hats, Boonie type and/or team ball cap – (both are preferred)
  - Underwear – 3
  - Socks NOT COTTON – 3
  - Belt, Black   1 (2 preferred)
  - Boots
  - Civilian Clothing: 1 set (pants, shirt, and socks)
- Toiletries:
  - Toothbrush
  - Toothpaste
  - Razor with blades
  - Shave cream
  - Soap
  - Shampoo
  - Deodorant: (unscented attracts less insects)
- Sleep gear:
  - Sleeping bag
- Miscellaneous:
  - Water: 4 quarts if travel by ground. Restricted for commercial air travel. (See discussion in Section 4 regarding water and air travel)
  - Rations/Food: at least 2 MREs (Meals Ready to Eat) or similar "heater meals"
  - Flashlight: (it doesn't have to be big, just reliable and water tight)
  - Batteries: (don't buy "heavy duty" they last ½ the time of regular batteries)

- Mug and spoon (any travel type mug, plastic, or metal)
- Jump bag:
    - Rain jacket and pants
    - Gloves, work type
    - Eye protection/safety glasses (required for work in/around aircraft)
    - Hearing protection: (soft ear plugs for work in/around aircraft and day sleeping)
    - Headlamp (if not LED type, a spare bulb is recommended)
    - Batteries, spare
    - Medical equipment, personal/work: (stethoscope/EMT scissors/hemostat/gloves etc.)
    - Water: 2 quarts if travel by ground. Restricted for commercial air travel. (See discussion in Section 4 regarding water and air travel)
    - Snacks: high energy, Snickers, Peanut M&M's,
    - First aid kit, individual type.
    - Wipes, (baby wipes) personal travel type packet
- On your person:
    - Federal ID, Federal credit card, immunization card and drivers license, etc. (wallet)
    - Phone, cell
    - Emergency contact card, team
    - Watch
    - Dog tags (some military pilots will not allow you aboard without dog tags)
    - Critical medications/allergy information bracelet or allergy dog tag.

Section 2: Objectives/Bag and Gear Selection

Objective

The objective in developing your personal gear is to enable you and your team to be self sufficient in nearly any conditions for approximately 3 days or 72 hours. After that time it is generally accepted that additional supplies will become available. To somewhat complicate this is the fact that team members are somewhat limited in how much weight we can carry and how many bags are allowed. Whatever you take, YOU must be able to move it.

A basic personal deployment kit should include: two bags, sufficient for 3 days, ideally including 6 quarts of water. (Current NTSB restrictions on water may require flexibility when on commercial aircraft. This is discussed in Section 4. Also, we assume some type of shelter will be available, hence personal tents/shelters will not be discussed here).

Recommended Equipment Bags/Luggage

One large, main bag: 6000–10 000 cubic inches or a bag with dimensions of approx. 15×30×15 inches to 16×36×16 inches or a similar-sized suitcase WITH WHEELS. This main bag will be checked for air travel and/or may be palletized for transport via military air or ground convoy; hence, it may not always be readily available to you.

One small bag, backpack style "jump bag/ready bag": 1200–3500 cubic inches. This jump bag will always stay with you, on the plane and in your immediate area of operation or in your vehicle.

Main Bag Considerations

With a minimum Fast Pack your main bag can run to 25–35 lbs. For the Comprehensive Pack out, your main bag may weigh 50–70+ pounds fully loaded, depending on how you outfit yourself. Wheels are very useful most of the time. Likewise, I have seen team bags come off the luggage belt in shreds, with straps broken, seams burst, or simply abraded through, not due to abuse, rather it was simply not the quality needed for this type of travel and weight. Standing in an abandoned airport with no power for 300 miles with your gear in a pile is the wrong time to figure out the $50–100 dollars you saved buying a "bargain" bag was a bad idea. It may be impossible to get a replacement for some time.

I have personally purchased and test packed and abused no less than ten main bags before some great ones emerged. They have ranged from $60-$300. You DO NOT have to spend $300 for a good bag.

I have below linked a few excellent bags. These are only suggestions to get you pointed in the right direction and provide visual examples of what we are discussing. The final decision is yours. I've tried a lot of bags that failed to support the weight or volumes loaded in them. I'm sure there are many more excellent bags not listed here yet to try.

Additionally, I've tried many bags that have excellent zippers, good wheels, and tough nylon that failed at the frame due to weight. As in, the bottom simply bends under the weight of the load. Avoid bags that don't have very rigid bottoms or full-length internal frames or rails that run the length of the bag to the wheel end. Some very excellent examples of good bags are listed below.

Main Bag Examples

High Sierra 36" Drop Bottom Rolling Duffel: This can usually be seen at Sierra Trading Post.com, Campmor.com, and Amazon.com. The High Sierra 36" Drop Bottom Rolling Duffel is a very nice bag with a lifetime warranty. This bag normally retails for near $200, but can sometimes be found for under $70 here. I have one with several deployments on it, as do several team members and it's a great bag for the money.

www.sierratradingpost.com
www.campmor.com

BlackHawk Enhanced Diver's Travel Bag with Wheels #21DT03BK: Several of the team members have these and are very happy with them. I've seen them for less than $150. This is an outstanding bag with a lifetime warranty (if you register it). There are two versions of this bag. The one with wheels is #21DT03BK.

www.blackhawk.com/

Cabelas Extreme Wheeled Duffel: This bag is utterly bombproof, has a lifetime warranty, and is expensive. Most agree it is worth it. You will likely never need another one in your lifetime.

www.cabelas.com

See also: L.L. Bean and Lands End also have some higher quality very rugged rolling duffels. While I believe they're high end enough to be suffiently rugged for deployment, the retail price of near $200 makes other bags a better value. These have lifetime warranties. Look for them on sale.

www.llbean.com
www.landsend.com

The North Face, MountainSmith, Mountain Hardware, and Eagle Creek are some of the finest rolling duffel bags available. They tend to be expensive at retail and come with lifetime warranties. Look for them on sale.

www.thenorthface.com
www.mountainsmith.com
www.mountainhardware.com
www.eaglecreek.com

Ready Bag/Jump bag

This can be a simple tactical-style backpack/daypack (preferred) or medium-size duffel. However, experience proves that having your hands free makes the backpack a better choice. It should be between 1200 and 3500 cubic inches. It will generally always be with you. You may carry it aboard for air travel and may check it at the aircraft door or put it under your seat or in the overhead bin. It will stay with you in your vehicle and be with you in your work area. Depending on circumstance, it should be able to hold at least 1 quart of your water supply. (Water transport is discussed in Section 4. Also, many bags now incorporate internal hydration systems, which are great for field work in conditions where you may be at risk of dehydration). It will also need to be able to accommodate sufficient gear for you to remain fairly comfortable and operational should your main bag be lost or delayed. Contents should include the basics: energy food/snacks, water, and basic comfort essentials such as a zip lock with dry socks, dry underwear, and baby wipes etc. It should contain basic protective essentials such as a rain poncho/parka, gloves, eye protection, hearing protection, sun block, along with the basics essential to perform your job such as stethoscope, medic scissors, personal protective equipment, etc., and a few other things that will be specifically outlined later.

Jump Bag Examples

Camelbak BFM, HAWG, and the Motherlode: These are excellent bags and have extensive field use. Several team members use the BFM and the comfort, versatility, and value is exceptional. They are worth the price and hold up very well. They can be seen at any police/military supply shops. Available nearly everywhere online, the best price on BFM is around $140 if you look.

www.camelbak.com

Maxpedition: Maxpedition offers a full line of pack options to meet any mission need. Good quality and customer service. Buy with confidence.

www.maxpedition.com

BlackHawk Tactical 3-Day Assault Pack: Several styles and sizes are available and all offer value and function. These packs run between $100 and $200 depending on style.

www.blackhawk.com

Spec Ops: Makes very good equipment, and is US made. The "T.H.E. Pack" (The Holds Everything Pack) is a very tough bag. This bag tends to fit smaller folks best. The team members who carry this pack are very happy with it and agree it is bombproof. This back can be found for about $100 if you are patient.

www.specopsbrand.com

The Kelty "Redwing": This is a very popular and very rugged non-"tactical" backpack and has year after year proved to be an excellent pack for both deployment and personal travel. These are also available at Dicks and REI and other outdoor equipment stores. They can be had for as little as $50.

www.kelty.com

www.REI.com

5.11products are also a good value and frequently on sale.

Section 3: Personal Equipment Checklist – Comprehensive

Checklist: **Bold** is your essential load out, i.e. "The Fast Pack" list. The rest is often useful but entirely optional. (*see reference notes for discussion of certain items)

Main Bag

- Clothing:
    - **Uniforms – 2 sets: (2 BDU blouses, 2 BDU pants, team shirts – name tagged and labeled*). (Depending on travel orders, you may be wearing one full set of uniform clothing)**
    - **Hats, Boonie type and/or team ball cap – (both are preferred)**
    - **Underwear – 3***
    - **Socks* – NOT COTTON – 3**
    - **Belt, Black – 1 (2 preferred)**
    - **Boots***
    - Sock Liners – 3 *
    - Compression bag, clothing type: (Eagle Creek makes some of the best)*
    - Shower shoes/flip-flops/Tevas etc. – 1
    - **Civilian Clothing: 1 set (pants, shorts, shirt, socks etc.)**
    - Sleepwear (scrubs, shorts, t-shirt etc.)
    - Swimwear (for co-ed shower facilities)
    - Tennis shoes or similar (allow your feet/boots some time off from each other)
- Cold weather clothing (optional and weather dependent):
    - Field jacket/ Parka, Polarguard or similar insulation (weather dependent)
    - Jacket/sweater, synthetic fleece
    - Pants, synthetic fleece
    - Gloves, synthetic fleece
    - Socks, synthetic: winter weight NOT COTTON
    - Thermal underwear, synthetic NOT COTTON
    - Hat/cap, wool or synthetic

- Toiletries: (a toiletries bag that hangs up is preferred)
  - **Toothbrush**
  - **Toothpaste**
  - **Razor with blades**
  - **Shave cream**
  - **Soap**
  - **Shampoo**
  - **Deodorant**: (unscented attracts less bugs)
  - Personal hygiene products
  - Handi wipes (travel pack)
  - Floss: (can double as high-strength sewing thread)
  - Foot powder (Gold Bond or similar works well for any/all hotspots or friction issues)
  - Moleskin
  - Toilet paper/paper towels: (several yards inside a zip lock to keep it dry)
  - Insect repellent: (3 M Ultrathon 2oz gel available at Wal-Mart or sporting goods store)
  - Sun block (REI brand is excellent, tasteless, odorless, greaseless and works well on lips)
  - Chapstick
  - Tums/antacids
  - Comb/brush
  - Washcloth/loofa*
  - Towel* (NOT COTTON)
  - Safety pins (3 large)
  - Small mirror: (unbreakable travel type)
  - Meds: Prescription and non-prescription pain relievers; (Tylenol, Advil, etc.)
  - Spare glasses in hard case
  - Spare contact lenses
  - Contact lens solution
  - Hearing protection: soft earplugs (essential for day sleepers during shift work)
- Sleep Gear:
  - **Sleeping bag***
  - Compression bag*
  - Mattress pad, foam or air*
  - Pillow*
  - Ground cloth (a military poncho doubles as an excellent ground cloth and shelter)
  - Space blanket
- Miscellaneous:
  - **Water* – 4 quarts. Restricted for air travel. (See discussion in Section 4 regarding water and air travel)**
  - **Rations/food: at least 2 MREs (Meals Ready to Eat) or similar "heater meals"**
  - **Flashlight/area light: it doesn't have to be big, just reliable and rugged/water tight**
  - **Batteries: don't buy "Heavy Duty" they last ½ the time of regular batteries**
  - **Mug and spoon: any travel type mug, plastic, or metal**
  - Rope: 50 ft. ("550 Paracord" is a great multiuse rope)

- Laundry bag
- Laundry detergent:* concentrate type
- Sewing/repair kit: small kit with 2–3 large safety pins
- Duct tape/gaffers tape: a 10 yard roll is about the size of a deck of cards
- Garbage bags:* 3 large, 45–55 gallon type
- Zip lock bags:* 3, one gallon freezer bags, 3, one-quart freezer bags
- Fire: Lighter, waterproof matches, magnesium starter, and striker, etc.
- Knife: Folding pocket type
- Leatherman type tool (optional)
- Strip plug* (optional; Wal-Mart $5 or less)
- Netting, mosquito type (optional)
- Chemical hand warmers: 2–4 (will dry out wet boots overnight)

Jump Bag

- Rain jacket and pants
- Work gloves
- Eye protection/safety glasses
- Hearing protection: soft ear plugs for work in and around aircraft and day sleeping
- Headlamp*: if not LED type, spare bulb is recommended
- Spare batteries
- Medical equipment, personal/work: (stethoscope/EMT scissors/hemostat/gloves, etc.)
- Water*– 2 quarts (if by ground, two Nalgene water bottles or hydration system or similar). Restricted for commercial air travel (see discussion in Section 4 regarding water and air travel)
- Snacks: high energy (Snickers, Peanut M&Ms, power bars, etc.)
- Notepad with pen or pencil ("Rite in the Rain" notepads are excellent)
- Sharpie/waterproof marker
- Team ball cap
- Zip-lock bag with the following:
  - Dry socks
  - Sock liners
  - Dry underwear
  - Rations/food: food for 24 hours (1–2 MREs, coffee/chocolate ("java juice/stomping grounds"))
- Zip-lock with the following:
  - Medications: prescription and non-prescription
  - Personal hygiene products
- Extra contact lenses/glasses
- Sun block
- Chapstick
- Hand wipes

- Band-Aids: fabric type
- Lighter/matches, waterproof
- Water purification tabs
- Sunglasses
- Sleep mask/bandana (for night shift day sleepers)
- Camera (charger and/or batteries)
- Reading material
- Playing cards/travel games
- Cell phone charger: car and wall or converter
- Trash bag – large 1: use as a bag cover, emergency rain gear or bivy
- Duct tape/gaffers tape: a 10 yard rolls is about the size of a deck of cards
- Rope: Paracord, 50 ft
- Chemlights/chemsticks – 3
- First aid kit, individual type
- Mask: particulate type, N-95
- Wipes: personal travel type packet.
- Zip ties
- Helmet (optional)
- Knee pads (optional)

On Your Person

- **Federal ID, federal credit card, immunization card**
- **Driver's license, professional licenses**
- **Emergency contact card, team/agency, etc.**
- **Dog tags (some military pilots will not allow you aboard without dog tags)**
- **Watch**
- **Critical medications/allergy information bracelet or allergy dog tag**
- Deployment orders/travel authorization (consider storing copy on jump drive)
- Money/credit cards
- Pocket size notebook/log book ("Rite in the Rain" recommended)
- Pen/Sharpie/waterproof marker
- Cell phone
- Cell phone carrier:* soft, unbreakable type. NOT PLASTIC
- Compass (optional)
- Whistle* (optional)

Before You Travel

- Make a photocopy of all important documents and cards (including your passport): lay the contents of your wallet on a photocopier and copy front and back. Leave a copy at your home in a secure place and a copy with someone you trust who you can contact if your wallet is lost or stolen. (If possible, email a copy to yourself)
- Print deployment orders and TA and itinerary (hard copy and digital copy to jump drive)

- Provide orders as needed to employer
- Leave team emergency contact information with your home base contact/family
- Make arrangements for pet care, home care, bills, mail pick-up, lawn care, etc.
- Refill critical prescriptions/meds
- Notify credit card carriers of pending travel

Section 4: Personal Equipment Issues and Considerations

Given the very nature of our mission, we are often working in less than ideal conditions. Plan on high heat, high humidity, and long hours. Laundry service or facilities may be unavailable as well. Clothes washed in a trash bag or buckets and hung to air dry may be the norm. At times uniforms may be worn for 2–3+ days, depending on how dirty it gets, how stinky one's teammates think they are and/or the lack of facilities. These conditions wear out the body too. Moisture and heat can break down the healthiest team member. As you build your kit, consider the following two issues.

Cotton Sucks: Cotton sucks up moisture and holds it. Once it's damp or wet, it tends to stay that way a long time, particularly in the heat and humidity we typically deploy in. It doesn't efficiently wick moisture away from the skin. With the exception of our BDUs, we have options in selecting high-performance synthetics for our base layer that are easily washed and dried. Synthetics air dry relatively quickly, even in high humidity. One can bucket wash good synthetics and line dry and wear within a few hours. If things get really pushed, one can very comfortably put on damp synthetics and they will dry within minutes while wearing them.

Skin Breakdown: Experience has shown serious skin breakdown related to retained heat and moisture that could have been avoided by selecting better undergarments. Obviously, this is a very personal choice but almost without exception, particularly in men, there have been significant issues related to this. Some effects were severe enough to render these individuals nearly immobile and essentially non-functional in the field. A quality synthetic undershirt can be very effective at controlling heat and moisture. In addition, it can quickly and easily be bucket or sink washed and air-dried. It will keep the "funk factor" down in your team shirt and BDU blouse and may extend the days between uniform washings. Additionally, a skin-drying agent such as Gold Bond powder can be effective in preventing moisture and heat issues.

Points to Consider

- Cotton will absorb up to 8% of its weight in water. Most synthetics will absorb less than 1%.
- A good synthetic will allow air to pass through (breathability) at five times the rate of cotton.
- Synthetics move moisture away from your skin. Cotton traps and holds it next to your skin.
- A synthetic t-shirt weighs about 60% of a cotton t-shirt.
- Synthetics wash easier, dry much quicker, and last much longer than cotton.

    Bottom Line: Synthetics dry quickly, maintain support, help control heat and moisture in the skin. They are easy to care for and they will take care of you.

*Following you will find a discussion of essential gear selection as noted in the checklists.

Underwear Suggestions: Nike Combat Gear, UnderArmor, and 5.11, among others, all make incredible stuff. All include an extensive line of under uniform clothing for military and police, as well as sport equipment for men and women. It's not cheap but it's worth every penny. Pieces can run from $16–20 to nearly $50 per item depending on what you choose. Currently I highly recommend the Nike Combat gear undershirts. Silky smooth, very cool, easy to wash and wear, and very well made. Many don't care for synthetic underwear, but most would not deploy without them. Other quality manufactures of this type of clothing include REI (lifetime warranty) Exofficio, and Duofold. Dicks Sporting Goods, Academy, RockCreek outfitters, REI, or any good hunting/outdoor/police/military supplier should carry what you need. Look for good quality stitching, very flat seams and NO COTTON CONTENT.

Additionally, when in a crunch, you can hand wash this stuff in the shower, ring it out, put in on and wear it. It will dry in 15 minutes and retain its shape, support, and comfort.

www.underarmor.com
www.nike.com
www.511.com
www.duofold.com
www.REI.com
www.exofficio.com

Socks: Quality Matters: Consider wearing socks that contain no cotton while in operations (after hours is fine). Cotton absorbs and holds moisture. Heat, friction, and skin maceration issues can be greatly reduced if not eliminated. Consider purchasing a good-quality combat-type boot sock. Advantages include lower friction, increased moisture transport away from the skin, fast drying, extended wear with no loss of shape or support, lower boot temperatures, and ease of cleaning. Good synthetic/synthetic wool blend socks can be hand washed and ready for wear by the start of your next shift. Extensive testing shows Darn Tough Boot Socks #1439 to be best socks you can buy. Any Darn Tough sock is worth owning. SmartWool and Thorlo boot socks are also great choices.

www.Darntough.com
www.smartwool.com
www.Thorlo.com

Sock Liners: These are optional, but again, heat and moisture control are issues here. Field experience has had NDMS personnel with rapidly developing, and at times severe foot breakdown to the point of needing wound care. Heat, moisture, and friction, even in well-fitting boots were the problem. A thin synthetic liner sock reduces all of these issues. Most significantly, it reduces skin maceration and friction. They are cheap insurance against issues and some injuries that can cause a lot of discomfort while deployed or possibly even render you immobile. Fox River Alturas liner socks #4478 are some of the best sock liners available. UnderArmor, Thorlo, Smartwool, etc. are some of the other many producers of excellent socks and liners. Any good sporting goods store should have some to choose from.

www.foxrivermills.com
www.underarmor.com
www.thorlo.com
www.smartwool.com

Boots: Quality Matters: No single piece of equipment will make or break your deployment faster than your boots. Your first deployment is NOT the time to break in your new boots or discover friction or discomfort issues. Wear them around the house and in the yard A LOT before you deploy. Boot selection is highly personal and I suggest you discuss this with your local "gear head" or drop me an email and we can discuss. jrmalloch@yahoo.com

Clothing Compression Bag: Eagle Creek Pack-It Compressor – 2 Pack clothing bag will allow you to pack your cloths in half the space. These are extremely rugged bags with a lifetime warranty. Item #40119. Generally found at any good outdoor/backpack supplier.
    www.eaglecreek.com

Washcloth and Towels: Again, cotton is nice but it's heavy and very slow to dry. McNett and MSR make very nice synthetics in washcloth and personal bath towel sizes. The MSR "Original" and the "Ultralight" seem too synthetic feeling. The "Personal" however, is a very nice soft towel that is light and dries quickly. All of the McNett products are excellent. See it at Dicks, Academy, REI etc. Also, consider a synthetic loofa instead of a washcloth, it's light, scrubs well, rinses, and dries fast.
    www.MSRcorp.com
    www.mcnett.com

Sleeping Bag/Sleep Kit: What you sleep in is a personal choice, but you need something. Cotton is not the best choice for all of the same reasons mentioned above. One thing to consider here is weight and size. This one item has the potential to take up the largest percentage of space in your main bag. Another consideration is temperature rating. Deployments in tropical heat are common and billeting may be in a Western Shelter with no AC or it may be on a warehouse floor, gymnasium, or similar, and the AC is freezing cold. Generally, a 30–40° bag will meet both needs. Add a sleeping sheet to your bag for increased comfort and range. (See www.seatosummit.com for sleep sheets.)

    Some of the finest bags available at any price are made by Wiggy's in Colorado. Wiggy's makes bags for spec-ops and military teams all over the world. They are warm even when damp, dry quickly, and are very durable and guaranteed forever. Anything can be custom made to your size for a very reasonable fee. They will sometimes offer excellent pricing to federal employees.

    Another good, readily available deployment sleeping bag is the Kelty Lightyear 3D 45, a very nice, <2 lb synthetic bag that gets very small and can be found for around $90. The links below will often have sales with great deals on mid- and high-end sleeping bags for as little as $50.
    www.wiggys.com 1–866-411–6465
    www.kelty.com
    www.Sierratradingpost.com
    www.REI.com (go to the outlet section)
    www.Campmor.com

Pillow: Personal choice here again. I like the Therm-a-rest compressible pillow. It compresses very small, is not an air pillow, rather a soft foam-filled pillow that's very comfortable. Sizes range from half size to full size pillows and work great. It has a soft flannel cover. The half size can be compressed to the size of a grapefruit and it goes in my compression bag with my sleeping bag. www.Campmor.com has them on sale from time to time for around $12. Retail is about $25 for the large. There are several similar choices available.

www.thermarest.com

Compression Bag for Sleep Kit: Quality Matters: This is what makes your giant sleeping bag small. Essentially, this is a thin nylon or similar bag with straps that compresses your sleeping bag into half its size and reduces the amount of space it consumes in your main deployment bag. Granite Gear makes some of the best and lightest. Sea to Summit, RockCreek outfitters, REI etc., have some great choices as well. It's a good idea to take your bag to one of these places and try out the size you need. If you get the right size, you might get your pillow and sheet in there as well.

Blowing out a lesser quality compression bag mid deployment leaves you with a sleeping bag that you now have to figure out how to pack in its uncompressed state. If you packed that 55 gal trash bag, you might be ok.

www.Granitegear.com
www.seatosummit.com
www.REI.com
www.rockcreek.com

Mattress, Sleep Type, Foam/Air: This will make that unexpected night on a gym or fire hall floor more bearable or can add an extra measure of comfort to your military cot. You don't have to spend a lot of money here unless you want to. There are many "closed cell" foam choices out there but one of the best is Therm-a-rest Z-lite. Compared to an inflatable, it is relatively bulky when folded, but will not puncture and go flat. It weighs about a pound. It's minimalist to be sure, but it's better than cement or the ground. High end would be the Therm-a-rest Prolight 3 or 4. This inflatable is premium and goes for around $100. It gets very small, weighs about a pound, and is very comfortable and so far very durable. Though I've never punctured one, I know the possibility exists. Another great choice is the Big Agnes. The AirCore is less than 1 lb, gets as small as a quart jar and is about $50. There is a long list of other choices beyond the three listed above, as well as quality manufactures such as REI.

www.Thermarest.com
www.bigagnes.com
www.REI.com

Soaps/Detergents etc.: Most carry soap, some don't carry detergent. I carry both, and have used it every time. I've extensively tested and now use the Sea to Summit Trek & Travel liquid soaps. These are excellent products that come packed in leak-proof bottles and are very versatile. The Trek & Travel Wilderness Wash does it all, shower/hair/shave/laundry. If you prefer, the Trek & Travel Laundry Wash does a great job combined with the other personal soaps, they've got it covered. If you prefer, a small 8oz Nalgene bottle with your detergent of choice will do the job. I do suggest unscented soaps and detergents as scents can attract insects.

www.Seatosummit.com
www.nalgene-outdoor.com

Garbage Bags: Choose large trash can size, 40 to 55 gallon size. Rolled up or folded into your pack, they take up little space. These are useful for an emergency rain poncho/bivy sack, to protect your gear from rain, to do laundry in, as an emergency shelter, as window covers for day sleepers, for suffocating a snoring bunkmate, etc. . .3–4 is sufficient.

Zip-Lock Bags, Heavy Duty: The 1 gallon size is useful for storing damp clothes/ damp towels when traveling, smaller bags are handy for holding small, loose items, like batteries, matches/lighters/coins/detergents/important documents/passports, etc., that you want to keep dry. The MRE zip lock is very useful for protecting your passport.

Strip Plug: Billeting/sleeping-quarters may have limited outlets. The team will need to charge equipment/radios/sat-phones etc. Western Shelters used for billeting have limited outlets near the ceiling. A 3 ft cord with strip will get some power down where you need it and give you more options for charging electronics as well.

Lights: Quality Matters: The choices are nearly unlimited. For $20–$50 you can purchase an utterly reliable, lightweight, and waterproof light that will allow you to work hands-free. It's a good idea to try to keep its battery type similar to your other gear if possible.

Petzl, PrincetonTec, Black Diamond, Pelican and many more make great lights. My personal favorite is the Petzl Tikka XP line. Your headlamp must be rugged and reliable. Quality is important. Your safety and your life could at some point depend on it.

My favorite area light is the Black Diamond Orbit. Any good camping supplier or police/ military supply house should have what you need.

www.petzl.com

www.blackdiamondequipment.com

Cell Phone Belt Holster/Carrier: From the moment you deploy until you return home, you will have a chance to break your cell phone holster every day. During loading and unloading trucks, climbing in and out of aircraft, in and out of vehicles, carrying heavy gear through airports, etc., are all places to break your cell phone carrier. A nylon or canvas type carrier is far less likely to break. The choices are nearly unlimited and can be found at Lowes, Home Depot, many sporting goods stores, and police/military and camping suppliers.

www.maxpedition.com

www.timbuk2.com

www.mountainsmith.com (see accessories section for example)

Water and Commercial Air Travel: Given current TSA restrictions, commercial travelers are restricted from bringing outside water through security. Your options include going without water, carry empty Nalgene bottles/hydrations systems and filling once through security, purchasing bottled water once through security or waiting until you are on the ground at your destination to procure water.

www.nalgene-outdoor.com

Summary

Effective gear does not have to be expensive but it does have to be carefully selected and functional. Learn from each other. Be prepared and motivated and ready to "Answer The Call".

Discussion Notes

Disclaimer

No list or gear guide is 100% comprehensive. All deployments, both national and international require consideration of items and issues not listed here. Additionally, new and better products are being released often and have not yet been tested. I have no personal, professional, or commercial affiliation with any of the products discussed herein. Feel free to email with comments/considerations and product reviews. jrmalloch@yahoo.com

Appendix 2

Re-Opening Your Business: A Post-Disaster Checklist

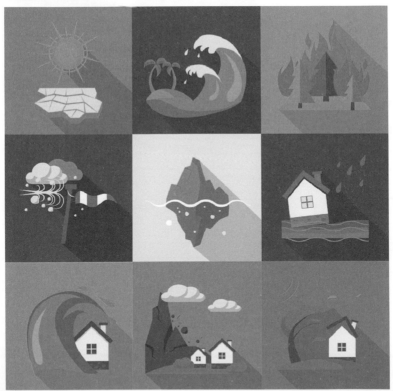

The Connecticut Small Business Development Center is funded in part through a cooperative agreement with the U.S. Small Business Administration, the Connecticut Department of Economic and Community Development, and the University of Connecticut.

✓Checklist for re-opening your business after a disaster

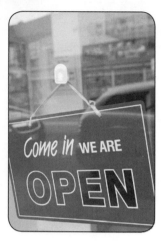

After a disaster, your natural instinct may be to reopen your business as soon as humanly possible. However, it's important to recognize that business after a disaster such as a flood or fire is anything but natural. Key suppliers, employees and customers are all affected. It's crucial to step back, take a deep breath, and reflect on all options available to you before throwing open the doors again.

The options available to you depend greatly on the financial health of your business. And having a good assessment of your business's status is the way to best analyze your position — and your choices moving forward. This way, you can determine whether:

- You can afford to reopen your business and have it be the same as it was before the disaster

- You can or should expand, downsize or even close your business.

The following areas of consideration and accompanying questions will help you make the best possible decisions for your business after a disaster. We hope it can help guide you during a difficult time.

✓ FIRST PRIORITIES

Looking inward	
	Were you happy running the business before the disaster?
	Were you making the profit you wanted?
	Did you prefer being your own boss?
	Have you considered other opportunities?
	Are you prepared for the potential extra demands that recovering your business will place on you, both personally and financially?

Assessing the damage	
	Is your facility operational?
	Can you reopen without significant repairs?
	Are your inventory, supplies and equipment recoverable?
	Have any of your staff been affected by the disaster?
	What are your chances for future success?

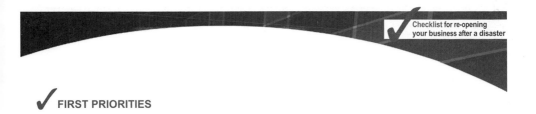

✓ FIRST PRIORITIES

Re-evaluate	
	Have you analyzed the potential demand for your product or services post-disaster?
	Have any of your key customers and/or suppliers been affected by the disaster, and if so, how will this impact your business?
	Has the disaster led to other businesses in your area closing — and if so — have you determined how this may impact your business?

Necessary tasks	
	Have you contacted your insurance company?
	Have you given your insurance company your preliminary damage assessment?
	Has your insurance company been able to tell you what your insurance payout is likely to be, when it will be made, and whether it will be in the form of cash or asset replacement, or a mix of both?
	Have you contacted your staff and key stakeholders (including local and government agencies) for support?
	Are you keeping staff and stakeholders, including key customers, suppliers and lenders/investors informed of what you are doing?
	Do you need to lay off staff for the time being?
	Do you need to postpone purchasing supplies or inventory?
	Can you cancel orders that you have already made?
	If customer orders have been lost, delayed or damaged, have you informed those customers?
	Do you qualify for financial assistance from the government and if so, have you applied for it?
	Have you restored your computer data backups and other necessary information?

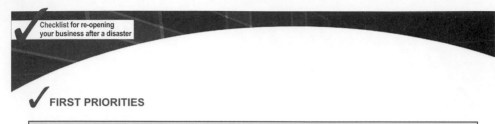

Checklist for re-opening
your business after a disaster

✓ **FIRST PRIORITIES**

	Analyzing financial status
	What is the current financial position of your business?
	Have you reconstructed the financial records of your business?
	If you cannot fully reconstruct your accounts, do you have access to historical financial statements or industry benchmarks?
	Have you determined how much cash your business currently has available by creating a cash flow statement?
	Have you created a balance sheet and a profit-and-loss statement from the beginning of the current fiscal year to the time of the disaster?
	Have you used information in the cash flow statement, profit-and-loss statement and balance sheet to determine the current financial health of your business?

	Creating a recovery plan
	Have you developed your recovery objective?
	Have you established a recovery team with clear responsibilities from the recovery plan?
	Can you support such team members in working off site?
	Are you aware of all the requirements to reopen your business? For example: • Do you need to arrange for the short-term lease of equipment until yours can be repaired/replaced? • Do you have adequate resources (staff, finances, etc.) to bring your business up to normal operating levels or to a level that reflects the current market conditions? • Do you know what it will cost to execute your recovery plan?
	Can you afford such a plan?
	Do you have a marketing strategy in place to promote the fact that you are open for business?
	Have you incorporated lessons from running your business prior to the disaster into your recovery plan?
	Have you incorporated your analysis of market conditions post-disaster into your recovery plan?
	Does your recovery plan reflect the financial goals you want to achieve (net profit margin, ROI, etc.)?

Additional recovery plan considerations

• *Adding new product lines or removing existing product lines*
• *Adding new services or reducing services*
• *Reducing operating costs*
• *Adopting new technologies and processes*
• *Relocating your business*

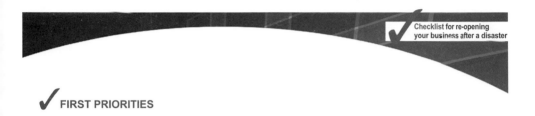

✓ FIRST PRIORITIES

Funding the reopening of your business
	Can you afford to reopen your business?
	Have you completed cash flow and profit-and-loss forecasts?
	Have you used these forecasts to run "what if" scenarios, to measure how your cash flow will be impacted by unexpected events?
	Do you intend to fund the reopening of your business from existing business sources, your own resources, other investors, banks, lenders or a mix?
	Do the forecasts and your financial statements show whether the business can afford to use internal or external sources of financing to fund the reopening? If not, can you adjust your recovery plan so that it is affordable?
	If you cannot afford your recovery plan, have you considered exiting the business?
	Have existing debt financing arrangements been reviewed to ensure the new needs of the business are adequately represented in the current finance facility and structure?

Sources of finance
	Even if you can fund the reopening of the business from existing sources, have you analyzed whether it is better to use external sources?
	If you are seeking debt financing, have you spoken to your bank about your recovery plan and your funding needs?
	What existing lines of credit does the business have access to, and can these lines of credit be accessed to fund the reopening of the business?
	If you do seek debt financing, what collateral do you have available to offer?
	If you are seeking debt financing, have you determined the reason you are seeking the money (i.e. to replace inventory or buy equipment), the length of the loan term and how much money you will need?
	Have you considered financing the reopening of your business from your own resources or from other investors?

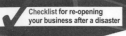
Checklist for re-opening
your business after a disaster

✓ FIRST PRIORITIES

Your business location	
	Given the potential change in market conditions, is your business in the right location?
	Are there any plans by local government or others that may impact the viability of the location of your business, such as changes that may restrict access?
	Have other businesses reopened or plan to reopen in your area?
	Is the size of your office or facility too large or small given the future potential of the business?

Business equipment	
	Do you have the necessary facility and equipment that your business needs to reopen?
	If not, will you receive such equipment from your insurance company, or will you have to purchase this equipment?
	If you have to purchase the equipment, have you analyzed whether it is better to purchase or lease it?
	Is the purchase of equipment (including maintenance costs and insurance) justified, given the possible change in market conditions?
	Is the necessary expertise readily available to install the equipment?

Inventory	
	If inventory or supplies are to be replaced, have you reviewed historical information to see what is slow-moving?
	For inventory identified as slow-moving, have you considered removing it from your product lineup?
	Have you made an assessment of whether or not the changed market conditions will impact the buying patterns of your customers?

Marketing	
	How do you intend to advertise that your business has re-opened?
	Is there any promotion of your local area by government or others?

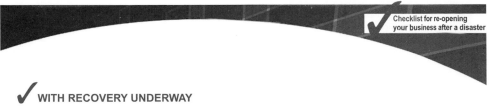

✔ WITH RECOVERY UNDERWAY

Business licenses
If you lost copies of your business license, permits or other official documents necessary to operate your business, have you approached the appropriate agency to get them replaced?

Record keeping
Have you considered what accounting system you are going to use to continue to keep your financial records up to date?
Are there any improvements you can make to your record keeping system, such as off-site backups?

Meeting statutory obligations
Has your ability to file and pay such returns/forms/obligations been delayed?
Do your reconstructed financial records give you the necessary information and evidence to be able to complete such returns?

Pricing
Have you completed a break-even analysis to determine whether the prices you charge are making you the profit you want to achieve?
Have you compared your pricing to your competitors'?

Lessons learned
Have you documented the lessons learned from your business recovery?
Have you considered putting a business continuity plan in place in case you go through another disaster?
Have you reviewed your insurance coverage to see whether it is adequate and whether there are any gaps in your coverage?

Giving thanks
Have you thanked everyone involved in assisting you?

Checklist for re-opening
your business after a disaster

CTSBDC *Locations*

AMERICA'S
SBDC
SMALL BUSINESS DEVELOPMENT CENTERS
CONNECTICUT
CELEBRATING 35 YEARS

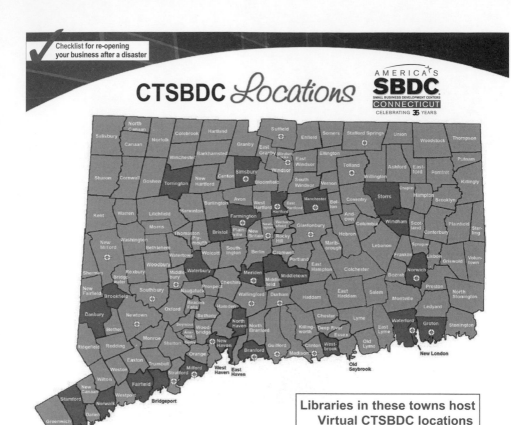

Libraries in these towns host Virtual CTSBDC locations

Branford
Clinton
Durham
Farmington
Glastonbury
Groton (2)
Guilford
Hartford
Manchester
Meriden
Middlebury
Milford
New Haven

New London
New Milford
Newington
Newtown
Norwich
Simsbury
Southbury
Stafford Springs
Stratford
Suffield
Tolland
Wallingford
Windsor Locks

CTSBDC Office Locations

Branford
Bridgeport
Bristol
Brookfield
Danbury
Fairfield
Farmington
Groton
Hartford (2)
Manchester
Meriden
Middletown (2)
Milford

New Haven
New London
North Haven
Norwalk
Norwich
Simsbury
Stamford (2)
Storrs (Lead Office)
Torrington
Waterbury
Waterford
Westbrook
Windham

Appendix 3

Disaster Recovery Toolkit for Small Businesses

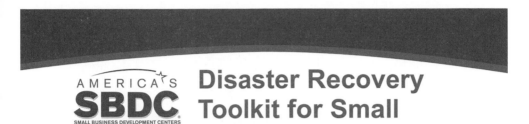

Disaster Recovery Toolkit for Small Businesses

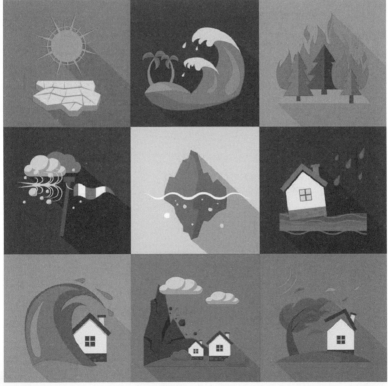

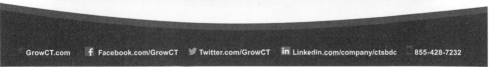

Table of Contents

This Disaster Recovery Toolkit for Small Business was modified by the Connecticut Small Business Development Center and originally created by the Kentucky Small Business Development Center and its author, CPA Australia. For questions, please contact CTSBDC at 1-860-486-4270 or online at http://GrowCT.com/.

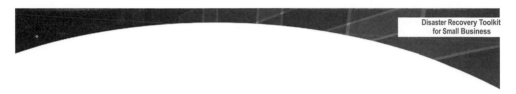

Introduction

Disasters can strike at any time: Tornadoes. Floods Hurricanes. Fires.
For a small business owner, what a disaster leaves in its wake can be devastating
— but it doesn't have to be. The purpose of this guide is to help business owners
assess the feasibility of reopening, what steps to take and how to reanalyze and
restructure your business after a disaster. It is the hope of the CTSBDC that the
recommendations and information in this guide can help you if the unexpected hits.

The time following a disaster is anything but business as usual. This time of transition is truly uncharted
territory for you, your employees and your customers. The faster you can return your business to some
level of normal operations, the quicker you can restore income, jobs, and the goods and services you
provide. Even if your business is not directly impacted by a disaster — whether natural, economic or
man-made — a resultant decline in sales will impact your business. The ability to resume operations,
if that's what you choose to do, and recover quickly is critical to your business survival.

Safeguard your business with PrepareCT

Your company keeps you so busy it's easy to put off thoughts of disruption and disaster. Until you're in one.

Stay ahead of emergency situations — connect with PrepareCT. Funded in part through a Cooperative
Agreement with the Small Business Administration, PrepareCT helps you create a disaster preparedness
plan through free one-on-one training, free workshops and free plan reviews by small business experts
eager to ensure you protect your business in event of catastrophe.

You've worked hard to create your small business. It's time to protect and enhance your investment.

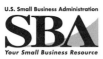

U.S. Small Business Administration

SBA

Your Small Business Resource

PrepareCT is funded in part through
a Cooperative Agreement with the
U.S. Small Business Administration.

PrepareCT is led by The Connecticut Small
Business Development Center (CTSBDC) in
partnership with 16 small business-focused
organizations throughout the state.

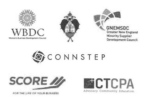

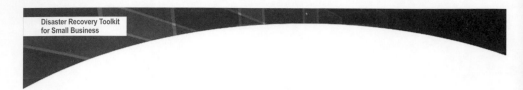

Disaster Recovery Toolkit
for Small Business

Business recovery post-disaster

Step 1: Decide if you should reopen at all

Research shows that up to 40 percent of businesses affected by a disaster may never reopen. The time it takes for a business to return to something resembling normal operating levels depends on a number of key considerations that should all be analyzed before you make your decision.

> Overall damage assessment
  • Can you operate from your existing location?
  • What inventory, supplies, equipment and other key assets are recoverable?
> Your insurance coverage and how quickly your claim can be processed
> What kinds of government assistance you might be able to access
> Feedback from employees, customers, suppliers and creditors/investors
> Your business's financial position
> How you will develop a plan to reopen your business

Evaluating your financial position

Businesses affected by a disaster should take the time to evaluate their financial position before making decisions on whether to reopen. Owners also need to figure out how they should operate in the new environment. Sizing up the financial position of your business is important for three reasons:

> Your business may have substantial costs associated with reopening. As a result, you need to know how you are going to pay for such expenses and if you can afford them.
> There may be a significant period of time before you can reopen. Therefore, you may have to rely on existing sources of cash and other assistance until that time.
> Knowing your financial position can assist you in making claims with your insurance company (i.e., business interruption insurance).

These assessments will help you to plan the direction in which you want to take your business.

Financial recovery

The first step in evaluating your financial position is to reconstruct your financial records *(see Reconstructing Financial Records after a disaster on Page 12)*. The initial focus of reconstructing accounts is to determine the cash position of the business, including cash in the bank, any receivables from existing debtors that are recoverable, insurance payouts, government assistance and other sources, with the exception of any cash payables, such as payments to suppliers or loan repayments.

Disaster Recovery Toolkit
for Small Business

Steps To Get Back In Business

Conduct Overall Damage Assessment

File Insurance Claim

Evaluate Financial Position

Study Your Market

Evaluate Historical Operations

Develop Plan to Reopen

Reopen or Exit the Business

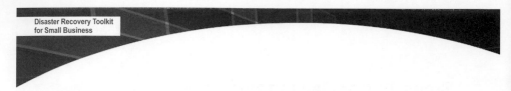

Recovery planning

Once you have established the financial position of your business, you are one step closer to reopening. The next step in reopening is to develop a recovery plan. A recovery plan should state what the business needs to reopen — such as processes or resources that are critical to reopening — along with your recovery objectives, including actions to achieve those objectives and the person(s) responsible for them. A recovery plan template is included in this toolkit. *(See Recovery Plan Template on Page 17)* Such a plan, together with cash-flow and profit-and-loss forecasts, will help you determine whether it is viable to reopen and how the business will finance the reopening.

In developing such a plan, it may be very difficult to make assumptions in a post-disaster environment. Past experiences may no longer be relevant and the market may have changed significantly, at least in the short term. Therefore, it is important to analyze your market again. If it is difficult to finance the planned reopening, the plan may have to be modified or you may have to consider exiting the business.

Checklist for re-opening your business after a disaster

Following a disaster, the immediate, gut reaction of many business owners is to reopen their business as soon as possible. However, a post-disaster environment is anything but business as usual for you, your employees, key suppliers and customers. It may therefore be prudent to reflect on your options before considering reopening. Knowing the financial position of your business will give the information you need to determine whether:

• You can afford to reopen your business the way it was before the disaster and how quickly you can reopen your business;
OR
• Whether you can or should expand, shrink or even close your business.

The period before reopening should also be seen as an opportunity to consider how your business operated before the disaster and to identify areas you would like improved, changed, or eliminated. You may also want to consider opportunities that you have always wanted to explore, but have yet to attempt.

This checklist leads you through these critical issues and highlights many other considerations you may need to make before and after reopening your business.

Disaster Recovery Toolkit
for Small Business

Preliminary Assessment	Yes/No
Should you reopen your business?	
• Were you happy running the business before the disaster?	
• Were you making the profit you wanted to make?	
• Do you prefer being your own boss?	
• Have you considered other opportunities?	
• Are you prepared for the potential extra demands that recovering your business will place on you, both personally and financially?	
Have you assessed the damage?	
• Is your facility operational?	
• Can you reopen from your current location without significant repairs?	
• Is your inventory, supplies and equipment recoverable?	
• Have any of your staff been affected by the disaster?	
How do your chances look for future success?	
Have you analyzed the potential demand for your product or services post disaser?	
Have any of your key customers and/or suppliers been affected by the disaster, and if so, how will this impact your business?	
Has the disaster led to other businesses in your area closing, and if so, have you determined how this may impact your business?	

Preliminary Actions	
• Have you contacted your insurance company?	
• Have you given your insurance company your preliminary damage assessment?	
• Has your insurance company been able to tell you what your insurance payout is likely to be, when it will be made, and whether it will be in the form of cash, asset replacement, or a mix of both?	
• Have you contacted your staff and other key stakeholders (including government and local agencies) for support?	
• Are you keeping staff and stakeholders — including key customers, suppliers and lenders or investors — up to date on what you are doing?	
• Do you need to lay off staff for the time being?	
• Do you need to postpone purchasing of supplies or inventory?	
• Can you cancel orders that you have made?	
• If customer orders have been lost or damaged or you simply cannot supply them on time, have you informed those customers?	
• Do you qualify for financial assistance from the government and, if so, have you applied for it?	
• Have you restored your computer data backups and other necessary information?	

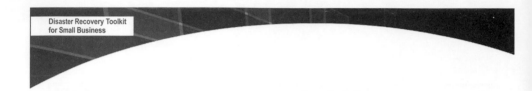

Financial position of the business	Yes/No
What is the current financial status of your business?	
• Have you reconstructed the financial records of your business?	
• If you cannot fully reconstruct your accounts, do you have access to historical financial statements or industry benchmarks?	
• Have you determined how much cash your business has available by creating a cash-flow statement?	
• Have you created a balance sheet and a profit-and-loss statement from the beginning of the current financial year to the time of the disaster?	
• Have you used your information in the cash-flow statement, profit-and-loss statement and balance sheet to analyze the current financial health of your business?	
Recovery Plan	
Have you developed your recovery objectives, actions and priorities?	
Have you established a recovery team with clear responsibilities from the recovery plan?	
Can you support such team members working off-site?	
Are you aware of all the requirements to reopen your business? For example, do you need to arrange for the short-term lease of equipment until yours can be repaired or replaced?	
Do you have adequate resources (staff, finances, etc.) to bring the business up to normal operating levels or to a level that reflects current market conditions?	
Do you know what it will cost to execute your recovery plan?	
Can you afford such a plan?	
Do you have a marketing strategy in place to promote the fact that you are open for business?	
Have you incorporated lessons from running your business prior to the disaster into your recovery plan?	
Have you incorporated your analysis of the post-disaster market conditions into your recovery plan?	
Does the recovery plan reflect financial goals you want to achieve (net profit margin, ROI, etc.)?	
Have you considered the following with respect to your recovery plan?	
> Adding new product lines or removal of existing product lines?	
> Adding new services or a reduction of services?	
> Reducing operating costs?	
> Adopting new technologies and processes?	
> Relocating your business?	

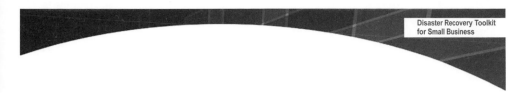

Funding the reopening of your business	Yes/No
• Can you afford to reopen your business?	
• Have you completed cash-flow and profit-and-loss forecasts?	
• Have you used these forecasts to run "what-if" scenarios to measure how your cash flow will be impacted by unexpected events?	
• Do you intend to fund the reopening of your business from existing business sources, your own resources, other investors, banks, lenders, or a mix?	
• Do the forecasts and your financial statements show whether the business can afford to use internal or external sources of financing to fund the reopening?	
> If not, can you adjust your recovery plan so that it is affordable?	
> If you cannot afford your recovery plan, have you considered exiting the business?	
• Where the business has existing debt-financing arrangements, have these been reviewed to ensure that the finance facility and structure fits the new needs of the business?	

Sources of finance	Yes/No
• Even if you can fund the reopening of the business from existing sources, have you analyzed whether it is more beneficial to use external sources of finance?	
• If you are seeking debt financing, have you spoken to your bank about your recovery plan and your funding needs?	
• What lines of credit does the business have access to and can these lines of credit be accessed to fund the reopening of the business?	
• If you do seek debt financing, what collateral do you have available to offer?	
• If you are seeking debt financing, have you determined how you will use the money (i.e., to replace inventory or buy equipment), the length of the loan term and how much you will need?	
• Have you considered financing the reopening of your business from your own resources or from other investors?	

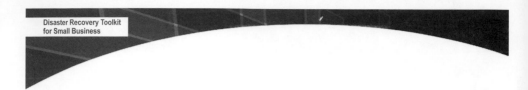

Disaster Recovery Toolkit
for Small Business

Physical requirements	Yes/No
Location	
• Given the potential change in market conditions, is your business in the right location?	
• Are there any plans by local government or others that may impact the viability of the location of your business, such as changes that may restrict access?	
• Have other businesses reopened or plan to reopen in your area?	
• Is the size of your office or facility too large or too small, given the future potential of the business?	
Major equipment	
• Do you have the plant and equipment that your business needs to reopen?	
• If not, will you receive such equipment from your insurance company or will you have to purchase it?	
• If you have to purchase the equipment, have you analyzed whether it is better to purchase or lease?	
• Is the purchase of the equipment (including maintenance costs and insurance) justified, given the possible change in market conditions?	
• Is the necessary expertise readily available to install the equipment?	
Inventory	
• If inventory or supplies are to be replaced, have you reviewed historical information to see what is slow-moving?	
• For inventory identified as slow-moving, have you considered removing those items from your product lineup?	
• Have you made an assessment of whether the changed market conditions will impact the buying patterns of your customers?	

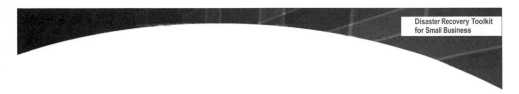

Disaster Recovery Toolkit for Small Business

Marketing	Yes/No
• How do you intend to advertise that your business has re-opened?	
• Is there any promotion of your local area by government or others?	

Pricing	Yes/No
• Have you done a breakeven analysis to determine whether the prices you charge are making the profit you need?	
• Have you compared your pricing to your competitors'?	

Lessons learned	Yes/No
• Have you documented lessons learned from your business recovery?	
• Have you considered putting a business continuity plan in place to help you in case you go through another disaster?	
• Have you reviewed your insurance coverage to see whether it is adequate and whether there are any gaps in your coverage?	

Other	Yes/No
Business licenses	
• If you lost copies of your business licenses, permits or other official documents necessary to operate your business, have you approached the appropriate agencies to get them replaced?	
Record keeping	
• Have you considered what accounting system you are going to use or continue to use to keep your financial records up to date?	
• Are there any improvements you can make to your record-keeping system, such as off-site backups?	
Meeting statutory obligations	
• Has your ability to file and pay such returns/forms/obligations been delayed?	
• Have your reconstructed financial records given you the necessary information and evidence to be able to complete such returns?	
Thank everyone	
• Have you thanked everyone involved in assisting you?	

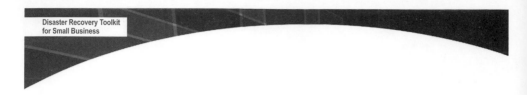

Reconstructing financial records after a disaster

One of the first steps you should take after a disaster is to attempt to reconstruct your financial accounts. These records will be your guide in making decisions on the future of your business. If you have not been able to salvage your financial records, you should seek documentation of past financial transactions. Such evidence will provide the foundation upon which you or your accountant can begin rebuilding the financial history of the business. Where such documents no longer exist or are incomplete, here are some resources that can be used to begin putting all the pieces back together:

Who has what?

Potential sources of information	
IRS: **800-829-4933**	Form 4506 - Request for copies of tax returns http://www.irs.gov/pub/irs-pdf/f4506.pdf
City/Town Clerk	Copies of property deeds.
Bank or Financial Institution	Past bank statements provide a great resource. For example, businesses may remember or make a good guess regarding transactions on a bank statement, even if the primary receipt of the transaction is gone.
Secretary of State: **502-564-3490**	Records pertaining to your business (articles of incorporation, annual reports, certificate of assumed names, etc.) are all available here.
Accountant / Financial Advisor	May have copies of financial statements and tax returns for your business.
Surviving Files	See if any files, including electronic files, can be recovered from the disaster. For electronic files — even though the hard drive may look bad – experts may be able to recover the data. First, consider how valuable the data is and if it can be found elsewhere.
Staff	Ask staff if they have records off-site; for example, any emails or other documents on their computers, flash drives or other storage devices.
Customers and Suppliers	Customers and suppliers may have invoices, purchase orders or receipts that they can share.
Off-Site Sources	Figure out if any files are kept off-site, such as with your company's IT or payroll vendors. In such situations, the provider may have business information you need.
Insurance Company	Speak to your insurance representative; he or she may have a list of assets owned by your business that you had previously given them.
Other Government Agencies	If the business has received government funding or grants, the awarding agency may have records.
Accreditation or Certification Bodies	If the business is subject to any other form of audit, certification or accreditation, these organizations may have records that could be helpful to you.
Attorney	They may have copies of contracts that the business has entered into in addition to articles of incorporation/organization or other founding documents.
Email Correspondence	The business, the business's internet service provider or staff members may have copies of emails and documents forwarded to clients, suppliers and other relevant parties that prove useful.

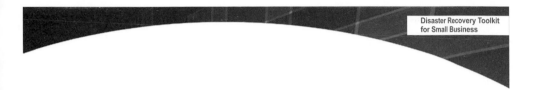

When it is not possible to fully reconstruct financial records, the information you have been able to find — combined with your knowledge of your business and industry — should give you a fairly comprehensive approximation of the company's financial position. If that is not successful, try applying industry benchmarks to the information that you have been able to reconstruct. Such benchmarks are available from your local Connecticut Small Business Development Center.

In addition to the reconstruction of records, consider temporary operation measures for the recovery phase, such as the recording of activities and transactions, managing cash flow and working with key clients, suppliers and the government. Following the reconstruction of financial records, businesses will be in a position to evaluate their financial positions and — from there — consider how to re-establish their businesses and explore financing requirement options.

Analyzing the financial health of a business after a disaster

Analyzing the financial health of your business should be part of the planning process you follow before reopening your business after a disaster. Such analysis will assist you in determining if it is financially viable for you to reopen your business, to find areas where the business can be improved and where your business was doing well before the disaster.

Financial ratio analysis is a common method used to examine the financial health of a business. Under normal circumstances, it can predict the potential for success or failure, and measure the progress of growth. But after a disaster, circumstances are different. Analysis may not be effective in predicting future trends. However, this analysis will enable you to spot any trends that were emerging in your business prior to the disaster and to compare how your business performed against similar businesses in the same industry. This information will help you determine how you want your business to operate after reopening.

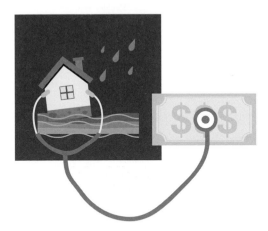

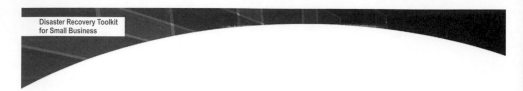

Disaster Recovery Toolkit
for Small Business

Financial ratios

There are many financial ratios a business can use to assess its financial health.
The main ratios, grouped into broad areas, are:

Liquidity ratios

Liquidity ratios assess your business's ability to meet its obligations. In general, it is better to have a high ratio in this category as an indication of sound business activities and an ability to withstand tight cash flow periods (which is likely following a disaster):

Current Ratio = Total Current Assets / Total Current Liabilities

The current ratio measures whether the business has enough current assets (cash in the bank, debtors, inventory and other assets that can be turned into cash quickly) to meet debts that are due in the next 12 months. A generally acceptable current ratio is 2 to 1, but this depends on the nature of the business.

Quick Ratio = (Current Assets - Inventory) / Current Liabilities

The quick ratio (also known as the acid test) helps answer a fundamental question for a business affected by a disaster: If the business does not have any sales income, could it meet its current obligations without having to sell inventory at below-market prices? The higher the ratio, the better for your company.

Solvency ratios

These ratios indicate the extent to which the business is able to meet all debt obligations from sources other than cash flow. Commonly used solvency ratios are:

Leverage ratio = Total Liabilities / Equity

The leverage ratio indicates the extent to which the business is reliant on debt financing versus owner's equity. Generally speaking, the higher the ratio, the more difficult it will be to obtain additional credit.

Debt to Assets = Total Liabilities / Total Assets

This ratio measures the percentage of assets being financed by liabilities. Generally speaking, this ratio should be less than 1, indicating that there are enough total assets to meet all debt obligations.

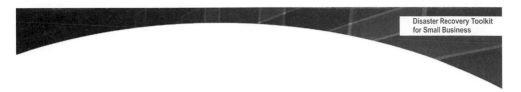

Profitability Ratios

These ratios measure your business performance and ultimately indicate the level of success of your operations. You can use these ratios to help determine whether the pricing of your products and services before the disaster were adequate to achieve a profit, and met the profit you wanted to achieve, in addition to comparing your results to industry averages. These ratios can guide you in your pricing policy upon reopening.

Gross Profit Margin = Gross Profit / Net Sales

The gross margin ratio measures the percentage of sales dollars available to pay the overhead expenses of the business after purchasing or manufacturing the inventory sold.

Net Margin Ratio = Net Profit / Net Sales

The net margin ratio measures the percentage of sales dollars left after all expenses (including stock), except income taxes. This ratio will provide an opportunity to compare your business's return on sales with the performance of other businesses in your industry.

Management Ratios

If you are assessing your financial health before the disaster, management ratios monitor how effectively you were managing your working capital. For example, if the length of time it took to collect your receivables is longer than the time you were taking to pay your payables, then there was a cash-flow issue. You were paying money out before you were receiving money for goods or services. This indicates that when you reopen your business, you should seek longer terms of credit from suppliers and try to reduce the time it takes to collect your receivables.

Days Debtors = (Debtors / Net Sales) x 365

Days Creditors = (Creditors / Inventory) x 365

Balance Sheet Ratios

These ratios indicate how efficiently your business is using assets and equity to make a profit.

Return on Assets = (Net Profit Before Tax / Total Assets) x 100

This ratio measures how efficiently profits are being generated from the assets employed in the business. This ratio will only have meaning when compared to other businesses. A low ratio in comparison with industry averages indicates an inefficient use of business assets and something to be watched upon reopening your business.

Return on Investment = (Net Profit Before Tax / Net Worth) x 100

The return on investment, or ROI, is perhaps the most important ratio of all. It tells the owner whether or not all the effort put into the business has been worthwhile. If the ROI is less than the rate of return on an alternative, low-risk investment such as a bank savings account, the owner may consider that option rather than funding the reopening of the business.

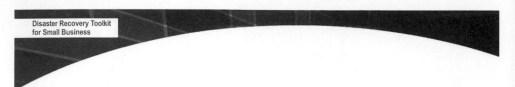

Comparing performance to other businesses

To compare the ratios of your business prior to the disaster to similar businesses in your industry, you need to access your industry benchmarks. They may be available from your accountant, industry association or your local small business development center. They may be available from your accountant or industry association; the CTSBDC can also provide you with this data. See the sample report below for more details on what this financial comparison would look like.

Company Benchmark Information		
	All	**Small Company**
Company Count	2944	2498
Income Statement and Balance Sheet		
Gross Margin	29.3%	34.8%
Operating Expenses	26.8%	32.3%
Operating Income	2.4%	2.5%
Net Income	1.1%	0.9%
Cash	9.2%	9.9%
Accounts Receivable	13.9%	9.8%
Inventory	8.4%	7.8%
Accounts Payable	11.9%	10.6%
Financial Ratios		
Quick Ratio	0.98	0.74
Current Ratio	1.44	1.16
Current Liabilities to Net Worth	52.5%	77%
Current Liabilities to Inventory	x3.08	x3.61
Total Debt to Net Worth	x1.03	x1.75
Days Accounts Receivable	25	16
Inventory Turnover	x17.03	x18.96

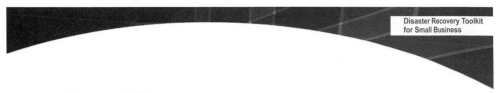

Action Planning Guide

Recovery Plan Template				
Critical Business Activity	**Recovery Action**	**Resource Requirements/ Outcomes**	**Recovery Time Objective**	**Who?**
Production Services Halted	> Reassess financial position of business, including cash flow, due to loss of revenue > Review expenses and develop a plan of action to reduce fixed and variable overhead > Negotiate with suppliers to prevent buildup of materials and reduce costs > Source alternate production site > Diversify product range and services offered	> Put aside cash reserves to cover costs > Reduce costs where possible > Research new products and services -identify alternate production site	2 weeks	Owner

This recovery plan template is designed to guide you through the process of identifying critical business activities that have been impacted by the disaster, the actions necessary to restore those activities and the identified costs, requirements, timeline and personnel responsible for these activities.

Checklist for Managing in Times of Financial Difficulty

This checklist is designed to guide businesses on how they can manage through difficult times. Difficulties can be caused by external factors such as a natural, economic or man-made disasters, a decrease in consumer confidence, rising fuel prices, increased competition, difficulty accessing finances and/or increasing interest rates; or they could be caused by internal factors such as poor risk-management, failure to manage cash flow properly or low profit margins.

Regardless of the causes, small businesses need to take action when the going gets tough. While there is no single cure-all, there are many steps a business owner can take to position the business for future growth. This checklist provides some tips and suggestions.

Taking stock of your business

Adopting a risk-management mindset is key. The first step is to take stock. Business owners need to identify and manage any weaknesses in their business or their industry's performance, while being aware of any new opportunities that might emerge.

To take stock of your business, you should:

Understand your customers

Any business begins and ends with the requirements and behaviors of the customer. If your customers aren't satisfied, the rest does not matter. It is therefore fundamental to understand your customers, including their paying habits. You need to understand why your customers buy your product or service. Is it a luxury or is it a discretionary product? Do you deal in mature products or staple items? Are your customers fickle and price sensitive, or are they long-standing and faithful?

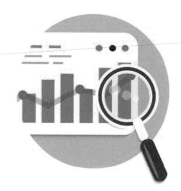

Measure, measure, measure

Some indicators quickly tell you how your business is tracking. They could be as simple as the value of daily sales, your cash balance, your receivables balance, or the value of orders and invoices you owe to suppliers. Or they could be an activity indicator such as total billable hours, an occupancy or usage factor, the value of sales booked for next week or an average sales value. Create a graph showing these indicators and update it daily or at least weekly. It will quickly show trends as they emerge.

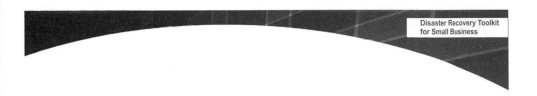

Take action with a purpose and for the right reasons

Develop strategies that aim to boost your cash position and/or profitability (you can be making a profit but still go out of business because you lack sufficient cash), without starving the business of the essential investment in inventory or marketing. Keep looking for underlying improvements in the business; don't just cut costs. In this way, your corrective actions will also put your company on better footing for longer-term success.

Change your attitude

Don't just do what you've always done. Remember, what you did last week may well have contributed to the unsatisfactory situation you find yourself in today. Consider new angles to old problems. Work on the parts of the business you can influence. Learn from others in the industry and be prepared to be flexible. Prepare financial statements and benchmark the information that emerges from them against industry averages Get someone else to have a look at your business, either your CPA or a trusted business consultant. Review your current position. Identify your problem areas and your strengths before trying to trade your way out of difficulty.

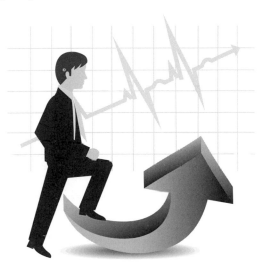

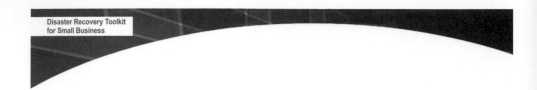

Disaster Recovery Toolkit
for Small Business

By working with a CTSBDC business advisor, you receive full access to unique tools that you can't get anywhere else. Gain a 360° perspective on your business and diagnose your problems, map opportunities, evaluate competencies and set your agenda to inspire new ideas of action with GrowthWheel® and the CTSBDC.

Improving the cash position of your business

The importance of financial management cannot be overemphasized, especially when business conditions become difficult. While profits may be the measure of success, it is cash that determines business survival. It is very important for the viability of your business to convert your customers' outstanding debt into cash. Here are some tips:

- **Prepare regular cash-flow forecasts.** If your business is having cash-flow difficulties, you should be preparing such forecasts on a regular basis. They will show the likely extent of any crisis — and how long it might last.

- **Monitor your entire cash cycle.** If you are in a difficult cash position, skew promotions toward those services or products which consume less resources or which can be turned into cash more quickly. In other words, generate cash through sales, but don't undersell your products or services. You must make a profit.

- **Measure and reward staff members who exhibit the right behavior.** For example, sales commissions should only be paid on receipt of payment, not necessarily when a sale is made. This will encourage sales staff to focus on making sales to customers who are most likely to pay.

- **Make full use of your terms of credit — this amounts to an interest-free loan.** Don't pay your suppliers too early or outside of your agreed credit terms. Be seen as a solid, dependable customer. Having a good reputation will give you better scope for negotiating deals and favorable credit terms.

- **Don't let personal draws get out of hand.** Ideally, the owners should take a modest but regular wage and leave the remaining cash in the business. Keep fringe benefits or withdrawals of stock to a minimum.

- **Don't hide your problems from the bank.** Keep the line of communication open. Demonstrate that you are on top of your business and understand your cash flow. Show you can provide financial information should you need to ask for temporary relief on loans.

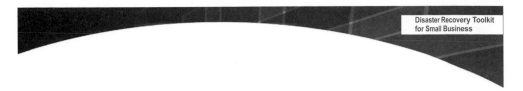

Ideas to improve business profitability

A profitable business is generally a successful business and your margin is a measure of that success. Here are some ways to boost profitability:

- **Prepare financial statements on a regular basis.** These will give you the information you need to determine overall profit margin and where costs can be saved. Financial statements can also be used to determine the margin on individual products and to compare how your business is performing against industry averages.

- **Focus on boosting profit. Retained profit is an important source of cash to meet your obligations and it can also be used for investments.** To maximize profit, you need to focus on sales that give you the highest margin, not just "sales." The only exception to this rule is when you deliberately set out to achieve another goal, such as liquidating inventory to make room for profitable products.

- **If at all possible, don't discount prices on lower-margin products or services.** Use an alternative strategy, such as bundling in support services for a higher price. This is an especially valuable strategy with slow-moving lines, as it justifies their investment.

- **Understand the profit contributions of each of your products, and your main customers.** This will show you where to best focus your efforts and identify opportunities for improvement.

- **Don't discount unless you can achieve the same or better gross profit margin.** It may require large increases in sales to generate the same amount in gross profit. While some price discounting may be required to get shoppers' attention, a much better approach is to deliver the discount through, for example, an add-on product. This should deliver more dollars of gross profit to the business. See the effect of discounting on gross profit on next page.

Disaster Recovery Toolkit
for Small Business

The effect of discounting

Present Gross Profit Margin	10%	15%	20%	25%	30%	35%	40%
If you cut your price by:	To achieve the same gross profit margin, you will need to increase sales by:						
5%	100%	50.0%	33.3%	25.0%	20.0%	16.7%	14.3%
6%	150%	66.7%	42.9%	31.6%	25.0%	20.7%	17.6%
8%	400%	114.3%	66.7%	47.1%	36.0%	29.6%	25.0%
10%	N/A	200.0%	100.0%	66.7%	50.0%	40.0%	33.3%
12%	N/A	400.0%	150.0%	92.3%	66.0%	52.2%	42.9%
15%	N/A	N/A	300.0%	150.0%	100.0%	75.0%	60.0%
20%	N/A	N/A	N/A	400.0%	200.0%	133.3%	100.0%

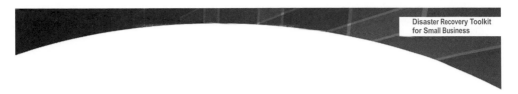

Controlling costs

Costs need to be controlled to a level that is consistent with your business's needs. Don't just cut costs. Longer-term and recurring savings are better than short-term wins. Once the easy savings are made, focus on improving sales and gross profit — both will have a larger impact on the success of your firm.

- **Identify the expenses that keep you in business.** For example, building maintenance costs, advertising, staff training skills. Keep them at sustainable levels. Remember the old saying, "Penny wise, pound foolish."

- **Look at costs carefully, but don't criticize every individual transaction.** Often a review of the business's processes can eliminate the need for certain costs completely. For example, total interest costs might be reduced by changing credit cards, by negotiating a lower rate with your bank or by reducing the amount of debt being used.

- **Measure the success of each promotional activity or campaign.** For example, direct-mail advertising is considered more cost effective than ads in papers or magazines, and is more measurable. This does not necessarily mean cutting your promotional/advertising spending, it just means increasing its efficiency.

- **Be flexible in your staffing arrangements.** Review staff availability against customer demands. For example, a core crew of full-time, permanent staffers supplemented with a group of seasonal, part-time workers may help you through busy periods. However, make sure you are familiar with appropriate legal requirements for such hiring.

- **Don't forget that your staff members are a key resource.** Replacing staff can be very costly. Correct motivation and incentives are key to creating an environment where people want to stay and succeed.

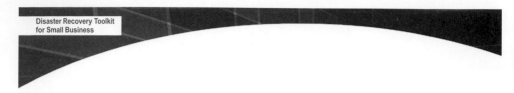

Cut the time needed to collect accounts receivables

Keep in regular contact with customers about unpaid invoices.
You would be surprised how many businesses don't follow up with late payers.

*   Keep in touch with your customers by asking questions such as:

    *   Were you happy with the product/service?

    *   Did we provide you with the right paperwork?

    *   When might we expect to be paid?

This is particularly important if you are discounting sales, as you have less gross profit margin to generate the cash you need to run your business.

*   **Negotiate periodic payments, if that helps your customer clear overdue amounts.** But make sure they stick to their side of the deal. For example, you might accept 90 percent of the old balance if it's paid by a certain time.

*   **Perform credit checks and establish and agree on proper commercial terms for future dealings with customers, including realistic credit limits.** Some customers may not be worth the effort if they continue to pay late and cause extra administration costs.

*   **Make sure your invoicing and accounts-receivable processes are well managed.** Don't let poor or sloppy processes — such as not preparing accounts receivable aging reports — contribute to customers' delayed payments.

*   **Encourage your customers to pay immediately** with discounts for cash sales, for example.

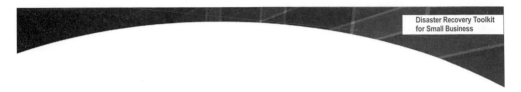

Control inventory

An essential principle is to have the right level of inventory to satisfy the needs of your customers
and to have room for new items.

- **Keeping inventory levels low reduces the amount of money you have tied up,** thereby freeing cash for other uses. It also helps to keep your storage and merchandising costs down and reduces your risk of carrying unsaleable stock.

- **Get rid of slow-moving and obsolete inventory.** Either put it all in a clearance bin so you can convert it to cash or write it off and destroy it to clear storage space. Carrying too much inventory means you are tying up cash. Removing it will help you focus on the inventory that generates the cash and margins that keep you in business.

- **Maintain necessary inventory** in order to maintain sales momentum and ensure customers are never disappointed over the products that you offer.

- **Tighten the purchasing of inventory.** Knowing your historical sales by product will help you buy the right amount. Not carrying enough inventory may discourage customers, as you may not be immediately able to satisfy their needs.

- **Negotiate deals with suppliers but avoid volume-based discounts.** When money is tight, there is no point investing in next month's inventory without good reason. Instead of volume discounts, try to negotiate discounts for prompt settlement (unless your cash position is poor) or negotiate for smaller and more frequent deliveries from your suppliers to smooth out your cash flow.

- **Don't let discount prices drive your inventory-buying decisions.** Buy inventory you can sell at a profit in a reasonable time frame.

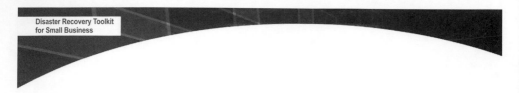

Disaster Recovery Toolkit
for Small Business

Improve sales

Focus on the additional profit from sales. Don't think that additional discounted sales are the measure of success.

- **Don't chase just any sale; chase profitable sales.** The only exception to this rule should be when you deliberately set out to achieve another goal, such as getting rid of dead stock or building market share.

- **Create added value with your offers.** For example, provide a gift or bonus with certain purchases or a discount on a second item. This tactic is especially effective if you can bundle slow-moving or dead stock at a discount together with a full-price item. You are delivering customer value while making a sale of an item you might not have otherwise sold.

- **Encourage companion selling and upselling by your sales personnel.**

- **Use in-store signs to highlight the Product of the Week, or Today's Special.** This is a very low-cost way of generating traffic and interest in a retail environment. It might get customers into the habit of coming back tomorrow for the Special of the Day. The best-run businesses use these ideas during the good times as well as the bad in order to maximize their profits and minimize risk. Using them can help your business to emerge in a much-improved market condition — which will likely lead to long-term growth.

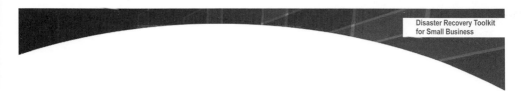

Disaster Recovery Toolkit
for Small Business

Checklists: Building it back up

	To improve the cash position of your business:
	Prepare regular cash-flow forecasts.
	Generate cash through sales but do not undersell your products or services.
	Only pay sales commission when payment is received.
	Negotiate extended terms of credit with suppliers.
	Take modest personal draws and wages.
	Don't hide problems from the bank. Tell your bank early if you need. money to overcome a cash flow problem.

	To improve the profitability of your business
	Prepare financial statements on a regular basis and use them to analyze performance and benchmark your business against industry averages.
	Understand the profit you generate on each item of product or service you sell.
	Concentrate on improving sales of your most profitable products and services.
	Don't discount prices on lower-margin products and services.
	Don't discount on your most profitable products or services unless the discount encourages increased sales that lead to at least the same profit.

	To control costs
	Identify the expenditures that are essential to keep your business running. Don't cut these costs.
	Look at costs carefully, but don't criticize every transaction.
	Conduct a review of business processes to see whether some expenses can be eliminated completely.
	Use measurable, direct-response marketing.
	Review staffing arrangements.
	Work to retain good staff members. Replacing staff can be expensive.

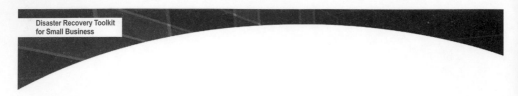

To promptly collect accounts receivables	
	Keep in regular contact with customers, particularly customers with outstanding invoices.
	Prepare an accounts receivable aging report.
	Negotiate periodic payments to help customers clear past due balances.
	Before you sell to a customer on credit, perform a credit check and agree on proper commercial terms of credit.
	Encourage immediate payments by offering discounts on cash sales.

To control inventory	
	Keep the right amount of stock - too much or not enough can damage your business.
	Identify slow moving and dead stock and try to sell it. If you can't sell it, write it off and destroy it.
	Identify items you simply must never run out of.
	Negotiate deals with suppliers, but avoid volume-based discounts.
	Tighten the purchasing of inventory by knowing when to buy. To do this, you need to know the historical sales by item.

To improve sales	
	Focus on the most profitable sales. Don't just chase any sale.
	Create added value by bundling a gift or training with your item.
	Use companion selling and upselling.
	Use in-store signs to highlight the product of the day/week.

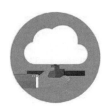

Cloud Storage

What is it, how does it work, and why do I need it?

Reconstructing financial records or important documents, of course, is much easier with cloud storage, which saves your data away from your business, safe and sound. Let's say your much-needed data is a key to your house. Cloud storage is like giving a trusted neighbor a copy of your house key. It's a backup if you lose your key. You can still get to what you need.

Cloud storage — like that trusted neighbor — is a disaster must. It stores your data off site, on multiple backup servers all over the world. Cloud storage providers keep data available and accessible, and the servers' physical environment protected, operational and maintained.

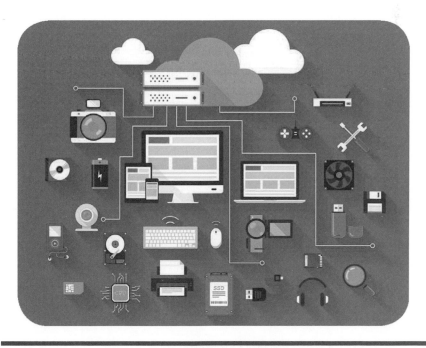

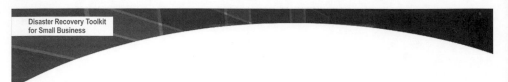

Disaster Recovery Toolkit
for Small Business

Cyber Security

Small Businesses' vulnerability to cyber security threats are increasingly of concern, and are not limited to a particular industry or business operation. Fox Business Small Business Center reports that Symantec's 2013Internet Security Threat report, saw more heightened and sustained criminal activity against small businesses. "Targeted attacks against small businesses almost doubled last year – it was up 91%. And it lasted three times longer than what we saw in 2012". According to Symantec, longer attacks hurt small businesses more than they do large enterprises. "Frankly, there's more to steal from [SMBs] than consumers, and they're a lot less secure than a lot of large enterprises," said a company spokesperson.

Before a Cyber Attack

You can increase your chances of avoiding cyber risks by setting up the proper controls. The following are things you can do to protect yourself, your family, and your property before a cyber incident occurs.

- Only connect to the Internet over secure, password- protected networks.

- Do not click on links or pop-ups, open attachments, or respond to emails from strangers.

- Always enter a URL by hand instead of following links if you are unsure of the sender.

- Do not respond to online requests for Personally Identifiable Information (PII); most organizations – banks, universities, companies, etc. – do not ask for your personal information over the Internet.

- Limit who you are sharing information with by reviewing the privacy settings on your social media accounts.

- Trust your gut; if you think an offer is too good to be true, then it probably is.

- Password protect all devices that connect to the Internet and user accounts.

- Do not use the same password twice; choose a password that means something to you and you only; change your passwords on a regular basis.

- If you see something suspicious, report it to the proper authorities.

The extent, nature, and timing of cyber incidents are impossible to predict. There may or may not be any warning. Some cyber incidents take a long time (weeks, months or years) to be discovered and identified. Familiarize yourself with the types of threats and protective measures you can take by:

- Signing up for the United States Computer Emergency Readiness Team (US-CERT) mailing list to receive the latest cybersecurity information directly to your inbox. Written for home and business users, alerts provide timely information about current security issues and vulnerabilities. Sign up at https://www.us-cert.gov.

- Becoming a Friend of the Department of Homeland Security's Stop. Think. Connect. Campaign and receive a monthly newsletter with cybersecurity current events and tips. Sign up at https://www.dhs.gov/stopthinkconnect.

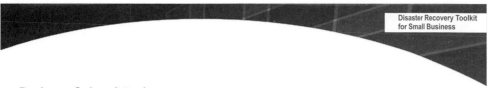

During a Cyber Attack

Immediate Actions
- Check to make sure the software on all of your systems is up-to-date.
- Run a scan to make sure your system is not infected or acting suspiciously.
- If you find a problem, disconnect your device from the Internet and perform a full system restore.

At Home

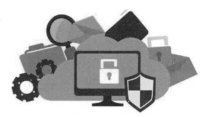

- Disconnect your device (computer, gaming system, tablet, etc.) from the Internet. By removing the Internet connection, you prevent an attacker or virus from being able to access your computer and perform tasks such as locating personal data, manipulating or deleting files, or using your device to attack others.
- If you have anti-virus software installed on your computer, update the virus definitions (if possible), and perform a manual scan of your entire system. Install all of the appropriate patches to fix known vulnerabilities.

At Work

- If you have access to an IT department, contact them immediately. The sooner they can investigate and clean your computer, the less damage to your computer and other computers on the network.

- If you believe you might have revealed sensitive information about your organization, report it to the appropriate people within the organization, including network administrators. They can be alert for any suspicious or unusual activity.

At a Public Place (library, school, etc.)

- Immediately inform a librarian, teacher, or manager in charge. If they have access to an IT department, contact them immediately.

- Immediate Actions if your Personally Identifiable Information (PII) is compromised:

PII is information that can be used to uniquely identify, contact, or locate a single person. PII includes but is not limited to:
- Full Name
- Social security number
- Address
- Date of birth
- Place of birth
- Driver's License Number
- Vehicle registration plate number
- Credit card numbers
- Physical appearance
- Gender or race

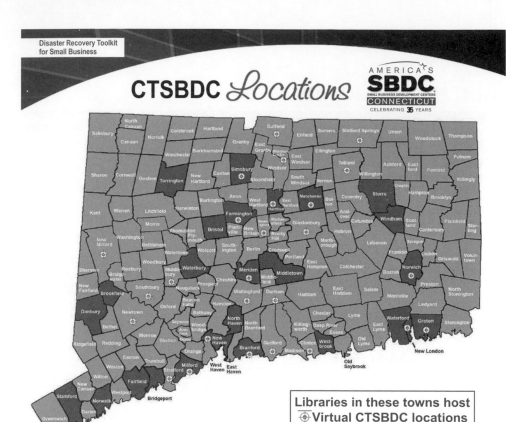

Disaster Recovery Toolkit for Small Business

CTSBDC *Locations*

AMERICA'S **SBDC**
SMALL BUSINESS DEVELOPMENT CENTERS
CONNECTICUT
CELEBRATING 35 YEARS

Libraries in these towns host ⊕Virtual CTSBDC locations

Branford	New London
Clinton	New Milford
Durham	Newington
Farmington	Newtown
Glastonbury	Norwich
Groton (2)	Simsbury
Guilford	Southbury
Hartford	Stafford Springs
Manchester	Stratford
Meriden	Suffield
Middlebury	Tolland
Milford	Wallingford
New Haven	Windsor Locks

CTSBDC Office Locations

Branford	New Haven
Bridgeport	New London
Bristol	North Haven
Brookfield	Norwalk
Danbury	Norwich
Fairfield	Simsbury
Farmington	Stamford (2)
Groton	Storrs (Lead Office)
Hartford (2)	Torrington
Manchester	Waterbury
Meriden	Waterford
Middletown (2)	Westbrook
Milford	Windham

Appendix 4

SALT Triage Scheme

SALT triage scheme. LSI = lifesaving interventions.

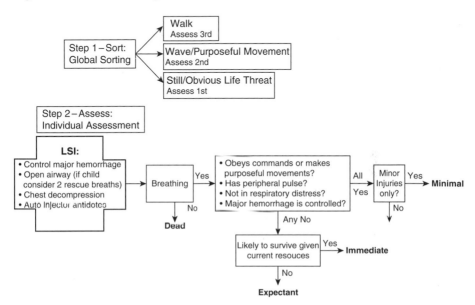

Appendix 5

Checklist for Trauma Anesthesia

Adapted by V. Behrens, R. Dudaryk, N. Nedeff, J.M. Tobin, A.J. Varon; Ryder Trauma Center

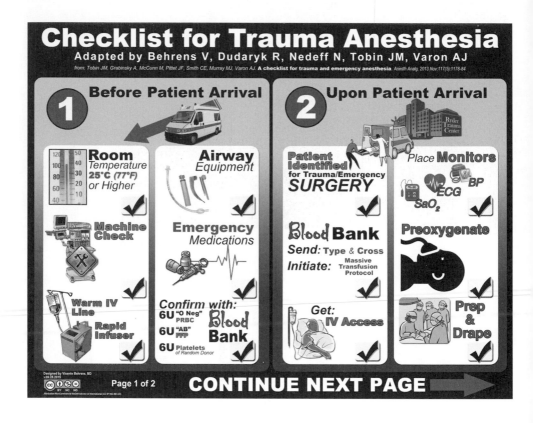

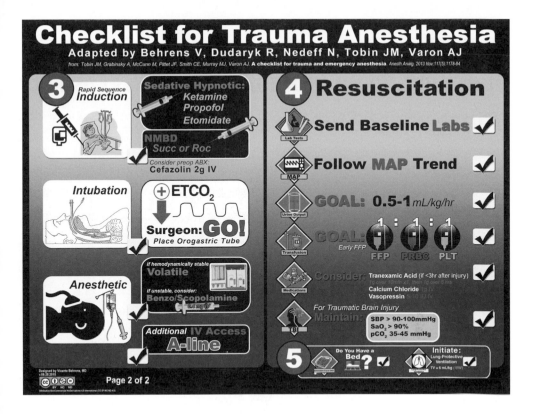

Appendix 6

Operating Room Procedures for Mass Casualty Management Step By Step

American Society of Anesthesiologists Committee on Trauma and Emergency Preparedness

Objective

To be able to manage the flow of patient care in the ORs during a mass casualty situation.

Steps (Indicate Date and Time for Each Item)

☐ **Refer to facility's operations manual**

Open up appropriate annex.

☐ **Activate call-in tree**

Assign an individual to activate. Use clerical personnel or automatic paging system, if available.

☐ **Assess status of operating rooms**

Determine staffing of ORs 0–2, 2–12, and 12–24 hours. Hold elective cases.

☐ **Alert current ORs**

Finish current surgical procedures as soon as possible and prepare to receive trauma.

☐ **Assign staff**

Set up for trauma/emergency cases.

☐ **Anesthesia coordinator should become OR medical director**

Work with OR nursing manager to facilitate communication and coordination of staff and facilities.

☐ **Report OR status to hospital command center (HCC)**

Enter telephone, email address of HCC.

☐ **Ensure adequate supplies**

Coordinate with anesthesia techs/supply personnel to ensure adequate supplies of fluids, medications, disposables, other.

☐ **Contact PACU**

Accelerate transfer of patients to floors/ICUs in preparation for high volume of cases.

☐ **Anesthesiologist should act as liaison in emergency department (ED)**

Send an experienced practitioner to the ED to act as a liaison (your eyes and ears) and keep communications open to anesthesia coordinator.

☐ **Consider assembly of stat teams**

Combination of anesthesia, surgical, nursing, respiratory personnel to triage, as needed.

☐ **HAZMET/WMD event**

Review special personal protective procedures, such as DECON and isolation techniques. Consider if part of the OR or hallways should be considered "hot" or should have ventilation altered. Good resources include CHEMM/REMM websites.

☐ **Coordinate with blood bank**

Verify blood availability.

☐ **Coordinate with other patient care areas**

ICUs, OB, peds, etc. to ensure continuity of care for new and existing patients.

Developed by the Committee on Trauma and Emergency Preparedness

Family Disaster Checklist and Plan

Your Family Disaster Supplies Kit

Disasters happen anytime and any-where. And when disaster strikes, you may not have much time to respond.

A highway spill of haz-ardous material could mean instant evacuation.

A winter storm could confine your family at home. An earthquake, flood, tornado or any other disaster could cut off basic services—gas, water, electricity and telephones—for days.

After a disaster, local officials and relief workers will be on the scene, but they cannot reach everyone immediately. You could get help in hours, or it may take days. Would your family be prepared to cope with the emergency until help arrives?

Your family will cope best by preparing for disaster *before* it strikes. One way to prepare is by assembling a Disaster Supplies Kit. Once disaster hits, you won't have time to shop or search for supplies. But if you've gathered supplies in advance, your family can endure an evacuation or home confinement.

To prepare your kit

- Review the checklist in this brochure.
- Gather the supplies that are listed. You may need them if your family is confined at home.
- Place the supplies you'd most likely need for an evacuation in an easy-to-carry container. These supplies are listed with an asterisk (*).

SUPPLIES

T here are six basics you should stock in your home: water, food, first aid supplies, clothing and bedding, tools and emergency supplies and special items. Keep the items that you would most likely need during an evacuation in an easy-to-carry container— suggested items are marked with an asterisk (*). Possible containers include

a large, covered trash container,

camping backpack,

or a duffle bag.

Water

Store water in plastic containers such as soft drink bottles. Avoid using containers that will decompose or break, such as milk cartons or glass bottles. A normally active person needs to drink at least two quarts of water each day. Hot environments and intense physical activity can double that amount. Children, nursing mothers and ill people will need more.

❑ Store one gallon of water per person per day (two quarts for drinking, two quarts for food preparation/sanitation)*

❑ Keep at least a three-day supply of water for each person in your household.

Food

Store at least a three-day supply of non-perishable food. Select foods that require no refrigeration, preparation or cooking and little or no water. If you must heat food, pack a can of sterno. Select food items that are compact and lightweight.

*Include a selection of the following foods in your Disaster Supplies Kit:

❑ Ready-to-eat canned meats, fruits and vegetables

❑ Canned juices, milk, soup (if powdered, store extra water)

❑ Staples — sugar, salt, pepper

❑ High energy foods — peanut butter, jelly, crackers, granloa bars, trail mix

❑ Vitamins

❑ Foods for infants, elderly persons or persons on special diets

❑ Comfort/stress foods — cookies, hard candy, sweetened cereals lollipops, instant coffee, tea bags

First Aid Kit

Assemble a first aid kit for your home and one for each car. A first aid kit* should include:

❑ Sterile adhesive bandages in assorted sizes
❑ 2-inch sterile gauze pads (4-6)
❑ 4-inch sterile gauze pads (4-6)
❑ Hypoallergenic adhesive tape
❑ Triangular bandages (3)
❑ 2-inch sterile roller bandages (3 rolls)
❑ 3-inch sterile roller bandages (3 rolls)
❑ Scissors
❑ Tweezers
❑ Needle
❑ Moistened towelettes
❑ Antiseptic
❑ Thermometer
❑ Tongue blades (2)
❑ Tube of petroleum jelly or other lubricant

❑ Assorted sizes of safety pins
❑ Cleansing agent/soap
❑ Latex gloves (2 pair)
❑ Sunscreen

Non-prescription drugs
❑ Aspirin or nonaspirin pain reliever
❑ Anti-diarrhea medication
❑ Antacid (for stomach upset)
❑ Syrup of Ipecac (use to induce vomiting if advised by the Poison Control Center)
❑ Laxative
❑ Activated charcoal (use if advised by the Poison Control Center)

Contact your local American Red Cross chapter to obtain a basic first aid manual.

Tools and Supplies

- ❑ Mess kits, or paper cups, plates and plastic utensils*
- ❑ Emergency preparedness manual*
- ❑ Battery operated radio and extra batteries*
- ❑ Flashlight and extra batteries*
- ❑ Cash or traveler's checks, change*
- ❑ Non-electric can opener, utility knife*
- ❑ Fire extinguisher: small canister, ABC type
- ❑ Tube tent
- ❑ Pliers
- ❑ Tape
- ❑ Compass
- ❑ Matches in a waterproof container
- ❑ Aluminum foil
- ❑ Plastic storage containers
- ❑ Signal flare
- ❑ Paper, pencil

- ❑ Needles, thread
- ❑ Medicine dropper
- ❑ Shut-off wrench, to turn off household gas and water
- ❑ Whistle
- ❑ Plastic sheeting
- ❑ Map of the area (for locating shelters)

Sanitation

- ❑ Toilet paper, towelettes*
- ❑ Soap, liquid detergent*
- ❑ Feminine supplies*
- ❑ Personal hygiene items*
- ❑ Plastic garbage bags, ties (for personal sanitation ases)
- ❑ Plastic bucket with tight lid
- ❑ Disinfectant
- ❑ Household chlorine bleach

Clothing and Bedding

*Include at least one complete change of clothing and footwear per person.

- ❑ Sturdy shoes or work boots*
- ❑ Rain gear*
- ❑ Blankets or sleeping bags*

- ❑ Hat and gloves
- ❑ Thermal underwear
- ❑ Sunglasses

Special Items

Remember family members with special needs, such as infants and elderly or disabled persons.

For Baby*
- ❑ Formula
- ❑ Diapers
- ❑ Bottles
- ❑ Powdered milk
- ❑ Medications

For Adults*
- ❑ Heart and high blood pressure medication
- ❑ Insulin
- ❑ Prescription drugs
- ❑ Denture needs
- ❑ Contact lenses and supplies
- ❑ Extra eye glasses

- ❑ **Entertainment** - games and books
- ❑ **Important Family Documents**
  Keep these records in a waterproof, portable container.

- Will, insurance policies, contracts, deeds, stocks and bonds
- Passports, social security cards, immunization records
- Bank account numbers
- Credit card account numbers and companies
- Inventory of valuable household goods, important telephone numbers
- Family records (birth, marriage, death certificates)

SUGGESTIONS AND REMINDERS

- ■ Store your kit in a convenient place known to all family members. Keep a smaller version of the Disaster Supplies Kit in the trunk of your car.

- ■ Keep items in air tight plastic bags.

- ■ Change your stored water supply every six months so it stays fresh.

- ■ Rotate your stored food every six months.

- ■ Re-think your kit and family needs at least once a year. Replace batteries, update clothes, etc.

- ■ Ask your physician or pharmacist about storing prescription medications.

CREATE A FAMILY DISASTER PLAN

To get started...

Contact your local emergency management or civil defense office and your local American Red Cross chapter.

- Find out which disasters are most likely to happen in your community.
- Ask how you would be warned
- Find out how to prepare for each.

Meet with your family.

- Discuss the types of disasters that could occur.
- Explain how to prepare and respond.
- Discuss what to do if advised to evacuate.
- Practice what you have discussed.

Plan how your family will stay in contact if separated by disaster.

- Pick two meeting places:
  1) a location a safe distance from your home in case of fire.
  2) a place outside your neighborhood in case you can't return home.
- Choose an **out-of-state** friend as a "check-in-contact" for everyone to call.

Complete these steps.

- Post emergency telephone numbers by every phone.
- Show responsible family members how and when to shut off water, gas and electricity at main switches.

- Install a smoke detector on each level of your home, especially near bedrooms; test monthly and change the batteries two times each year.
- Contact your local fire department to learn about home fire hazards.
- Learn first aid and CPR. Contact your local American Red Cross chapter for information and training

Meet with your neighbors.

Plan how the neighborhood could work together after a disaster. Know your neighbor's skills (medical, technical). Consider how you could help neighbors who have special needs, such as elderly or disabled persons. Make plans for child care in case parents can't get home.

Remember to practice and maintain your plan.

The Federal Emergency Management Agency's Community and Family Preparedness Program and the American Red Cross Community Disaster Education Program are nationwide efforts to help people prepare for disasters of all types. For more information, please contact your local emergency management office and American Red Cross chapter. This brochure and other preparedness materials are available by calling FEMA at 1-800-480-2520, or writing: FEMA, P.O. Box 2012, Jessup, MD 20794-2012. Publications are also available on the World Wide Web at:

FEMA's Web site: http://www.fema.gov   American Red Cross Web site: http://www.redcross.org

Local sponsorship provided by:

FEMA L-189
ARC 4463

Federal Emergency Management Agency

EARTHQUAKE • TORNADO • WINTER STORM • FIR

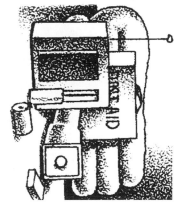

Your
Family Disaster Supplies Kit

HURRICANE • FLASH FLOOD • HAZARDOUS MATERIALS SPIL

HURRICANE · FLASH FLOOD · FIRE · HAZARDOUS MATERIALS SPILL · EARTHQUAKE · TORNADO · WINTER STORM

Your
Family Disaster Plan

W here will your family be when disaster strikes? They could be anywhere—

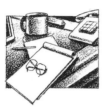

at work

at school

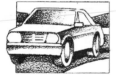

or in the car.

How will you find each other? Will you know if your children are safe?

Disaster can strike quickly and without warning. It can force you to evacuate your neighborhood or confine you to your home. What would you do if basic services—water, gas, electricity or telephones—were cut off? Local officials and relief workers will be on the scene after a disaster, but they cannot reach everyone right away.

Families can—and do—cope with disaster by preparing in advance and working together as a team. Follow the steps listed in this brochure to create your family's disaster plan. Knowing what to do is your best protection and your responsibility.

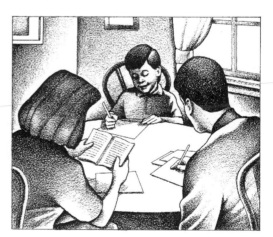

Keep enough supplies in your home to meet your needs for at least three days. Assemble a Disaster Supplies Kit with items you may need in an evacuation. Store these supplies in sturdy, easy-to-carry containers such as backpacks, duffle bags or covered trash containers.

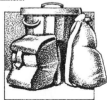

Include:

- A three-day supply of water (one gallon per person per day) and food that won't spoil.
- One change of clothing and footwear per person, and one blanket or sleeping bag per person.
- A first aid kit that includes your family's prescription medications.
- Emergency tools including a battery-powered radio, flashlight and plenty of extra batteries.
- An extra set of car keys and a credit card, cash or traveler's checks.
- Sanitation supplies.
- Special items for infant, elderly or disabled family members.
- An extra pair of glasses.

Keep important family documents in a waterproof container. Keep a smaller kit in the trunk of your car.

Locate the main electric fuse box, water service main and natural gas main. Learn how and when to turn these utilities off. Teach all responsible family members. Keep necessary tools near gas and water shut-off valves.

Remember, turn off the utilities only if you suspect the lines are damaged or if you are instructed to do so. *If you turn the gas off, you will need a professional to turn it back on.*

4 Steps to Safety

1

Find Out What Could Happen to You

Contact your local emergency management or civil defense office and American Red Cross chapter — be prepared to take notes:

- ❑ Ask what types of disasters are most likely to happen. Request information on how to prepare for each.
- ❑ Learn about your community's warning signals: what they sound like and what you should do when you hear them.
- ❑ Ask about animal care after disaster. Animals may not be allowed inside
- emergency shelters due to health regulations.
- ❑ Find out how to help elderly or disabled persons, if needed.
- ❑ Next, find out about the disaster plans at your workplace, your children's school or daycare center and other places where your family spends time.

2

Create a Disaster Plan

Meet with your family and discuss why you need to prepare for disaster. Explain the dangers of fire, severe weather and earthquakes to children. Plan to share responsibilities and work together as a team.

- ❑ Discuss the types of disasters that are most likely to happen. Explain what to do in each case.
- ❑ Pick two places to meet:
  1. Right outside your home in case of a sudden emergency, like a fire.
  2. Outside your neighborhood in case you can't return home. Everyone must know the address and phone number.
- ❑ Ask an out-of-state friend to be your "family contact." After a disaster, it's often easier to call long distance. Other family members should call this person and tell them where they are. Everyone must know your contact's phone number.
- ❑ Discuss what to do in an evacuation. Plan how to take care of your pets.

Fill out, copy and distribute to all family members

Family Disaster Plan

Emergency Meeting Place_____
                                    outside your home

Meeting Place_____ Phone_____
                  outside your neighborhood

Address_____

_____

Family Contact_____
                                            (name)

Phone (   )_____ Phone (   )_____
                  day   evening

Complete This Checklist

- Post emergency telephone numbers by phones (fire, police, ambulance, etc.).
- Teach children how and when to call 911 or your local Emergency Medical Services number for emergency help.
- Show each family member how and when to turn off the water, gas and electricity at the main switches.
- Check if you have adequate insurance coverage.
- Teach each family member how to use the fire extinguisher (ABC type), and show them where it's kept.

- Install smoke detectors on each level of your home, especially near bedrooms.
- Conduct a home hazard hunt.
- Stock emergency supplies and assemble a Disaster Supplies Kit.
- Take a Red Cross first aid and CPR class.
- Determine the best escape routes from your home. Find two ways out of each room.
- Find the safe spots in your home for each type of disaster.

Practice and Maintain Your Plan

- Quiz your kids every six months so they remember what to do.
- Conduct fire and emergency evacuation drills.

Year	Drill Date
_____	_____
_____	_____
_____	_____

- Replace stored water every three months and stored food every six months.
- Test and recharge your fire extinguisher(s) according to manufacturer's instructions.

- Test your smoke detectors monthly and change the batteries at least once a year.

Jan. ❑	July ❑
Feb. ❑	Aug. ❑
Mar. ❑	Sep. ❑
Apr. ❑	Oct. ❑
May ❑	Nov. ❑
June ❑	Dec. ❑

  Change batteries in _____ each year.
  (month)

NEIGHBORS HELPING NEIGHBORS

Working with neighbors can save lives and property. Meet with your neighbors to plan how the neighborhood could work together after a disaster until help arrives. If you're a member of a neighborhood organization, such as a home association or crime watch group, introduce disaster preparedness as a new activity. Know your neighbors' special skills (e.g., medical, technical) and consider how you could help neighbors who have special needs, such as disabled and elderly persons. Make plans for child care in case parents can't get home.

HOME HAZARD HUNT

During a disaster, ordinary objects in your home can cause injury or damage. Anything that can move, fall, break or cause a fire is a home hazard. For example, a hot water heater or a bookshelf can fall. Inspect your home at least once a year and fix potential hazards.

Contact your local fire department to learn about home fire hazards.

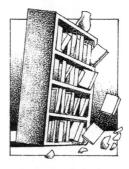

EVACUATION

Evacuate immediately if told to do so:

- Listen to your battery-powered radio and follow the instructions of local emergency officials.
- Wear protective clothing and sturdy shoes.
- Take your Disaster Supplies Kit.
- Lock your home.
- Use travel routes specified by local authorities — don't use shortcuts because certain areas may be impassable or dangerous.

If you're sure you have time:

- Shut off water, gas and electricity before leaving, if instructed to do so.
- Post a note telling others when you left and where you are going.
- Make arrangements for your pets.

IF DISASTER STRIKES

If disaster strikes

Remain calm and patient. Put your plan into action.

Check for injuries

Give first aid and get help for seriously injured people.

Listen to your battery powered radio for news and instructions

Evacuate, if advised to do so. Wear protective clothing and sturdy shoes.

Check for damage in your home...

- Use flashlights — do not light matches or turn on electrical switches, if you suspect damage.
- Check for fires, fire hazards and other household hazards.
- Sniff for gas leaks, starting at the water heater. If you smell gas or suspect a leak, turn off the main gas valve, open windows, and get everyone outside quickly.
- Shut off any other damaged utilities.
- Clean up spilled medicines, bleaches, gasoline and other flammable liquids immediately.

Remember to...

- Confine or secure your pets.
- Call your family contact— do not use the telephone again unless it is a life-threatening emergency.
- Check on your neighbors, especially elderly or disabled persons.
- Make sure you have an adequate water supply in case service is cut off.
- Stay away from downed power lines.

The Federal Emergency Management Agency's Community and Family Preparedness Program and the American Red Cross Community Disaster Education Program are nationwide efforts to help people prepare for disasters of all types. For more information, please contact your local emergency management office and American Red Cross chapter. This brochure and other preparedness materials are available by calling FEMA at 1-800-480-2520, or writing: FEMA, P.O. Box 2012, Jessup, MD 20794-2012.
Publications are also available on the World Wide Web at:
FEMA's Web site: http://www.fema.gov
American Red Cross Web site: http://www.redcross.org

Ask for: *Are You Ready?, Your Family Disaster Supplies Kit* and *Food & Water in an Emergency.*

September 1991
FEMA L-191
ARC 4466

Local sponsorship provided by:

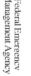

Federal Emergency Management Agency

EARTHQUAKE • TORNADO • WINTER STORM • FIRE

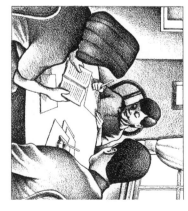

Your
Family Disaster Pl

HURRICANE • FLASH FLOOD • HAZARDOUS MATERIALS SPILL

ASA COMMITTEE ON TRAUMA & EMERGENCY PREPAREDNESS (COTEP):
FAMILY PREPAREDNESS CHECKLIST

🏠 SHELTER	🏃 EVACUATE
Supplies (at least 3 days)	**Supplies (72 hours or more)**
• Medications • Food and water (one gallon per person/per day) • Pet care • Batteries	• Medications • Food and water (one gallon per person/per day) • Pet care • Batteries
First aid & Disaster Kit	**Communications (battery powered radio)**
Communications (battery powered radio)	**Clothing (weather/climate appropriate)**
Security Plan	**Transportation & Fuel**
Sanitation/Hygiene Plan	• Pre-planned routes & alternatives
Cash	**Utilities**
	• Shut off water & electricity if instructed
Utilities	**"Go Bags"**
• Ability to safely shut off • Establish alternative power & lighting	• Documents/supplies • Maps/Compass • Flashlight • First aid & Disaster kit • Cash
	Meeting Place
	• Right outside home • Outside neighborhood
	Critical Documents *(in water proof container)*
	• Identity (passport, drivers license) • Marriage license/divorce decree • Birth certificates • Medical license • Insurance documents • Financial records and deeds • Irreplaceable photos

Make sure every member of the family knows the plan, that you post in an accessible place and you practice yearly. For more details: www.ready.gov

Appendix 8

Powered Air Purifying Respirator Placement

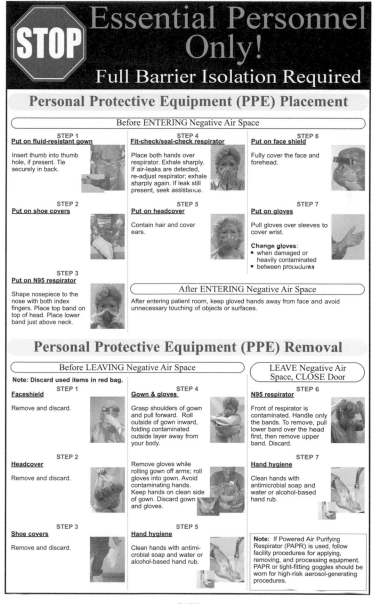

Association for Professionals in Infection Control and
Epidemiology- Minnesota Chapter

Minnesota Department of Health, Infectious Disease Epidemiology, Prevention, and Control
651-201-5414, 1-877-676-5414, TTY 651-201-5797, www.health.state.mn.us

STOP Essential Personnel Only!
Full Barrier Isolation Required

Personal Protective Equipment (PPE) Placement for
High Risk Procedures with Powered Air Purifying Respirator (PAPR)

Before ENTERING Negative Air Space

STEP 1
Put on shoe covers

STEP 3
Put on head cover if half-hood is used

Hair must be covered. Head cover is not needed if full hood is used.

STEP 5
Attach PAPR hose to hood; place hood over head

Fully cover the face and chin.

STEP 2
Attach PAPR hose to power pack

Turn power pack on. Verify air flow to hood.

STEP 4
Put on power pack

Place power pack on mid-back and secure belt clasp around waist.

Turn on power pack.

STEP 6
Put on fluid-resistant gown and gloves

Insert thumb into thumb hole. Tie securely in back. Pull gloves over sleeves to cover wrist.

Personal Protective Equipment (PPE) Removal

Before LEAVING Negative Air Space

Note: Discard used items in red bag.

Following completion of patient cares and while still in negative air space:

STEP 1
Remove and discard shoe covers

STEP 2
Remove and discard gown & gloves

Grasp shoulders of gown and pull forward. Roll outside of gown inward, folding contaminated outside layer away from your body.

Remove gloves while rolling gown off arms; roll gloves into gown. Avoid contaminating hands. Keep hands on clean side of gown. Discard gown and gloves.

STEP 3
Perform hand hygiene

Clean hands with antimicrobial soap and water or alcohol-based hand rub.

Put on a new pair of gloves

LEAVE Negative Air Space, CLOSE Door

Note: When using a PAPR, an assistant is required during PPE removal to assure proper removal and minimize contamination of equipment.

STEP 4
Gloves

Assistant:
Put on gloves.

STEP 5
Unfasten battery pack

Assistant:
Support battery pack while wearer unfastens pack.

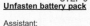

STEP 6
Remove hood and head cover

Discard head cover. Continue holding hood.

Assistant:
Continue supporting battery pack.

STEP 7
Detach hose from hood

Hold hood and hose away from body to avoid contaminating clothing.

Hand hose to assistant.

Place PAPR hood in designated receptacle for reprocessing or disposal.

(Step 7, continued)

Assistant:
Place hose and power pack in designated receptacle for reprocessing.

STEP 8
All personnel remove and discard gloves and perform hand hygiene

Clean hands with antimicrobial soap and water or alcohol-based hand rub.

Decontaminate power pack, hose, and hood per facility procedures before reuse.

 Association for Professionals in Infection Control and Epidemiology- Minnesota Chapter

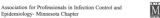 Minnesota Department of Health, Infectious Disease Epidemiology, Prevention, and Control
651-201-5414, 1-877-676-5414, TTY 651-201-5797, www.health.state.mn.us
12/2006

Appendix 9

Quick Reference Guides for Mass Decontamination

The following pages are designed to be stand alone, quick reference checklists and supporting graphics that concisely capture information to aid first responders in a mass decontamination situation for a HAZMAT/WMD incident. This section is meant to be printed double-sided so that the supporting graphics are on the reverse side of the checklist.

Guidelines for HAZMAT/WMD Mass Casualty Decontamination

INCIDENT COMMANDER'S OVERVIEW CHECKLIST

- ☐ Determine wind direction and establish safe area for decontamination set up.
- ☐ Establish a visible command post.
- ☐ Conduct scene safety assessment, to include secondary devices.
- ☐ Protect yourself.
- ☐ Approximate number of casualties.
- ☐ Determine type/state (liquid, solid or gas) of the hazard.
- ☐ Assess risks and determine need for decontamination.
- ☐ Conduct Decontamination Triage to prioritize victims.
- ☐ Communicate decontamination process to the victims (e.g., remove garments down to underwear immediately).
- ☐ Notify medical facilities.
- ☐ Establish perimeter/zones.
- ☐ Set up decontamination site.
- ☐ Execute decontamination.
- ☐ Observe victims for delayed symptoms.
- ☐ Perform Secondary decontamination (as necessary).
- ☐ Transport casualties to medical facility (as necessary).

When responders are unable to determine if actual chemical agent exposure has occurred, and in those situations where actual exposure appears unlikely, decontamination should be deferred PENDING OBSERVATION AND/OR SCENE INVESTIGATION. If symptoms develop, individuals should be treated followed by prompt field decontamination by the most expeditious means available.

Mass Decontamination Process

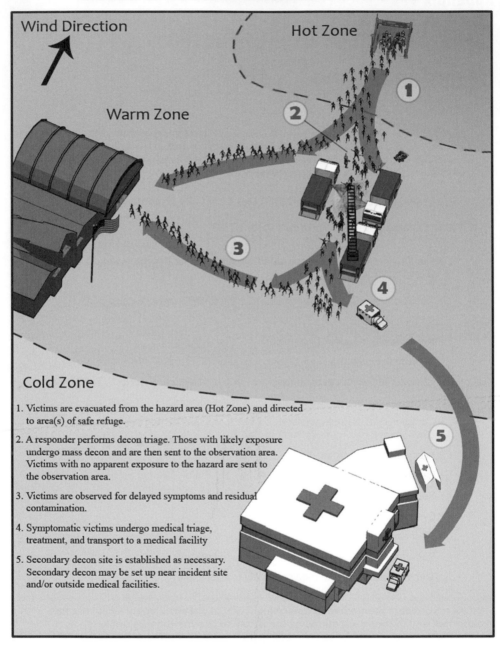

Wind Direction

Hot Zone

Warm Zone

Cold Zone

1. Victims are evacuated from the hazard area (Hot Zone) and directed to area(s) of safe refuge.

2. A responder performs decon triage. Those with likely exposure undergo mass decon and are then sent to the observation area. Victims with no apparent exposure to the hazard are sent to the observation area.

3. Victims are observed for delayed symptoms and residual contamination.

4. Symptomatic victims undergo medical triage, treatment, and transport to a medical facility

5. Secondary decon site is established as necessary. Secondary decon may be set up near incident site and/or outside medical facilities.

Guidelines for HAZMAT/WMD Mass Casualty Decontamination

INITIAL SIZE-UP CHECKLIST

- ☐ Communicate the incident to first responders.
- ☐ Conduct scene safety assessment.
- ☐ Do not rush into the incident scene – protect yourself.
- ☐ Local law enforcement should check for possible secondary devices near decontamination site.
- ☐ Look for signs and symptoms of exposure and utilize detectors, if available.
- ☐ Estimate how many suspected victims are involved.
- ☐ Determine whether mass decontamination is required.
- ☐ Determine what resources are needed and readily available for mass decontamination.
- ☐ Determine the impact of weather conditions on decontamination operations (temperature, wind speed, wind direction).
- ☐ Decontamination should be set up upwind from the incident. If the temperature is below 65°F, consider cold weather decontamination.
- ☐ Alert hospitals to prepare for victims exposed to contamination.

Guidelines for HAZMAT/WMD Mass Casualty Decontamination

VICTIM CONTROL/DECONTAMINATION TRIAGE CHECKLIST

☐ *Ensure all responders are properly protected.*

☐ Gain control of the victims as rapidly as possible (public address systems, instructional signs) and direct victims to area(s) of safe refuge to begin decontamination or for observation.

☐ In multi-lingual communities, use multi-lingual or illustrated signs to provide instructions to victims.

☐ Perform decontamination triage by separating and prioritizing victims into categories in preparation for mass decontamination (see Decontamination Triage Tree on reverse).

❖ Non-ambulatory
❖ Ambulatory and symptomatic
❖ Ambulatory, non-symptomatic, exposed to contaminant
❖ Ambulatory, non-symptomatic, no obvious exposure to contaminant

Note: it is possible that the severity of conventional injuries may require that certain victims receive an elevated priority, regardless of whether they are showing obvious signs/symptoms of exposure.

☐ ENCOURAGE VICTIMS TO REMOVE AS MUCH CLOTHING AS POSSIBLE, BUT AT LEAST REMOVE OUTER GARMENTS DOWN TO UNDERWEAR. Cutting and/or unbuttoning is preferred to pulling clothing over the head.

☐ If clothes must be lifted over the head, instruct victims to do so carefully by placing hands and arms inside the garment and using the hands to pull the head opening away from the face and head as much as possible.

HAZMAT/WMD

Known Agent
- Perform Decon as Needed

Unknown Agent

Solid, Biological or Radiological Particles
- **Contact with Material** → Remove Clothing → Wet Decon → Observe for Delayed Symptoms
- **No Contact with Material** → Observe for Delayed Symptoms

Liquid
- **Contact with Material/ Symptoms** → Remove Clothing → Wet Decon → Decon with Soap → Observe for Delayed Symptoms
- **No Contact with Material/ No Symptoms** → Observe for Delayed Symptoms

Gas
- **Contact with Material** → Remove Clothing → Wet Decon → Observe for Delayed Symptoms
- **No Contact with Material** → Observe for Delayed Symptoms

Unknown or Combination
- If liquid not ruled out, follow liquid decontamination procedures

Guidelines for HAZMAT/WMD Mass Casualty Decontamination

DECONTAMINATION SETUP CHECKLIST

☐ *Ensure all responders are properly protected.*

☐ Local law enforcement should check for possible secondary devices near the selected decontamination site(s).

☐ Establish Hot/Warm/Cold zones. Set up barriers or police tape to delineate zones. Post signs directing victims on where to go and what to do.

☐ **If not already accomplished,** instruct victims to remove as much clothing as possible. Cutting and unbuttoning is preferred to pulling clothing over the head. Collect clothing in the Warm zone.

☐ Set up decontamination site upwind of the hot zone. Ideally, it should be uphill from the hot zone, easily accessible for responders, and have good drainage.

☐ Suggested setup: Ladder Pipe Decontamination System (or other expedient system) to dispense high-volume, low-pressure water (~60 psi) with wide fog pattern.

Note: Decontamination of exposed and/or symptomatic victims should not wait for set up of decontamination tents or additives such as soap,

☐ Establish victim observation area(s) and secondary decontamination area(s) as necessary.

Ladder Pipe Decontamination System Method

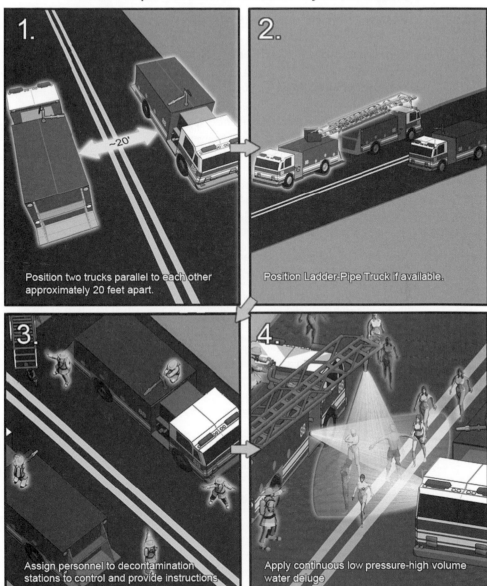

1. Position two trucks parallel to each other approximately 20 feet apart.

2. Position Ladder-Pipe Truck if available.

3. Assign personnel to decontamination stations to control and provide instructions to victims

4. Apply continuous low pressure-high volume water deluge

Guidelines for HAZMAT/WMD Mass Casualty Decontamination

MASS DECONTAMINATION EXECUTION CHECKLIST

☐ Instruct victims to move to specific areas depending on medical and decontamination triage status.

☐ **If not already accomplished,** instruct victims to remove as much clothing as possible.

☐ Establish a method for collecting and tracking personal items (e.g., bag labeled with victim name/number).

☐ Based on decontamination triage prioritization, instruct victims to move through the decontamination corridor. Wash time should be between 30 seconds and three minutes. Do not <u>delay the high-volume, low pressure water shower to create a soap-water solution</u>

☐ Instruct victims to:

❖ Tilt head back.
❖ Raise and spread arms and spread legs to expose armpits and groin.
❖ Walk through shower system slowly, and periodically turn 90 degrees (1/4 turn).
❖ When the contamination involves chemical vapor, biological or radiological materials, victims should apply gentle friction by using their hands, a cloth, or a sponge to aid in removal of contamination.
❖ Rubbing should start with the head and proceed down the body to the feet.
❖ When the contamination is a liquid chemical agent, DO NOT apply friction without the aid of soap as this may spread the hazard over the body and increase medical risk.

☐ After passing through decontamination corridor, provide victims with clothing/cover.

☐ Use some means to identify victims that have been decontaminated.

☐ Direct symptomatic patients to additional treatment or secondary decontamination area(s) as appropriate.

☐ Direct non-symptomatic victims to observation area(s).

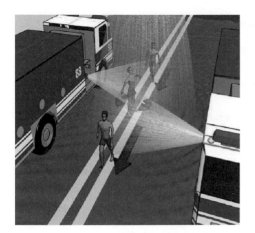

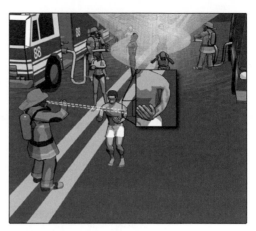

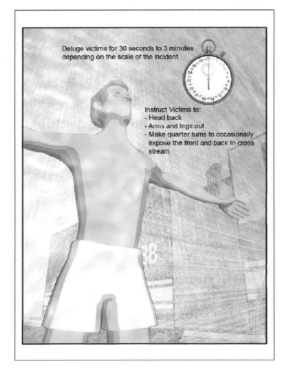

Guidelines for HAZMAT/WMD Mass Casualty Decontamination

COLD WEATHER DECONTAMINATION (<65°F) CHECKLIST

- ☐ Conduct some form of decontamination regardless of temperature conditions.
- ☐ Remove clothing outdoors
- ☐ If victims are outdoors in very low temperatures **(<36°F)** , use a dry method of decontamination (e.g., removal of clothing, blotting) instead of water for liquid contamination.
- ☐ After dry decontamination, victims should be moved inside or to a heated area for water/soapy water high-volume, low-pressure water shower and to mitigate the effects of cold weather.
- ☐ Physically identify decontaminated victims (e.g., tag around neck).
- ☐ Observe for signs of hypothermia, delayed symptoms and completeness of decontamination.
- ☐ Follow all other General Rules for Mass Casualty Decontamination

Temperature Decontamination Guide

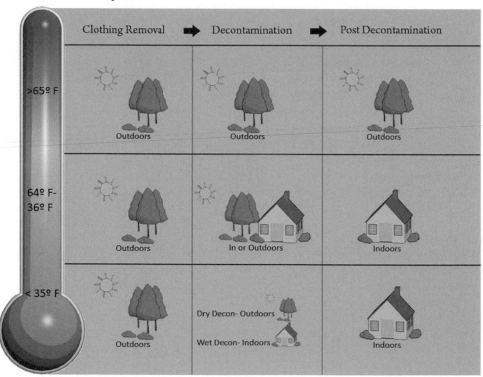

Guidelines for HAZMAT/WMD Mass Casualty Decontamination

POST DECONTAMINATION CHECKLIST

☐ Observe victims for delayed symptoms and completeness of decontamination.

☐ Perform secondary decontamination as necessary.

☐ Transport symptomatic victims to medical facilities for assistance.

☐ Arrange for clothing/cover and possible recovery of personal effects.

☐ Collect contaminated personal items for possible decontamination.

☐ Provide follow-up information to the victims (e.g., symptoms to watch for).

☐ Provide instructions to victims prior to release (e.g., care, follow-up).

☐ Decontaminate all responders, equipment, and incident site.

☐ Conduct medical check on all responders.

☐ Complete victim and first responder documentation and accountability.

Appendix 10

Draft Connecticut Acute Care Hospital Pediatric Disaster Preparedness Checklist

(1) Hospital-based incident command generally is informed by three goals

- Chain of command
- Span of control
- Common language

See Monteiro article[1] for Hospital Incident Command System[2,3] chart with highlighted pediatric portions of the system model. Checklist items for incident command pertinent to children include:

Present?	HICS Chart Items With Recommended Pediatric Components
	Pediatric Medical/Technical Specialist Who Reports to Incident Commander • Works within the incident command group to identify potential pediatric care related concerns and strategies
	Pediatric **Inpatient**# Leader Who Reports to Medical Care Branch Director Pediatric **Outpatient** Leader Who Reports to Medical Care Branch Director Pediatric **Mental Health Leader**^ Who Reports to Medical Care Branch Director Pediatric **Casualty Care Leader*** Who Reports to Medical Care Branch Director Pediatric **Clinical Care Support Leader** Who Reports to Medical Care Branch Director
	Food Services Unit Leader who Reports to Infrastructure Branch Director • Responsible for nutritional needs of children
	Victim Decontamination Unit Leader who reports to HazMat Branch Director • Responsible for providing age-appropriate communication and assistance while pediatric patients are undergoing decontamination
	Access Control Unit Leader who reports to Security Branch Director • Responsible for security of pediatric patients (injured and well) and enforcing disaster credentialing identification/reunification policies as they relate to access control.

Family Care Unit Leader who reports to Logistics Section Chief
- Helps coordinate issues of reunification and psychosocial issues of family
- (not victims)

^ Mental health leader may be a psychiatrist, psychologist, social worker or child life specialist
* Casualty care is Emergency Medicine in HICS
#If a hospital does not have inpatient pediatrics, then a transfer and contingency care plan is desirable

(2) Strategies for operational continuity

Present?	Planning consideration
	• Overstaffing: Influx of staff /convergent volunteerism • Emergency credentialing plan such as The Emergency System for Advance Registration of Volunteer Health Professionals (ESAR-VHP)
	• Understaffing: Staff may be unable or unwilling to come to work at the hospital

	• Stranded staff plan
	   • Lodging/'Hoteling'
	   • Food
	   • Hygiene
	   • Communications
	   • Family and pets of staff policy
	   • Reimbursement plan for staff who work overtime/protracted hours
	   • Medical needs of stranded staff

	• Staff education for personal disaster preparedness strategy
	• Pediatric Disaster Formulary • Equipment quickly available, in pediatric sizes when applicable (*See appendix. For the purposes of the checklist, facilities should have all listed equipment or a reasonable alternative*)
	• "Push" Notification Strategy (Everbridge and/or AmCom system, Mass-texting, automated phone messages, etc.) for staff
	• Backup phone tree staff notification strategy with responsible person to activate the tree.
	• "Pull" Notification Strategy, e.g. website with information for staff and the general public
	• *Memoranda of Understanding* with local, state and regional hospitals[4]

(3) Pediatric principles of surge capacity[4]

Present?	Planning consideration
	• Alternate care site for low-acuity patients (e.g. lobby or cafeteria), with triage/assess/discharge for worried well

- Policy for treating children with family and care-givers[5]
- Child-proofing of the alternate care site
- Supervisory plan with ratios of caregivers to children of 1:4 for infants, 1:10 for preschool age children, and 1:20 for older children.
- Pre-vetted, predetermined staff for the surge capacity site (e.g. child life, volunteers, preschool teachers, other educators, nursing assistants/ CNAs)
- Plan for rapid discharge and admission of patients to generate surge capacity
- Plan for unidirectional flow of disaster patients through the emergency department
- Rapid registration protocol
- Family tracking, family unity and family reunification plans (computerized system, GPS locators, etc.)
- Plan to activate additional support staff, including social work, mental health providers, chaplains, and child life
- Plan to mobilize surge capacity equipment, medication, and patient supplies (gowns, clothes, bedding)

(4) Development of staff safety and decontamination protocols/infection control

Present?	Planning consideration
	• Stockpile of N95 respirators and fit-testing policy for staff
	• Have a supply of PAPRs available for staff
	• Have a stock of PPE available for staff

	• Decontamination policy for children including means to counter hypothermia, provide for modesty, and identify disrobed patients
	   • Presence of temporary (pop-up) decontamination venue
	   • Presence of permanent (brick-and-mortar) decontamination venue

	• Plan to cohort patients with potentially transmissible infectious agents • Policy about parents/family members staying with child with infectious disease
	• Provision of surgical masks to patients with potentially transmissible agents
	• Provision of linens, dressings and gowns for coverage of infectious rashes
	• Provision of hand sanitizer to children and families
	• Antibiotics, antivirals, and antidotes for potential disaster agents available in pharmacy

(5) Sheltering in place

Present?	Planning consideration
	• 96 hour self-sufficiency disaster plan: Food, generators, supplies, medication, and redundant/resilient communications infrastructure • Plan for controlled degradation of care and environment after 72 hours.
	• Alternate medical record plan if electronic medical record fails
	• Plan for sheltering uninjured/well children
	• Available toys, games, and other distractions for children

(6) Evacuation strategies

Present?	Planning consideration
	• Potential receiving facilities for child disaster victims identified with memoranda of understanding
	• Evacuation routes and alternate routes identified
	• Evacuation tabletop drill or full scale exercise conducted
	• Family reunification plan for evacuation established

	• Evacuation devices for children (e.g. pediatric evacuation sleds) present
	   • Use of stairwells
	   • Infant aprons
	   • Plan to avoid hypothermia

	• Protocols for the transport of ventilated patients and patients on extracorporeal membrane oxygenation (if present at facility)

References

1. Monteiro S, Shannon M, Sandora T, Chung S. Pediatric aspects of hospital preparedness. *Clin Ped Emerg Med* 2009;**10**(3):218–227.

2. Yarmohammadian MH, Atighechian G, Shams L, Haghshenas A. Are hospitals ready to response to disasters? Challenges, opportunities and strategies of Hospital Emergency Incident Command System (HEICS). *J Res Med Sci* 2011;**16**(8):1070–1077.

3. Zane RD, Prestipino AL. Implementing the Hospital Emergency Incident Command System: an integrated delivery system's experience. *Prehosp Disaster Med* 2004;**19**(4):311–317.

4. Burke RV, Kim TY, Bachman SL, Iverson EI, Berg BM. Using mixed methods to assess pediatric disaster preparedness in the hospital setting. *Prehosp Disaster Med* 2014;**29**(6):569–575.

5. Markenson D, Reynolds S. The pediatrician and disaster preparedness. *Pediatrics* 2006;**117**(2): e340–362.

Appendix: Pediatric-Specific Disaster Surge Formulary To Support Surge

Instruments/Equipment

- Disposable BP cuffs – neonatal, infant, child, small adult
- Gastrointestinal system supplies
- Antireflux valve (10, 12, 14 Fr)
- Feeding tubes (5, 8 Fr)
- Sharps: needle/syringes
- Bulb syringes
- Safety syringes (21, 25)
- Filter needles
- Catheter tip syringe 60 ml
- Sharps container
- Luer lock syringes, 20 and 60 ml Syringes 1, 3, 5, 10 ml
- IV access/supplies IV start kits
- Stopcocks
- T-connectors
- IV start catheter (18, 20, 22, 24 G)
- Arm boards—infant, child
- Blood administration tubing
- IV filters (0.22 and 1.2 μm)
- Syringe pump tubing
- Microdrip tubing

IV solutions

- Glucose water
- Normal saline 10 ml
- Normal saline 1000 ml

Irrigation solutions

- Normal saline irrigation solution 2000 ml
- Sterile water irrigation solution 2000 ml

Miscellaneous

- Sterile lubricant
- Alcohol wipes
- Alcohol swab sticks
- Tongue blades
- Heel warmers
- Tape measure
- Body bag

- Disposable linen savers
- Safety pins
- Povodine iodine wipes
- Hydrogen peroxide
- Individual bottled drinking water

Child-Specific Supplies
- Formula
- Nipples
- Bottles
- Diapers
- Pacifiers
- Warmers/Warming Devices for Infants
- Blankets

Data from ©2009 Association for Healthcare Resource & Materials Management of the American Hospital Association.

Index